ONE Touch Radiology

For NEET/NEXT/FMGE/INI-CET

Mayur Arun Kulkarni MD, DNB (Radiology)
Director
Shree Diagnostics, Pune, Maharashtra
Radiology Faculty – Marrow App

CBSPD
Dedicated to Education

CBS Publishers & Distributors Pvt Ltd

• New Delhi • Bengaluru • Chennai • Kochi • Kolkata • Lucknow • Mumbai
• Hyderabad • Jharkhand • Nagpur • Patna • Pune • Uttarakhand

ONE Touch Radiology

For NEET/NEXT/FMGE/INI-CET

ISBN: 978-93-94525-58-0

First Edition: 2024

Published by **Satish Kumar Jain** and produced by **Varun Jain** for

CBS Publishers & Distributors Pvt Ltd
4819/XI Prahlad Street, 24 Ansari Road, Daryaganj, New Delhi 110 002, India.
Ph: +91-11-23289259, 23266861, 23266867 Website: www.cbspd.com
Fax: 011-23243014
e-mail: delhi@cbspd.com; cbspubs@airtelmail.in.

Corporate Office: 204 FIE, Industrial Area, Patparganj, Delhi 110 092
Ph: +91-11-4934 4934 Fax: 4934 4935
e-mail: feedback@cbspd.com; bhupesharora@cbspd.com

Branches

- **Bengaluru:** Seema House 2975, 17th Cross, K.R. Road, Banasankari 2nd Stage, Bengaluru-560 070, Karnataka
  Ph: +91-80-26771678/79 Fax: +91-80-26771680 e-mail: bangalore@cbspd.com
- **Chennai:** 7, Subbaraya Street, Shenoy Nagar, Chennai-600 030, Tamil Nadu
  Ph: +91-44-26680620, 26681266 Fax: +91-44-42032115 e-mail: chennai@cbspd.com
- **Kochi:** 68/1534, 35, 36-Power House Road, Opp. KSEB, Cochin-682018, Kochi, Kerala
  Ph: +91-484-4059061-65 Fax: +91-484-4059065 e-mail: kochi@cbspd.com
- **Kolkata:** Hind Ceramics Compound, 1st Floor, 147, Nilganj Road, Belghoria, Kolkata-700056, West Bengal
  Ph: +033-2563-3055/56 e-mail: kolkata@cbspd.com
- **Lucknow:** Basement, Khushnuma Complex, 7-Meerabai Marg (Behind Jawahar Bhawan), Lucknow-226001, Uttar Pradesh
  Ph: +0522-4000032 e-mail: tiwari.lucknow@cbspd.com
- **Mumbai:** PWD Shed, Gala No. 25/26, Ramchandra Bhatt Marg, Next to J.J. Hospital Gate No. 2, Opp. Union Bank of India, Noor B
  Mumbai-400009, Maharashtra
  Ph: +91-22-66661880/89 Fax: +91-22-24902342 e-mail: mumbai@cbspd.com

Representatives

- **Hyderabad** +91-9885175004
- **Jharkhand** +91-9811541605
- **Nagpur** +91-9421
- **Patna** +91-9334159340
- **Pune** +91-9623451994
- **Uttarakhand** +91-9716

Printed at : Goyal Offset Works Pvt. Ltd. Haryana

Preface

ear Students,

s the heroine in a Hindi movie 'Dabangg' says "Thappad se darr nahi lagta sahab, pyar se lagta hai!"

ften my students walk up to me and say "Padhai se darr nahi lagta sir, lekin images se lagta hai!"

This left me thinking as to what I can do for all of you so that you can overcome this fear and be onfident with X-ray/USG/CT/MRI images. Well, the best way out of a difficulty is through it – hence NE TOUCH RADIOLOGY for you!

Why this Book?

mages are the soul of Radiology. Although so many of these being asked so frequently in your exams, here wasn't a single comprehensive reliable source of good images available for students even now. NE TOUCH RADIOLOGY will be that source. You will find good quality, labeled, unambiguous images for your uick review and revision in this book.

Who is this Book for?

his book is for anyone who wants to learn and fall in love with Radiology. It is most relevant for hose who are preparing for their NEXT/NEET-PG/INI-CET/FMG examinations. However, if you are an ndergraduate student, carry it with you in your back-pack into your clinics and jump to Pneumothorax/ neumoperitoneum/Stroke when you get these cases and get the imaging part covered then and there.

How to use this Book?

his book has almost all the important images and relevant theory alongside it. But this is a concise book neant for quick review and not a descriptive textbook per se. Hence, I want you to use it along with your nline/Offline classes, like an add-on resource. Most of the images here are the same ones you will see in my Marrow modules as well as in my Offline classes. However, even if you have followed any other source – this ook will help you with spotter images and high-yield theory part. Also, when you are studying Medicine/ urgery/Orthopedics/Pediatrics/OB/GYN – keep this book handy so that you can go through the images f specific topics then and there.

How did I Write this Book?

very topic/image/table used in this book is based on a detailed review of recent examination pattern and ll the high-yield topics have been included in this book. This will be more than enough for all those who re preparing for NEXT/NEET-PG/INI-CET/FMGE.

My wife, Dr Kavita has been my pillar of support throughout this endeavor as during this period, he single-handedly played the role of both parents to Spruha and Hrida – two little angels in my life. No words can express my feelings for them. My parents have always blessed and pushed me to do better. r Swapnil Yewalkar, Dr Amit Shetty, Dr Saurabh Patil, Dr Tejas Mankeshwar, Dr Basavraj Biradar have nade important contributions to this book. My Marrow family of all faculties and friends have an equal hare of credit in my success.

Remember my dear friends – You are as Good as you think you are!

So, believe in yourself and give your best shot in whatever you do. And you will succeed for sure.

Let's Learn, Love and Rock Radiology together!

ove

Mayur Arun Kulkarni

Contents

LATEST QUESTION PAPERS

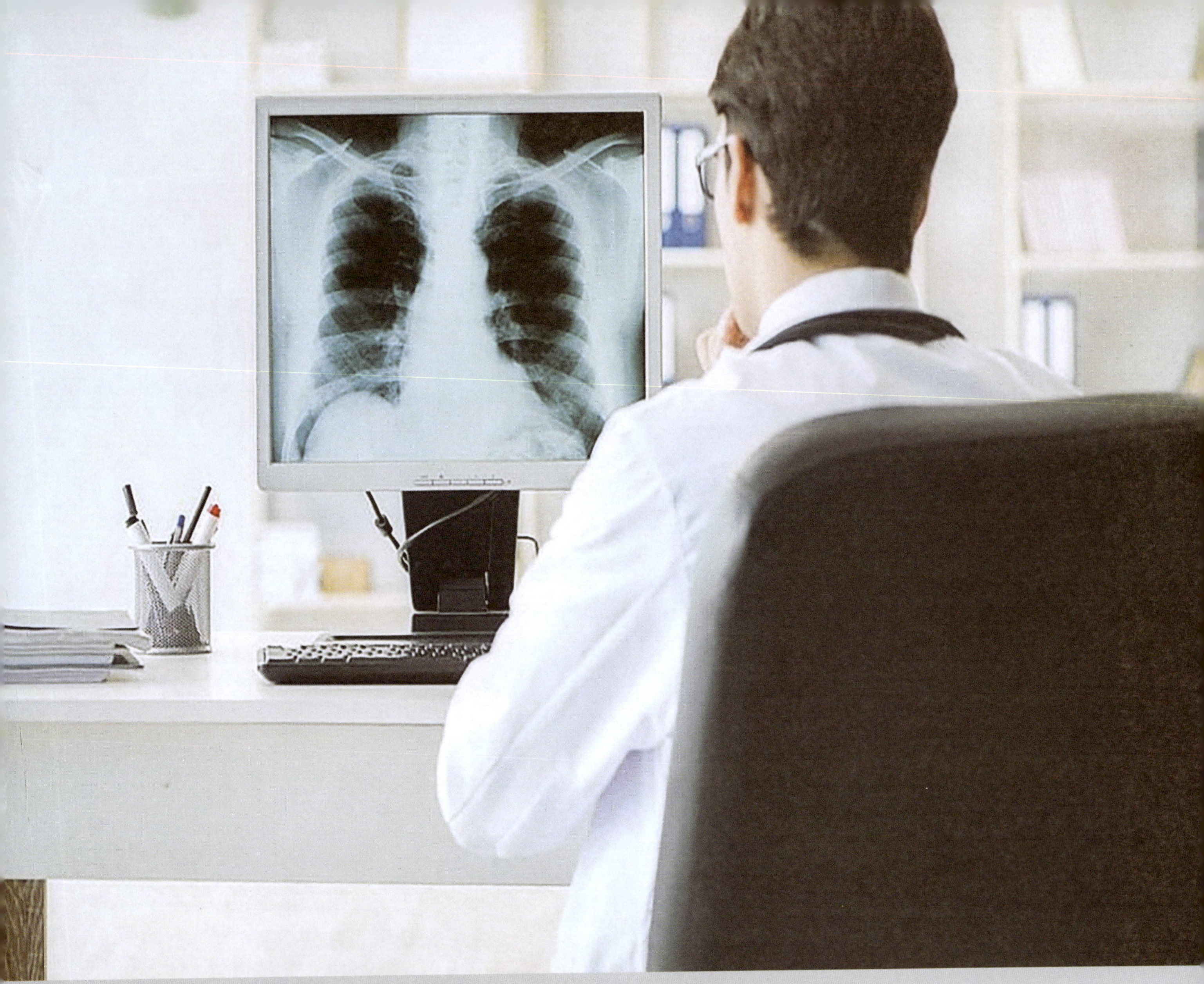

THEORY

1. GENERAL RADIOLOGY

X-RAYS

Radiation symbols

International Radiation Symbol "The Trefoil"	X-ray Radiation Hazard	High Level Sealed Source Ionizing Radiation Symbol IAEA and SO — 2007
	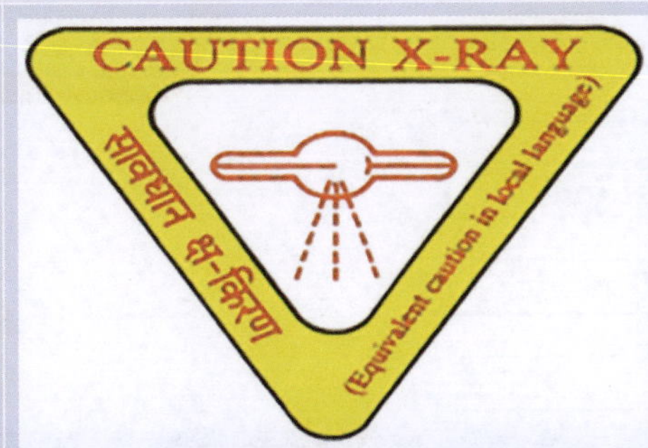	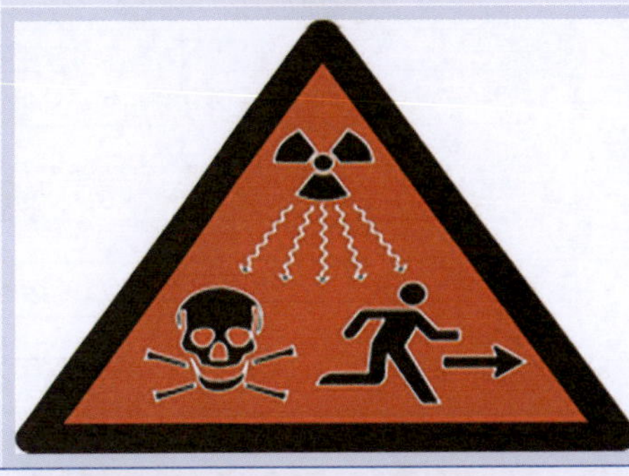

X-ray basics

Wilhelm Conrad Röntgen — Founding Father of Radiology

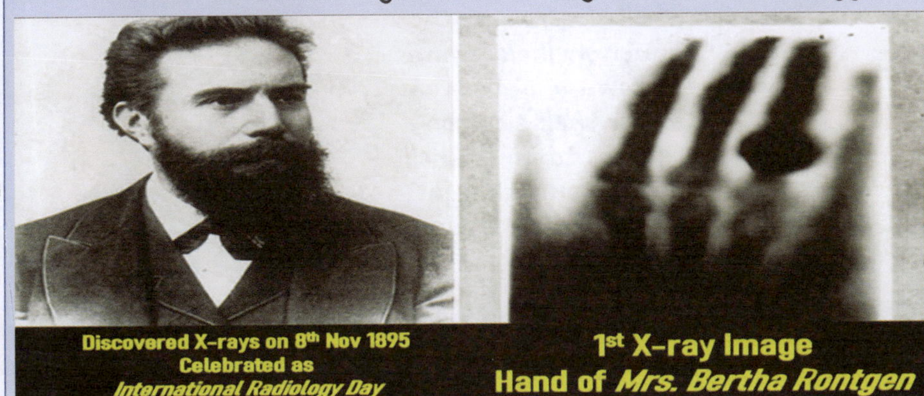

X-ray Tube — Structure

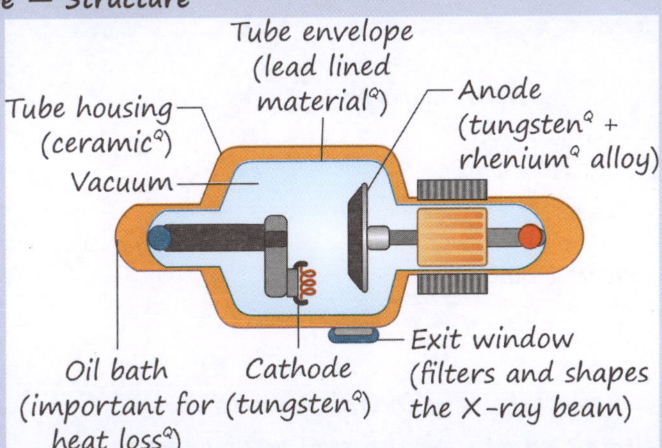

X-rays are a part of Electromagnetic spectrum[Q]

- Electromagnetic spectrum[Q]:
- All energy components are part of this spectrum.
- In increasing order of frequencies/energies this spectrum includes—radio waves (least frequency and energy),[Q] microwaves, infra-red, visible light, ultraviolet, X-rays and gamma rays (Maximum frequency and energy).[Q]
- All have same speed[Q]—speed of light—3×10^8 m/s
- All have same type of wave[Q]

X-ray specifics:

- Have relatively high frequency and high energy
- Wavelength = 0.01–10 nm
- Energy 100 eV – 100 keV

Tungsten:

- It is an important component of X-ray tube (Cathode filament)
- Symbol—W[Q]
- Atomic number—74[Q]
- Atomic mass number—184[Q]
- Classified as transitional metal[Q] in the periodic table

Contd...

X-ray basics

Electric current through cathode filament
↓
Cathode filament is heated
↓
Thermionic emission
↓
Cloud of electrons around cathode
↓
Electrons accelerated toward anode
↓
X-rays are produced

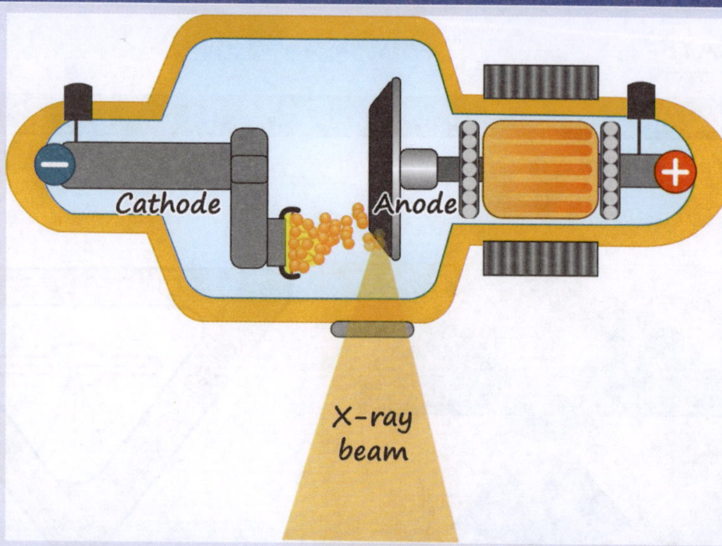

Mechanisms of X-ray Production

Continuous Spectrum—70–80%

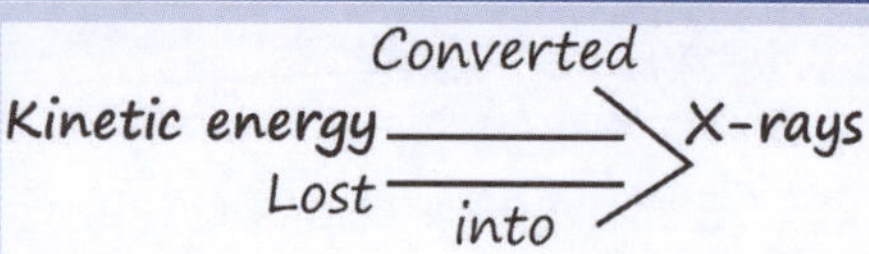

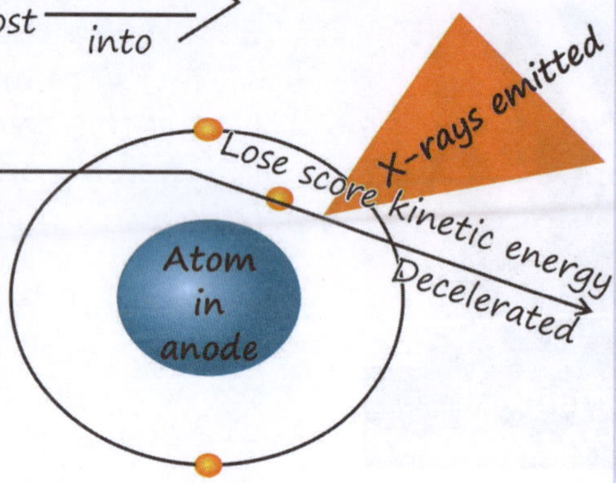

Accelerated electron is deviated/decelerated when it comes close to nucleus of an atom in the anode

Characteristic Spectrum—20–30%

When electron hits inner shell electron — the inner shell electron is thrown out. Then an outer shell electron jumps to inner shell — losing some energy emitted as X-rays

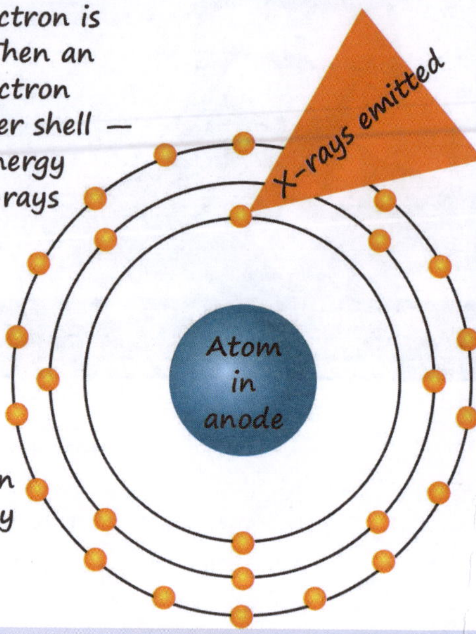

Used in mammography

Interaction of X-rays with matter

Occurs Inside the patient body

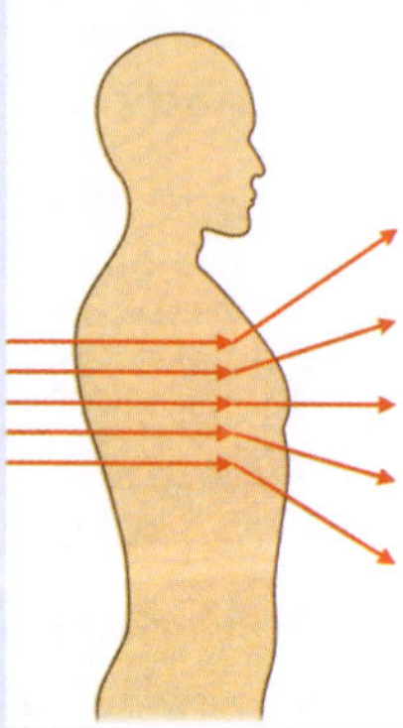

1. Compton effect — Overall most common
2. Photoelectric effect — Also seen in diagnostic radiology
3. Coherent scattering
4. Photodisintegration
5. Pair production

(3–5) Not seen in diagnostic radiology

Compton effect—Interaction of X-ray photon with outer shell electron[Q]

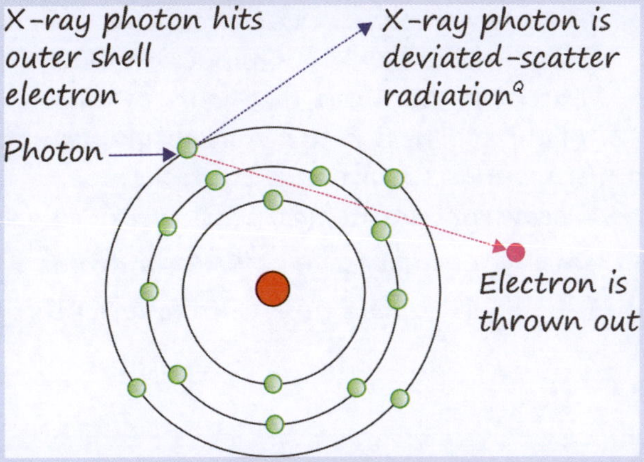

- Most common interaction of X-rays with matter[Q]
- It is a mid-energy phenomenon[Q]
- Most important outcome is scatter radiation[Q]. It causes image distortion, blurring and decreased diagnostic quality of the radiographic image
- Hence, to minimize scatter radiation, we try to minimize compton effect[Q]
- Minimizing compton effect—Using high energy X-rays[Q]

Photo-Electric Effect—Interaction of X-ray photon with inner shell electron[Q]

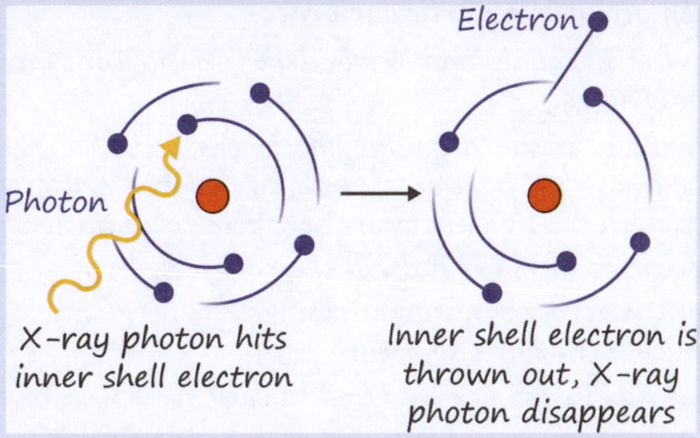

- Less common
- It is a low-energy phenomenon[Q]
- There is no scatter radiation[Q]—hence, image quality is better.
- Because there is no scatter radiation, we try to maximize photoelectric effect[Q]
- Maximizing photoelectric effect—
    - Using low energy X-rays[Q]
    - High atomic number target[Q]

Exposure Factors—Kilovoltage peak (kVp) and Milliampere second (mAs)

Kilovolt peak (kVp):

- Voltage applied across the cathode and anode in the X-ray tube.
- High kVp—results in higher penetrating power of X-rays[Q]
- kVp also affects radiographic contrast–
    - Low kVp—high contrast[Q]—called short scale contrast[Q]
    - High kVp—low contrast[Q]—called long scale contrast[Q]

Milliampere second (mAs)[Q]

- Combination of:
    - mAmp[Q]—current passed through the cathode filament
    - Time[Q]—time of exposure
- Determines the number of X-ray photons[Q] in the X-ray beam
- Directly affects the contrast—increased mAs—increased contrast[Q]

RADIATION UNITS

Radiation exposure

- Conventional unit—Rontgen[Q]
- SI unit—Coulomb/Kg[Q]

Absorbed dose

- Conventional unit—Rad[Q]
    - Rad—stands for radiation absorbed dose
- SI unit—Gray[Q]

Absorbed dose equivalent

- Conventional unit—REM[Q]
    - Rem—stands for rontgen equivalent man
- SI unit—Sievert[Q]

Radioactivity

- Conventional unit-curie[Q]
- SI unit-Becquerel[Q]

Acute radiation syndromes[Q]/Radiationsickness[Q]/Radiation toxicity[Q]

Concept—Acute Radiation Syndromes (ARS)—Why do they occur in a particular order?

Law of Bergonié and Tribondeau[Q]: Basic Concept in Radiobiology

Whatever tissue/organ/region in the body has the maximum proportion of undifferentiated cells/cells in active mitosis will be more sensitive to radiation.

Four stages of acute radiation syndromes

1. Prodromal stage: Nausea vomiting-diarrhea stage—lasts from few minutes to hours
2. Latent phase: Lasts few hours to days
3. Manifest illness phase: Actual symptomatic stage—lasts from days to weeks
4. Recovery/Death stage: Lasts weeks to years

Acute hematological syndrome/ Bone marrow syndrome—1st clinical syndrome to occur

Threshold dose: Around 1–2 Gray[Q]

Gastrointestinal syndrome:

- 2nd organ system affected
- Threshold dose is 6–10 Gray[Q]
- Symptoms are malaise, severe diarrhea, electrolyte imbalance

Cardiovascular[Q]/CNS syndrome[Q]:

Threshold dose is around 20 Gray[Q]

DETERMINISTIC AND STOCHASTIC EFFECTS OF RADIATION

Smart-Work strategy tip: Remembering the various properties of these effects can be difficult. Hence, let us study them in a comparative manner. Also try to remember their examples first so that using those examples we can remember the individual properties.

	Deterministic effects	Stochastic effects
Examples	• Acute radiation syndromes[Q] (discussed above) • Cataract[Q] • Skin changes[Q]—Erythema, ulceration • Sterility[Q] • Radiation myelitis • Fibrosis • Teratogenesis/Fetal death	• Radiation induced carcinogenesis[Q] • Genetic mutations[Q] • Chromosome aberrations[Q]
Onset	Acute[Q] and subacute[Q] effects	Chronic effects[Q]
Threshold dose	Yes[Q]	No threshold dose[Q]
Severity of effect	Directly proportional to dose[Q]	Not related to dose[Q]
Risk of occurrence	Nonlinear relationship with threshold[Q]	**Linear relationship with no threshold (LNT)**
	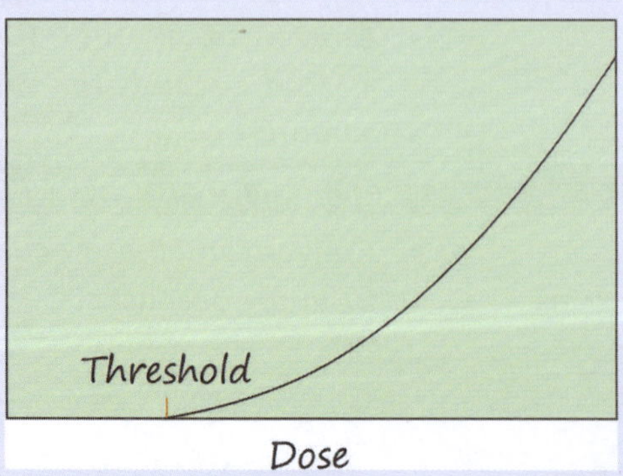	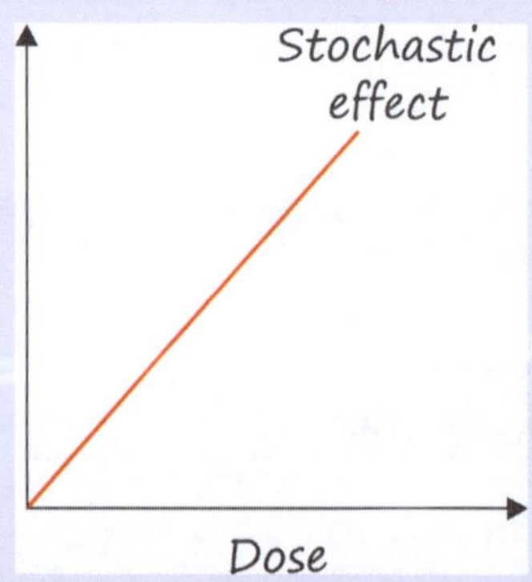

ADIATION EXPOSURE, PROTECTION AND GUIDELINES

Radiation exposures in various modalities

Modality	Radiation exposure in mSv	
PET	25	CT/PET/ Radionuclide studies
CT abdomen	10	CT/PET/ Radionuclide studies
CT thorax	8	CT/PET/ Radionuclide studies
Dynamic cardiac scintigraphy	6	CT/PET/ Radionuclide studies
Bone scan	4	CT/PET/ Radionuclide studies
CT head[Q]	3.5	CT/PET/ Radionuclide studies
Barium enema[Q]	7.2	Diagnostic procedures
Barium meal follow through	3	Diagnostic procedures
Barium meal	2.6	Diagnostic procedures
Barium swallow	1.5	Diagnostic procedures
MCU[Q]	1.2	Diagnostic procedures
Lumbar spine[Q]	1.0	Spot radiographs
Abdomen X-ray	0.7	Spot radiographs
Hip joint	0.4	Spot radiographs
Skull X-ray	0.06	Spot radiographs
CXR PA view[Q]	0.02	Spot radiographs
Limb X-rays[Q]/joint X-rays[Q]	<0.01	Spot radiographs

Permissible radiation exposure—recent guidelines

Recommended dose limits in planned exposure situations:

Type of Dose	Occupational exposure	Public exposure
Effective dose	20 mSv per year[Q], averaged over defined 5-year periods (100 mSv in 5 years) Or provision that the effective dose should not be exceeded 50 mSv[Q] in any single year with the total dose at end of 5 years should be <100 mSv.	1 mSv in a year[Q] A higher per year exposure may be allowed in a single year, provided that the average over defined 5-year periods does not exceed 1 mSv per year[Q]
Annual equivalent dose in:		
Lens of eye	150 mSv[Q]	15 mSv[Q]
Skin	500 mSv[Q]	50 mSv[Q]
Hands and feet	500 mSv[Q]	–
Pragnant radiation workers	**After declaration of pregnancy - 1 mSv dose to the embryo/fetus should not be exceeded[Q].**	

The ICRP and AERB guidelines are exactly similar with just one difference:

AERB–allows maximum exposure to occupational workers in any one year to be a maximum of **30 mSv**, provided that the total dose at end of 5 years should be <100 mSv

PYQ ALERT

Thermoluminescent dosimeter (TLD) Badge[Q]—NEET 2020 pattern question

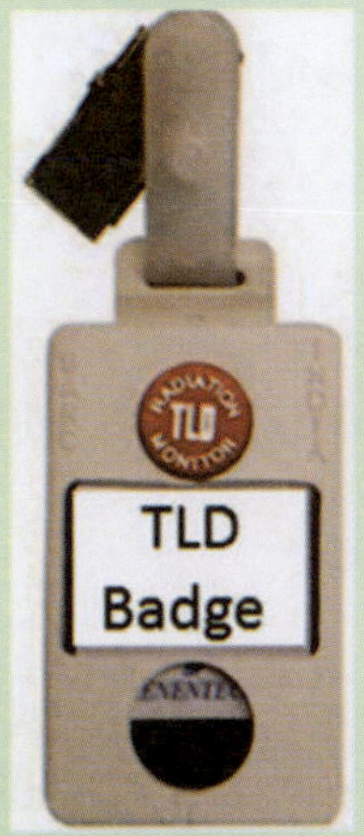

- Thermoluminescent dosimeter (TLD)[Q] is a passive radiation detection device that is used for personal dose monitoring or to measure patient dose.
- Composed of phosphor crystals[Q] [lithium fluoride (LiF)[Q], lithium borate ($Li_2B_4O_7$)[Q], beryllium oxide (BeO)[Q], and magnesium borate (MgB_4O_7)[Q]] that measure ionizing radiation primarily by trapping propagated gamma and neutron exposure.
- Incident energy is absorbed by some of the crystal's atoms thereby producing free electrons. Free electrons are trapped by the imperfect lattice structure of the crystal that is created due to doping impurities.
- The crystal is heated, the crystal vibrates to release the free electron back to its ground state. Trapped ionization is released as light, which is measured by photomultiplier tubes. This value is in ratio with the ionizing radiation captured by the phosphor, and represents the dosage administered to a person[Q], provided equipment was mounted properly.
- TLDs can measure doses between 0.01 mGy and 10 Gy[Q].

COMPUTED TOMOGRAPHY

Computed tomography is basically a fusion of two technologies:

1. **Tomography**[Q]: X-ray-based imaging technique developed to acquire sectional images of the body.
2. **Computers**[Q]: Brought in to deal with the complex mathematical algorithms and iterations in the image reconstruction.

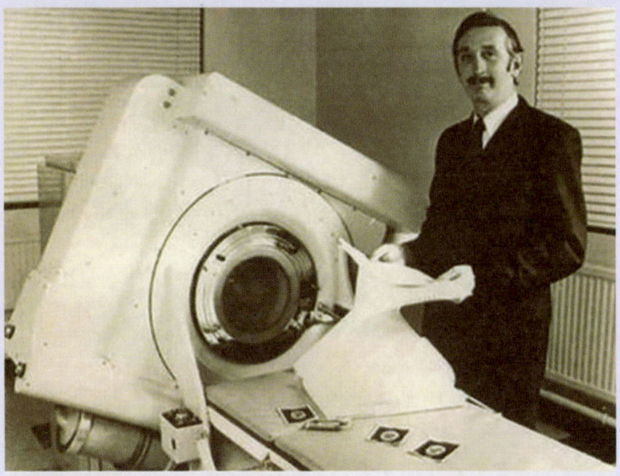

- Father of CT technology
- Invented the 1st generation CT scanner/EMI scanner
- Hounsfield Unit Scale (HU scale/CT value scale)
- Awarded Nobel Prize jointly with Allan Cormack in 1979

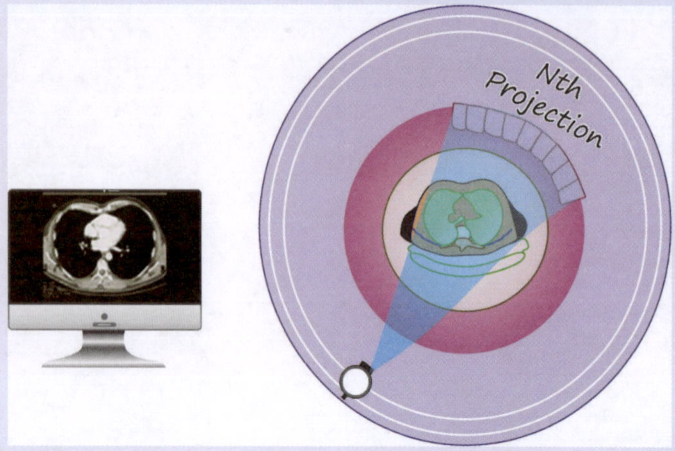

CT scan—basic principle: The internal structure of an object can be reconstructed from multiple projection of that object[Q].

BASIC PRINCIPLE OF CT SCAN

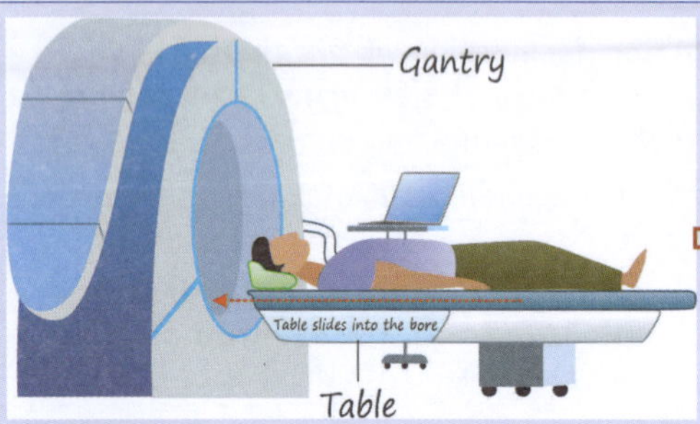

CT machine—has a gantry (tomographic unit) and tale (patient lies on this tale and it slides into the ore of the gantry)

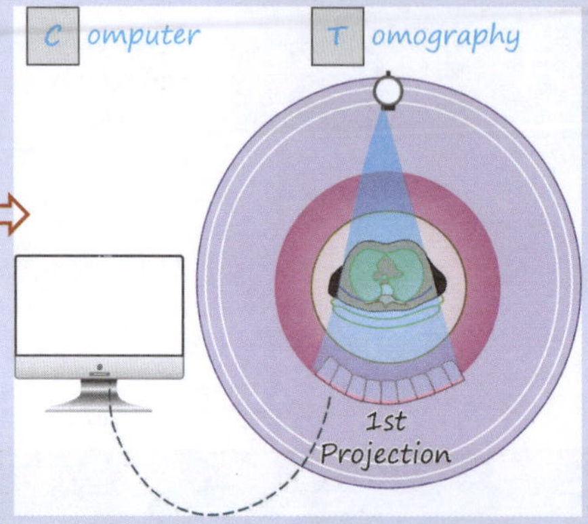

1st Projection data is obtained and transferred to computer

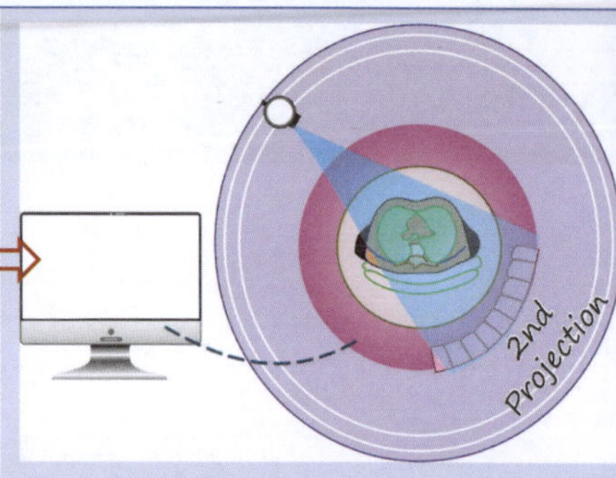

2nd Projection data is obtained (from a different angle) and transferred to computer

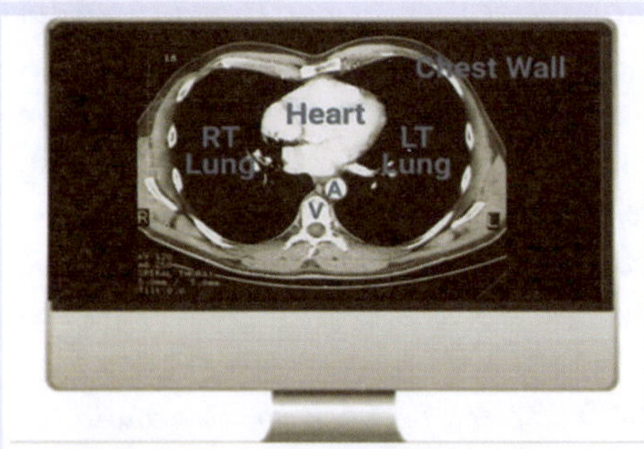

Computer reconstructs internal structure of body from all the projection data—using complex mathematical algorithms

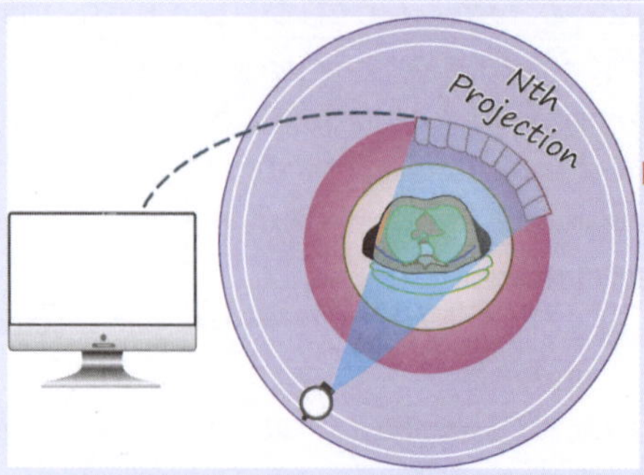

Nth Projection is obtained—all from different angles around the patient and transferred to computer

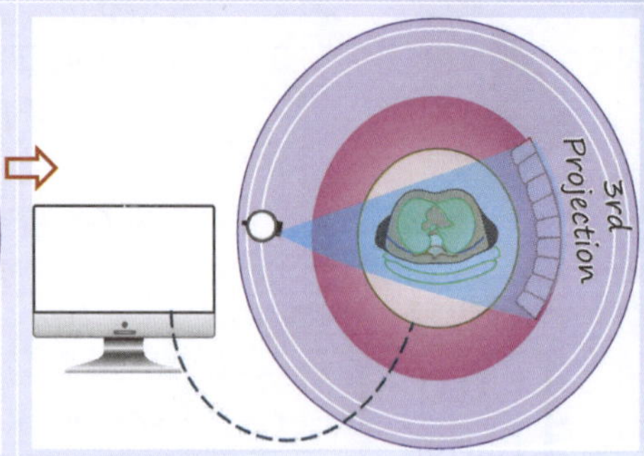

3rd Projection data is obtained (from another different angles) and transferred to computer

CT scan Miscellaneous

Hounsfield unit (HU) scale/CT value scale

Each tissue in the body is allotted a numerical value – it is "HU/CT value"

$$\text{HU Value} = 1000 \times \frac{\mu_x - \mu_w}{\mu_w}$$

- μ_x = Linear attenuation coefficient of a tissue "x"
- μ_w = Linear attenuation coefficient of water
- Main determinant of linear attenuation coefficient of a tissue is its desnsity[Q]

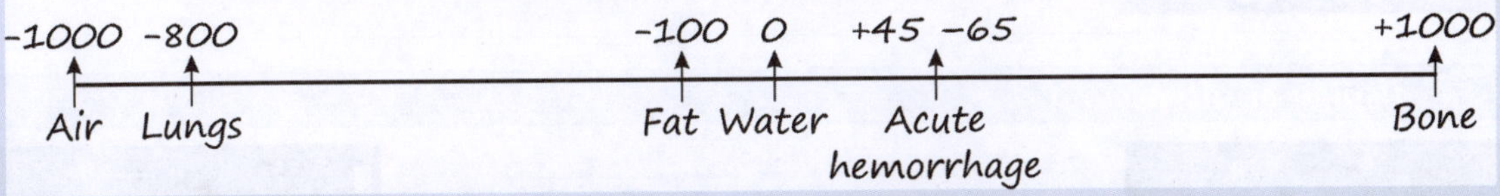

CT descriptive terminology

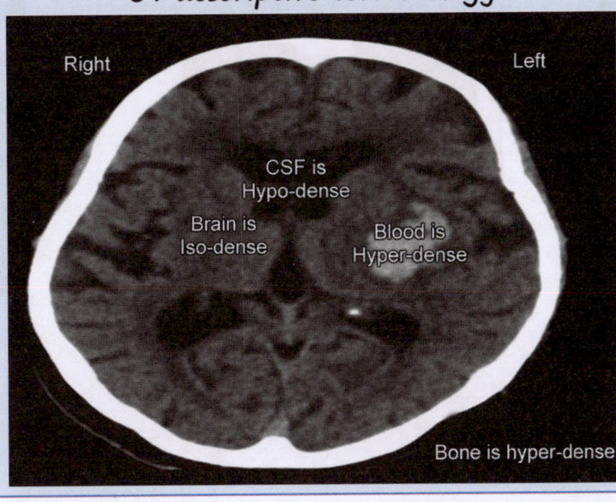

ULTRASOUND IMAGING

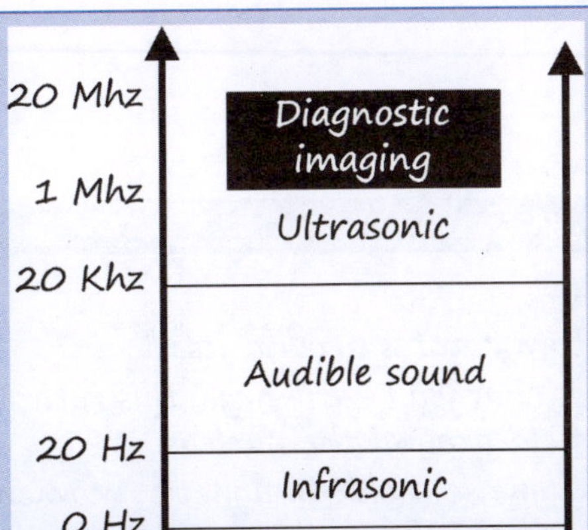

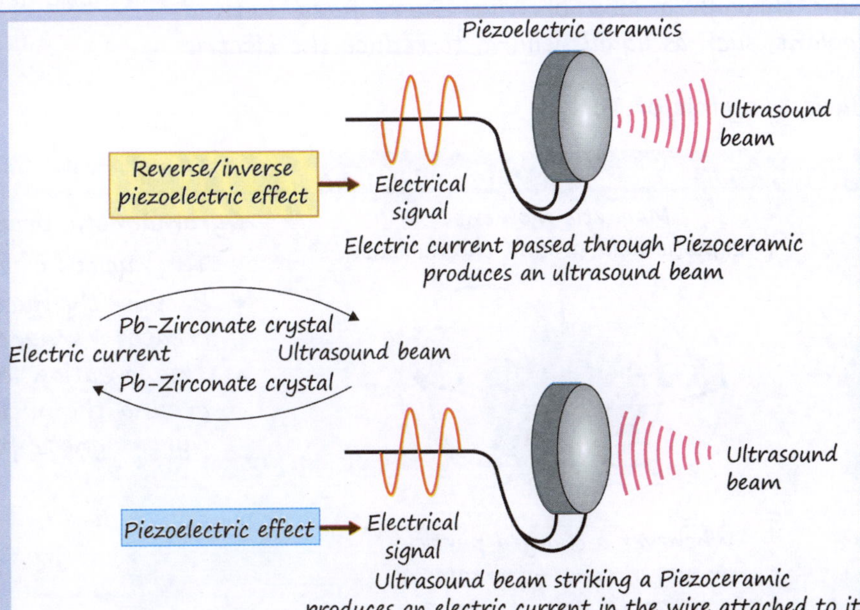

Contd...

Pulse-echo principle

Pulse–echo principle

Depth-location of organ can be determined

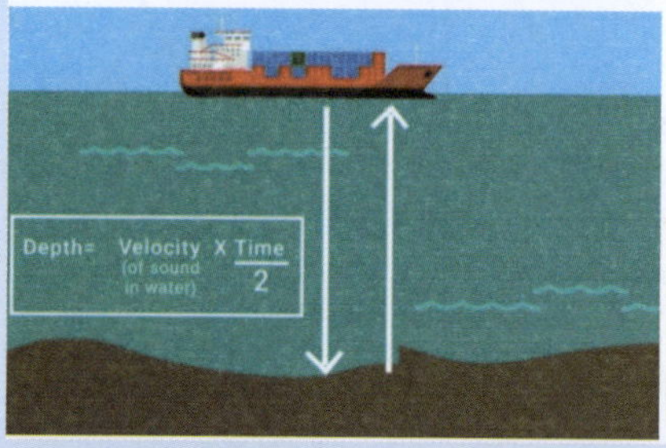

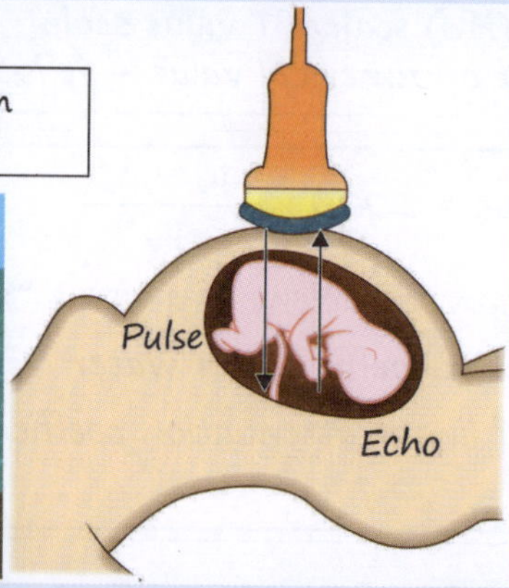

Sound emitted by probe (pulse)
↓
Hits an organ in the body and is reflected back (echo)
↓
Received by probe

In methods of display of ultrasound

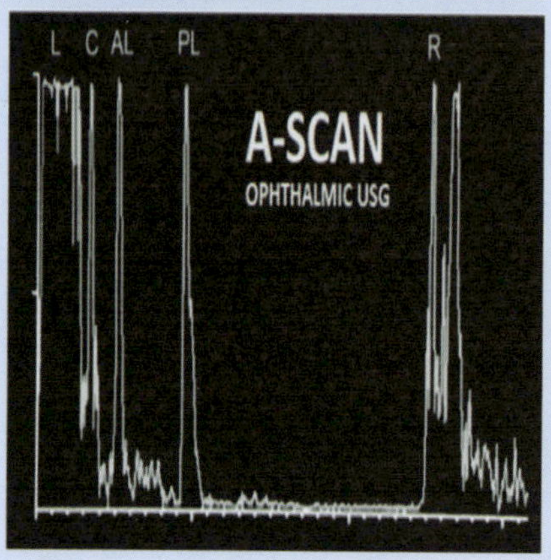

A-mode

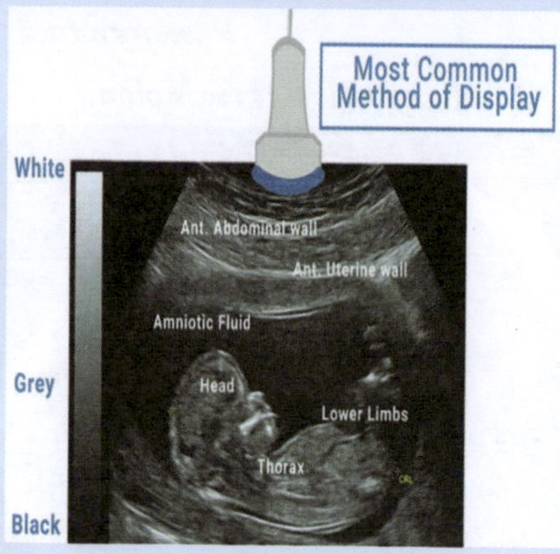

B-mode

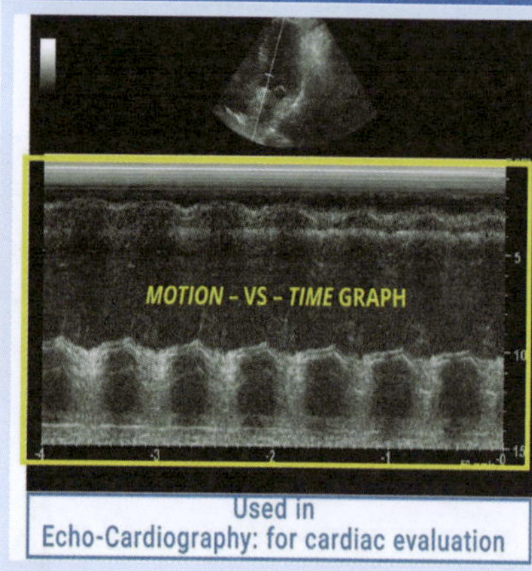

M-mode

MRI BASICS

MRI Magnet—is a Superconducting Magnet[Q]

The magnetic field is generated by a current, which runs through a loop of wire. Surrounded with a coolant, such as liquid helium, to reduce the electric resistance of the wire. At 4 Kelvin (-269°C) electric wire loses its resistance. Thus producing a permanent magnetic field.

Basic Principle of MRI

"Human MRI is based on Gyromagnetic property[Q] of Hydrogen nucleus"

Magnetic moment (magnetic field around the nucleus)

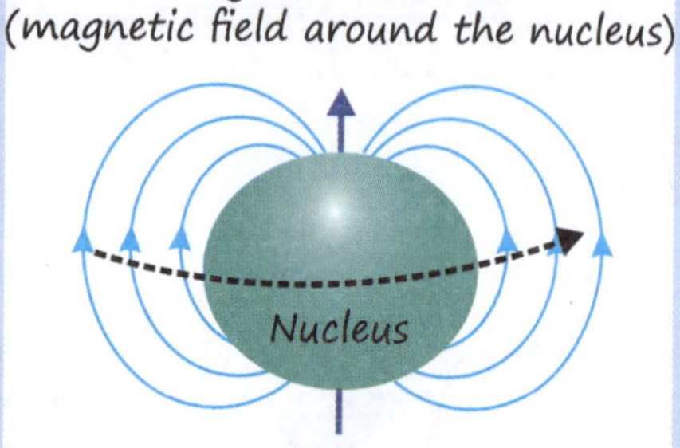

Whenever a charged particle moves in space—it creates a magnetic field around it

Gyromagnetic property:

- The nucleus of an atom rotates around itself.
- Because the nucleus is charged (+ve charge) this rotation creates a magnetic field around the nucleus.
- This creation of magnetic field (magnetic moment) around the nucleus created due to its rotation is called **Gyromagnetic property[Q].**

Contd...

"Human MRI is based on Gyromagnetic property[Q] of Hydrogen nucleus"

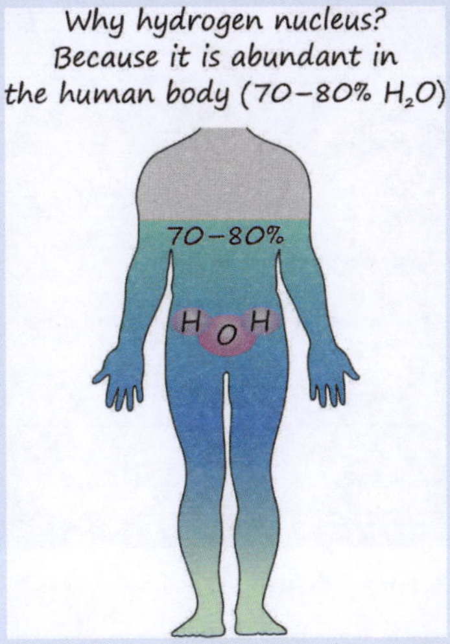

Why Hydrogen nucleus?

- Hydrogen has the highest Gyromagnetic ratio—suggests a strong gyromagnetic property.
- Hydrogen is very abundant in the human body (70-80% of body weight is formed by water)
- Hence, if we measure the signal arising from Hydrogen nuclei in the body—it will be a very strong signal—thus creating an excellent Image.

MRI Image Basics

T1W	T2W H_2O is Bright on T2W images
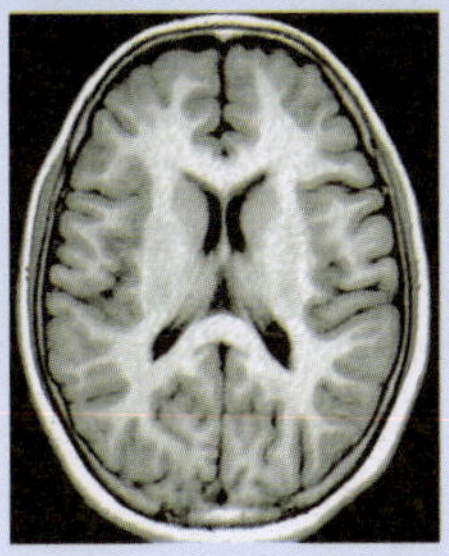	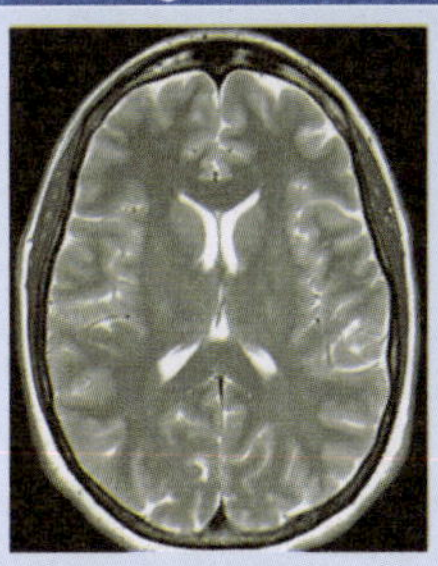

CSF signal intensity	T1W	T2W
	CSF is Hypointense (Black)	CSF is Hyperintense (White)
Gray matter and white matter	Anatomical image – So white matter appears white, gray matter appears gray.	Appearance of gray and white matter is opposite to their names

T2W	Fluid attenuated inversion recovery (FLAIR)
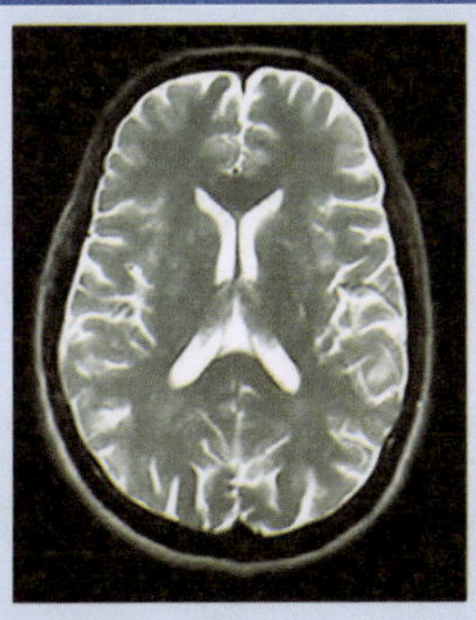	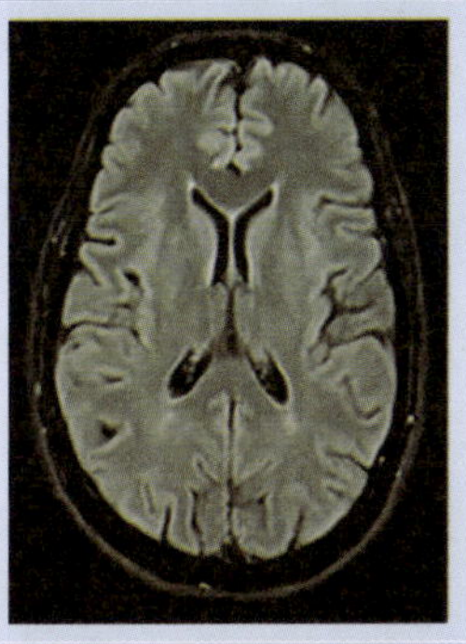
CSF/Water: Hyperintense Gray-White matter appearance (Opposite to their names) • Gray matter is hyperintense • White matter is hypointense	**CSF/Water**: Hypointense–Fluid signal is attenuated[Q]-hence the name: • Gray matter is hyperintense • White matter is hypointense
Better for depiction of pathology	Can detect even the smallest of lesions

MRI image gallery

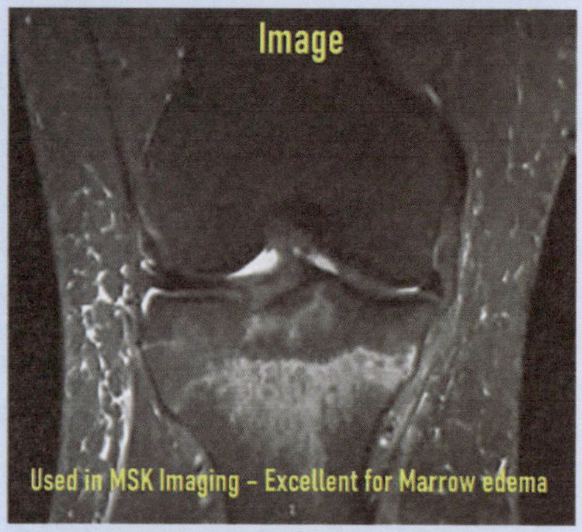

Short Tau inversion recovery (STIR)

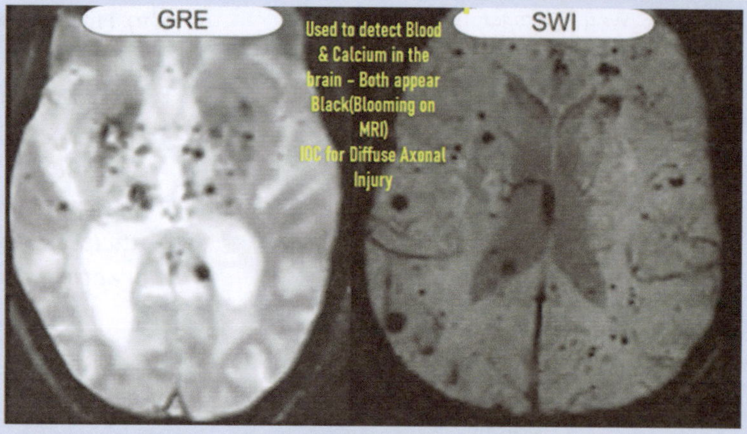

Blood sensitive sequences

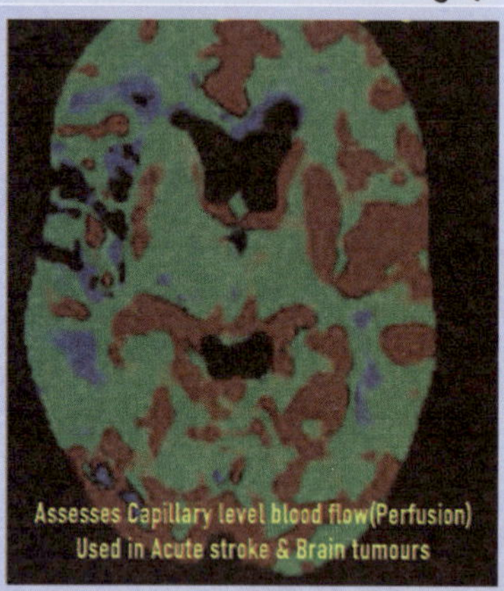

Perfusion weighted imaging (PWI)

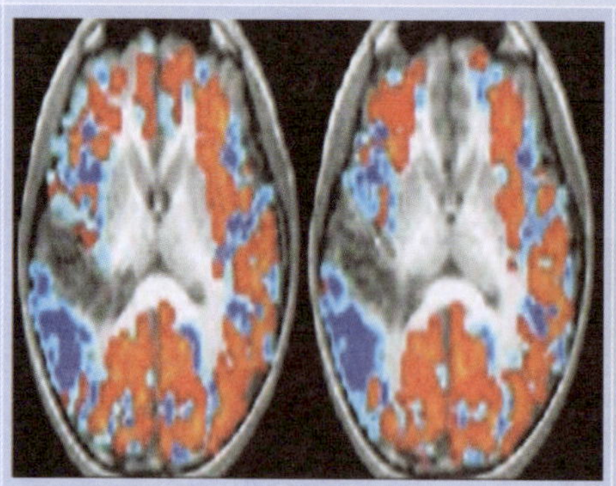
Functional MRI/Bold–Blood Oxygen Level Dependant Imaging Fat MRI acquisition–to detect functional centers of the brain

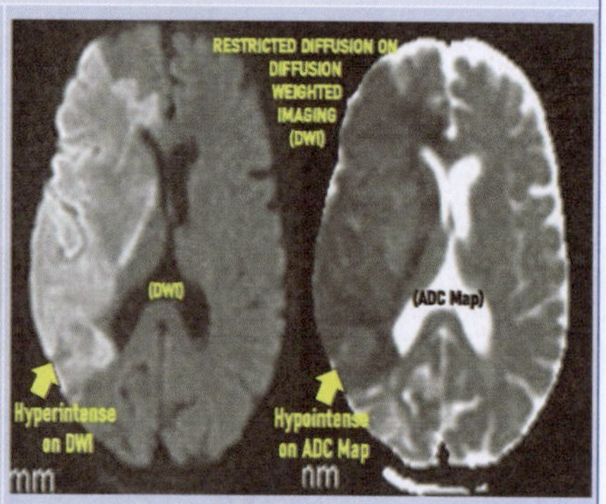

Diffusion weighted imaging (DWI)

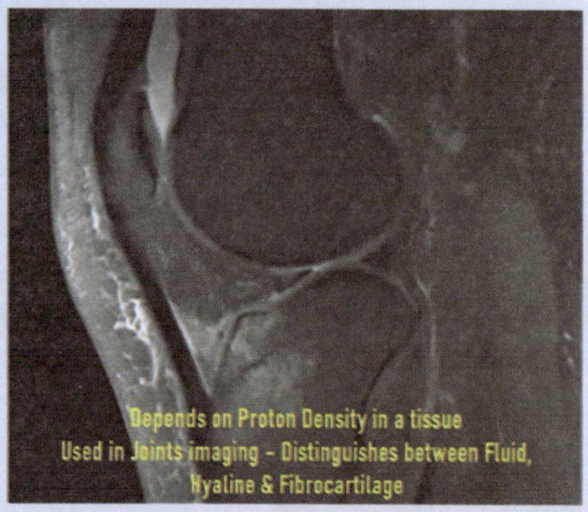

Proton density (PD) image

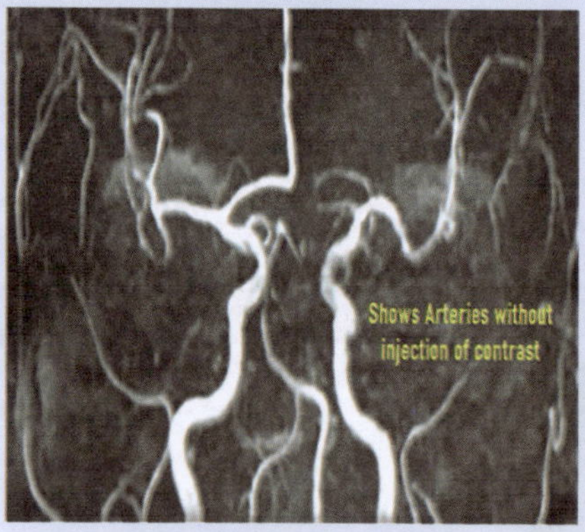

TOF–MRA: Time of flight MR angiography

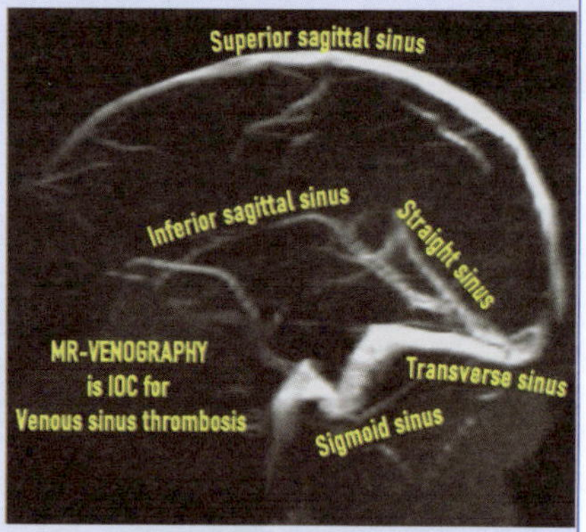

MR-Venography

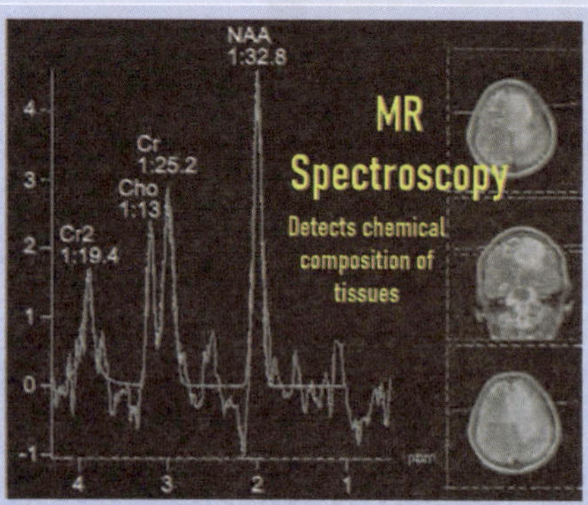

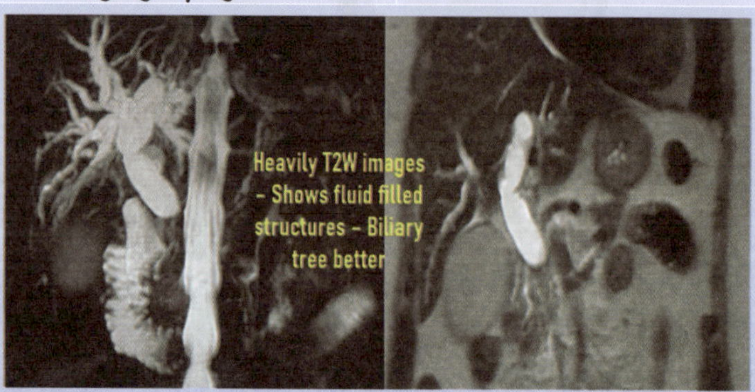

Magnetic Resonance Cholangio-Pancreaticography (MRC)

CONTRAINDICATIONS FOR MRI[Q]

Absolute contraindications[Q]:
- *Cardiac pacemaker*
- *Metallic foreign body of eye*
- *Ferromagnetic hemostatic aneurysm clips in CNS*

Relative contraindications[Q]:
- *Cochlear implants*
- *Claustrophobia*
- *Insulin pumps/Nerve stimulators*
- *1st trimester pregnancy*
- *Epidural catheters/CNS Ventricular catheters*
- *Spinal fixation devices*
- *Feeding tubes*
- *Prosthetic heart valves*
- *Orthopedic external fixators*

Faraday Cage[Q]—*is a shielding box used all around the MRI room to shield out stray electromagnetic interference. Made up of wood panels wrapped with copper[Q].*

CONTRAST MEDIA

Definition: *Any agent that is used to enhance the appearance of a particular structure/organ in the body.*

Classification

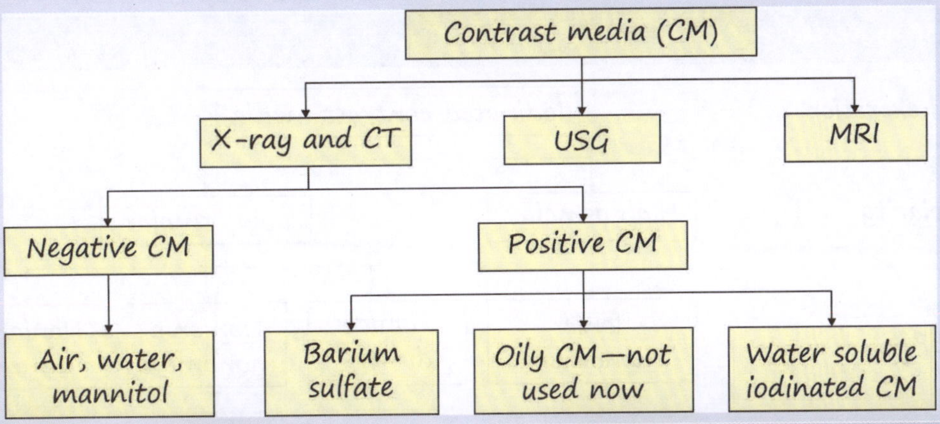

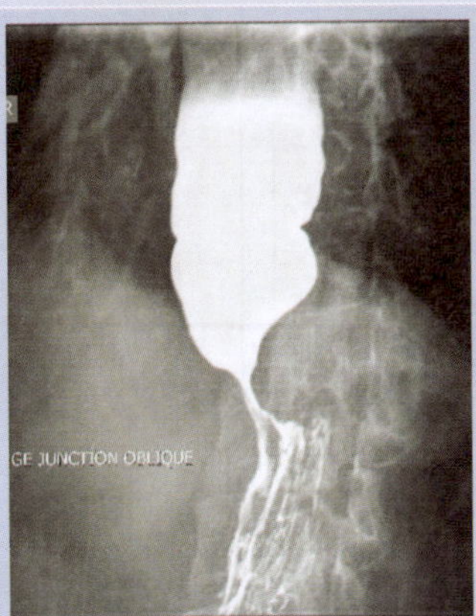

Positive CM
- *Attenuate more X-rays than soft tissues—hence, appear whiter*
- *Examples – Barium sulfate and Iodinated media*

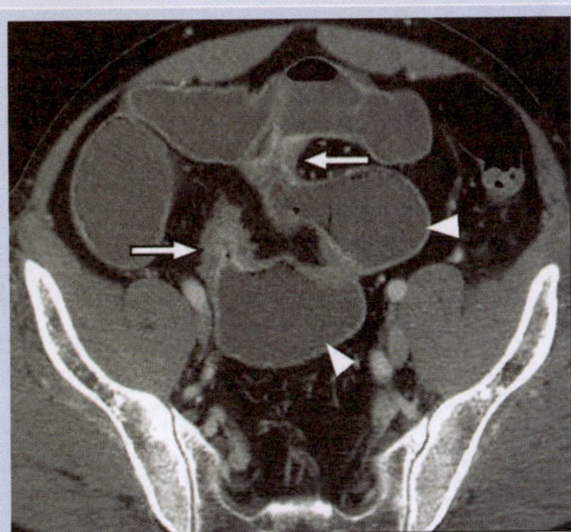

Negative CM
- *Attenuate less X-rays than soft tissues—hence, appear blacker*
- *Examples – Air, water, mannitol*

Barium – *Used as Barium sulfate ($BaSO_4$) suspension[Q]*

Why? – *Inert*
- *No damage/irritation to bowel mucosa*
- *Not absorbed*
- *No interference with normal digestion/absorption*

Contd...

Absolute contraindication: Perforation causes severe chemical peritonitis – may be fatal.

Relative contraindications: Hypersensitivity, left sided colonic obstruction. Vesicovaginal/Rectovaginal fistulas

Where? – It is used for bowel evaluation

Barium study	Used for
Barium swallow	Cricopharynx – Esophagus – Gastroesophageal junction
Barium meal	Stomach and Proximal duodenum
Barium meal follow-through	Small bowel
Barium enema	Large bowel

Iodine to particle ratio: Concept

Iodine – Numerator – Determines attenuation – Should be as high as possible

Particles – Denominator – Determines osmolarity – Should be as low as possible

Hence overall the I/P ratio must be as high as possible[Q]

Iodinated contrast materials

Renal excretion	Iodinated contrast media			
Osmolarity	High osmolar	Low osmolar		
Subtypes	Ionic monomers	Ionic dimers	Nonionic monomers	Nonionic dimers
Iodine: Particle ratio:	3:2	6:2	3:1	6:1
Examples	Trazograf Urografin Angiografin, Gastrografin Thalmic acid (conray), Urivision, Urovideo	Ioxaglic acid, Iocarmic acid	Amipaque, iohexol/ omnipaque Iopamidol, Ioversol Iopromide	Iotrol, Iotrolan, Iodixanol

Contrast Induced Nephropathy (CIN)

Diagnostic criteria: Impairment of renal function, measured as

- 25% increase in serum creatinine from baseline[Q] or
- 0.5 mg/dL (44 μmol/L) increase in absolute serum creatinine value[Q]
- Within 48–72 hours[Q] after intravenous contrast administration(following contrast exposure, serum creatinine levels peak between 2 and 5 days and usually return to normal in 14 days)

Markers of CIN:

- Serum creatinine[Q] – as described in in diagnosis
- Estimated GFR (eGFR)[Q] (estimated GFR [eGFR] <60 mL/min/1.73 m^2) – predictive marker of CIN
- Serum Cystatin C levels[Q]
- Plasma neutrophil gelatinase-associated lipocalin (NGAL), also known as human neutrophil lipocalin, is an early predictive biomarker

Contd...

Risk factors:	Prevention of CIN:
Most important risk factor - Pre-existing Chronic kidney disease[Q] • Elderly age • DM • Metabolic syndrome • Anemia • Hypovolemia/Dehydration • MM **Treatment of CIN** • Supportive Rx – sufficient in most cases. • Hemodialysis[Q] – rarely needed—can efficiently remove contrast from the blood stream	• Precontrast Renal function tests • Precontrast hydration using IV normal saline[Q] – is most important step • N-Acetyl cysteine[Q] –sulfhydryl groups that act as antioxidants and free radical scavengers High dose statins[Q] – Rosuvastatin • Bicarbonate therapy[Q] • Statins - Rosuvastatin

MRI contrast agents

T_1 Relaxation agents[Q]	T_2 Relaxation agents[Q]	Liver specific contrast agents
• **Gadolinium compounds[Q]**: Most commonly used MRI contrast medium[Q] • **Paramagnetic substances[Q]**: Affect the magnetic properties of adjacent molecules Act as extracellular contrast agent cause shortening of T_1 relaxation time[Q]—hence, appear bright on T1W MRI[Q] • **FDA approved agents:** ▪ Gd-HP-DO3A-Gadoteridol/ProHance ▪ Gd—DTPA—Magnevist ▪ Gd—DTPA—BMA—Omniscan	Superparamagnetic iron oxide (SPIO)[Q]/Ultrasmall—SPIO (USPIO)[Q]— undergoes selective phagocytosis by reticuloendothelial system cells[Q] (Kupffer cells)[Q] Uptake causes hypointense appearance on T2W images[Q] Specific for FNH—shows around 60–70% signal loss on T2W images[Q] Hepatic adenomas show only 15–20% signal loss.	Manganese—DPDP[Q] Gd—BOPTA[Q] Gd—EOB—DTPA[Q]

Nephrogenic systemic fibrosis (NSF)/Nephrogenic fibrosing dermopathy

- In renal failure patients
- Associated gadolinium compounds:
  - Omniscan/Gadodiamide[Q]—Most commonly implicated
  - Magnevist/Gadopentetate dimeglumine[Q]—2nd most common
  - OptiMARK/Gadoversetamide[Q]
- Subcutaneous edema and firm, indurated, erythematous skin plaques—progress to flexure contractures with restricted movements – progressive condition with no Rx.

Toll-like receptors (TLR)[Q] - TLR4 and TLR7 – involved in pathogenesis

2. RESPIRATORY SYSTEM IMAGING

CHEST RADIOGRAPH PROJECTIONS/VIEWS

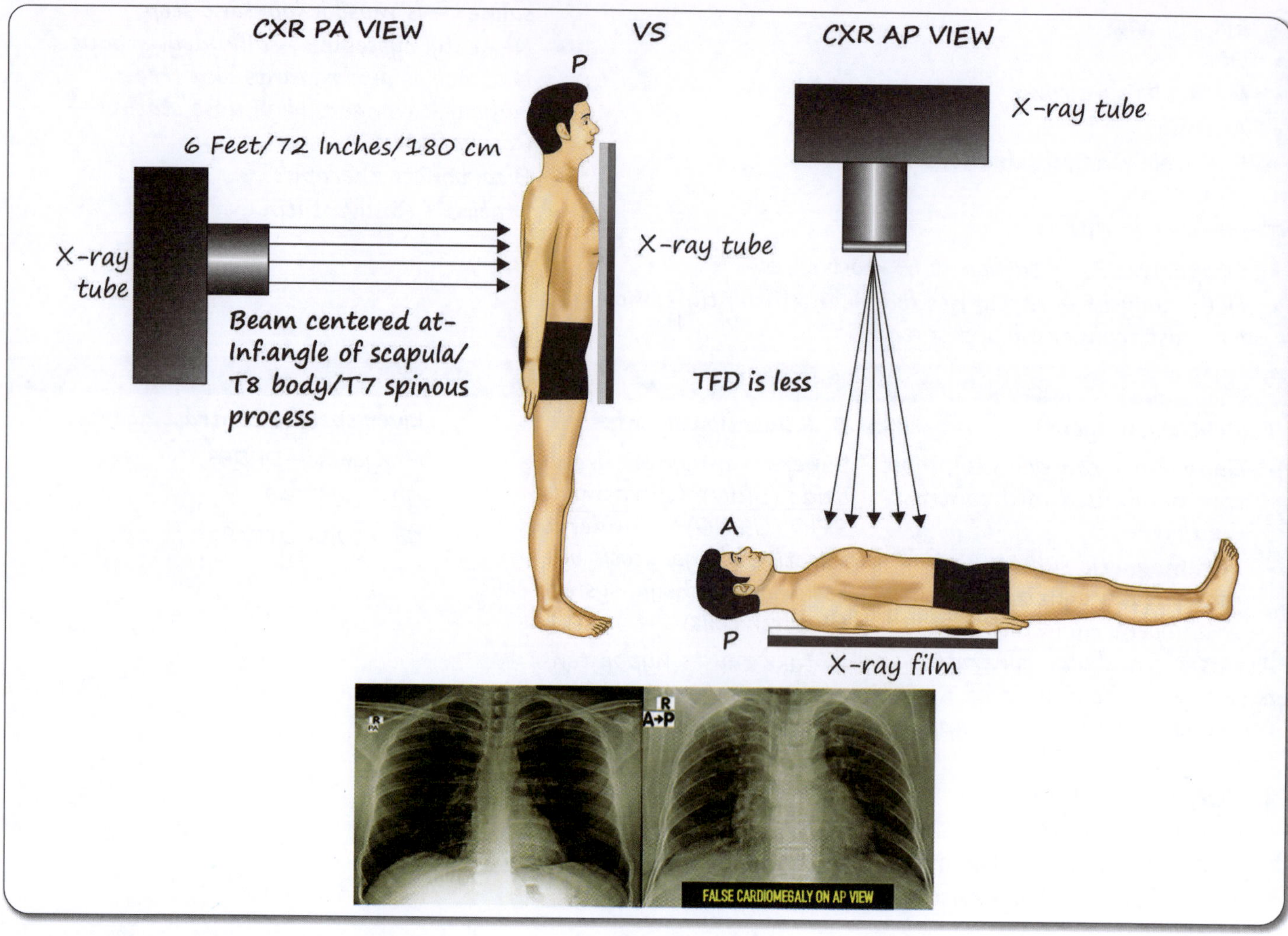

Other Chest Projections

Lateral decubitus view	• Best X-ray projection for detection of minimal pleural effusion[Q]
Lordotic view/apicogram	• Demonstration of lung apices[Q]–Pancoast tumor[Q] • Better for middle lobe pathologies[Q] (RML and Lingular segment)/ Interlobar pleural effusions[Q]
Paired inspiratory and expiratory views	• Diaphragmatic movement in palsy • Foreign body aspiration • Air trapping
Right posterior oblique	• Right side rib fractures/lesions • Shows the maximum area of right lung field
Left posterior oblique	• Left side rib fractures/lesions • Left Posterior Obliques (LPO) shows the left lung field
Right anterior oblique	• Evaluation of sternum[Q] • Evaluation of esophagus in barium swallow studies[Q] • Assessment of pulmonary artery, right ventricle, size of left atrium
Left anterior oblique	• Patient erect, rotated 45° with left anterior shoulder against cassette • Assessment of aortic window[Q] and aorta

CXR BASIC INTERPRETATION

Radiographic exposure

Good quality radiograph—margins of lower thoracic vertebral bodies should just be visible through the heart[Q] (Yellow arrows).

Patient centering/rotation

- Comparing distance between:
  - Midline anatomic landmark: The spinous process of upper dorsal vertebrae (Yellow dot)
  - Lateral anatomic landmarks: Medial end of clavicles on either side (Yellow vertical solid lines)
- Well centered X-ray: Equal distance on both sides
- Rotated X-ray: Distance unequal; whatever side the patient is rotated—distance more on that same side
- Rotation causes Unilateral radiolucency[Q] (blackness).

Identifying anterior and posterior end of ribs

- **Anterior ends of ribs (Blue dotted lines):**
  - Away from midline and
  - Obliquely oriented
- **Posterior ends of Ribs (Yellow dotted lines):**
  - Close to midline and
  - Horizontally oriented

Identifying inspiration versus expiration

- By counting of ribs seen above the diaphragm
- Criteria for good Inspiratory X-ray:
  - At least 6 anterior ends of ribs seen (Blue numbers on right)
  - At least 10 posterior ends of ribs seen (Yellow numbers on left)

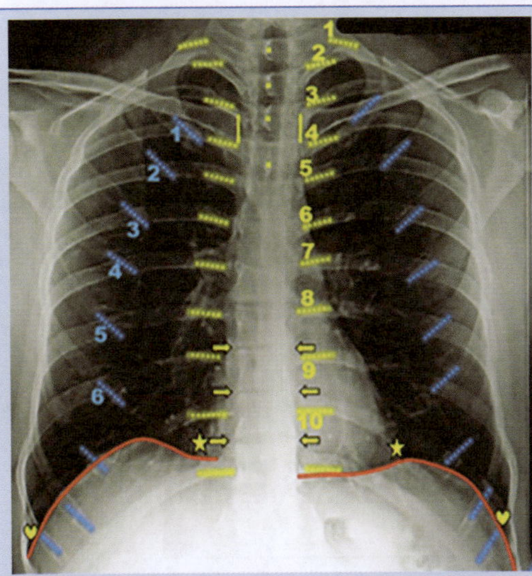

Diaphragm:

- Diaphragmatic contour is formed by the right and left domes of diaphragm (Red solid lines).
- Parts of Diaphragm **NOT SEEN** on a CXR PA:
  - Central tendon of diaphragm[Q]
  - Small medial most portion of left dome of diaphragm[Q]
- **Diaphragmatic levels:**
  - The left dome is always lower than the right[Q].
  - In few normal patients, both the domes may be at the same level.
  - A difference in the levels of the domes of diaphragm of >3 cm is significant[Q]—must be investigated for any abnormality.
- **Diaphragmatic angles:**
  - **Cardiophrenic angle (Yellow stars):** Sharp angle at the interface of heart and diaphragm. May not always be sharp as this is a common site for epicardial fat pads, or pericardial cysts which may obscure these angles.
  - **Costophrenic angle (Yellow hearts):** Sharp, acute angles at the junction point of Diaphragm and the chest wall laterally. Always sharp and acute. Blunting of these angles is seen in pleural effusions[Q].

Trachea: Vertical linear band like lucency in upper mediastinum

Identifying the Carina

Carina is the point where the trachea divides into the right and left bronchi. Carefully, tracing the tracheal lucency downward will bring you to the carina. To Identify, it is important clinically. Normal carinal angle is 60°–75°. Carinal widening occurs in enlarged left atrium (in mitral stenosis)[Q] and enlarged subcarinal lymph nodes[Q]

CXR–ADDITIONAL FINDINGS

Mediastinal margins on CXR

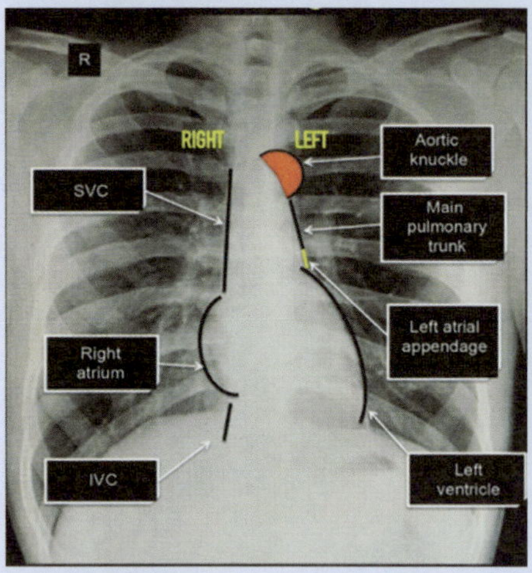

Trachea and main bronchi

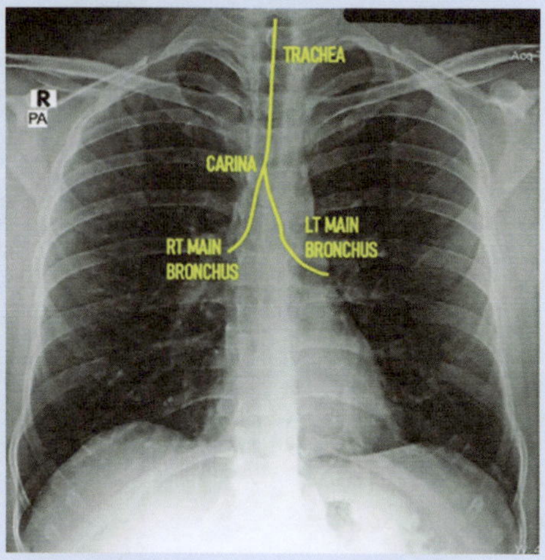

Hidden areas on CXR

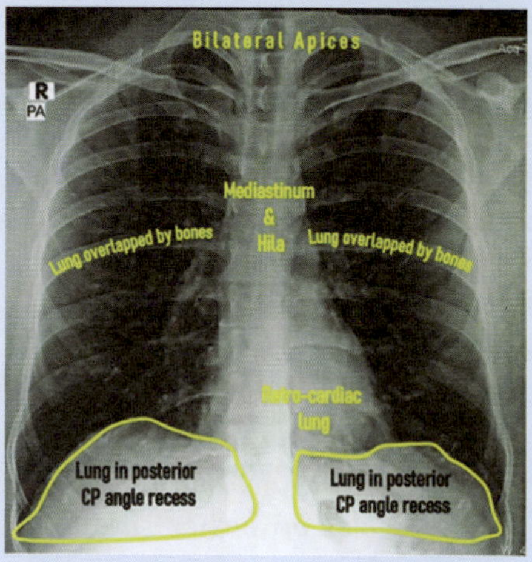

Hilar shadows on CXR

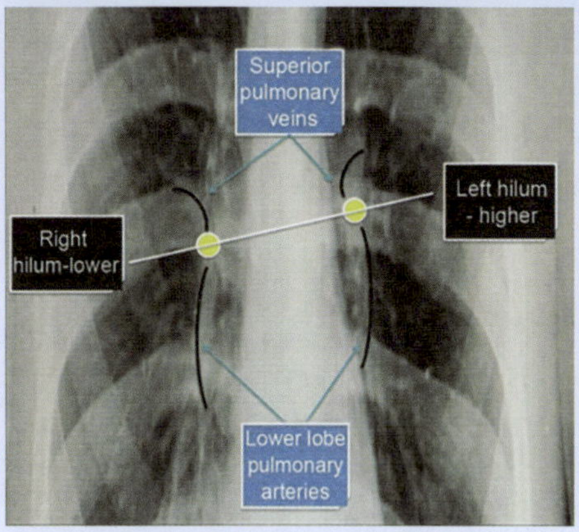

Normal Hilum:

Major contributors:

- Upper lobe pulmonary vein[Q] – forms the short indistinct upper limb of hilum
- Lower lobe pulmonary vein[Q] – forms the long prominent lower limb of hilum

Minor contributors:

- Central bronchi
- Lymph nodes

Lower lobe pulmonary vein[Q] – DOES NOT contribute to hilar shadows

Hilar point[Q]: Is where the upper and lower hilar limbs meet

Hilar level: Left hilum is always higher[Q] than left. They may be at same level – but right is NEVER higher.

Hilar shape: Is concave laterally[Q].

Cardiothoracic ratio on CXR

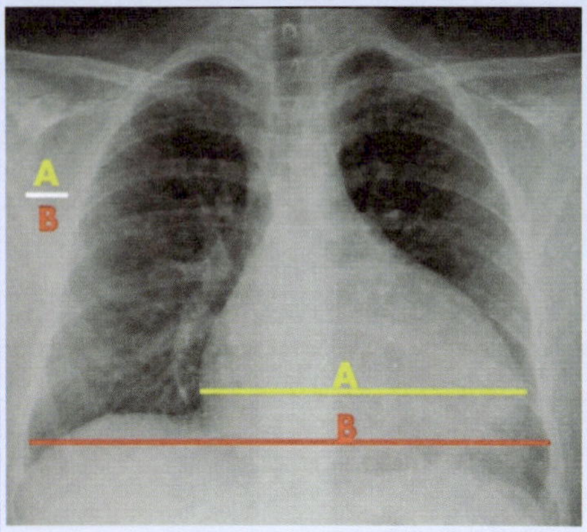

Cardiothoracic ratio

Diagnosis based on cardiothoracic ratio

On a CXR PA view	
<0.50	Normal
0.50–0.55	Borderline
>0.55	Cardiomegaly[Q]
On a CXR AP view/Pediatric CXR	
<0.60	Normal
>0.60	Cardiomegaly[Q]

Contd...

Lung fissures on CXR

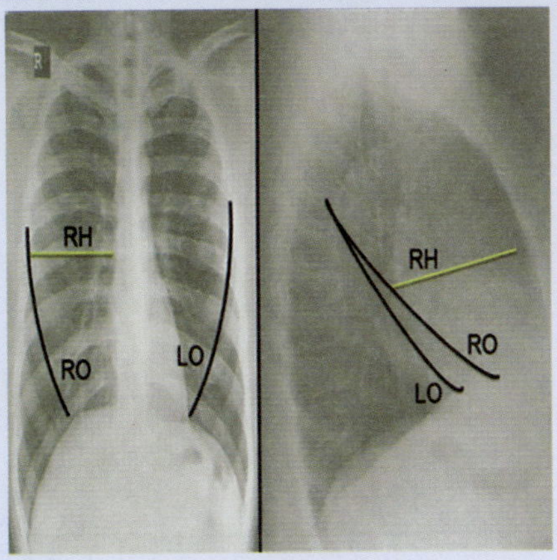

Main Fissures

Right lung has two fissures: Major/Oblique and Minor/Horizontal fissure

Left lung has just one fissure: Major/Oblique fissure

Major/Oblique Fissure

- On lateral film runs 'obliquely' from Posterosuperior to anteroinferior.
- Begins posteriorly at level of T4/T5 level, passes through the hilum and comes down anteroinferiorly.

Minor/Horizontal Fissure

Runs 'horizontally' on the right side from the hilum to the region of 6th rib in the midaxillary line.

Normal findings on lateral CXR

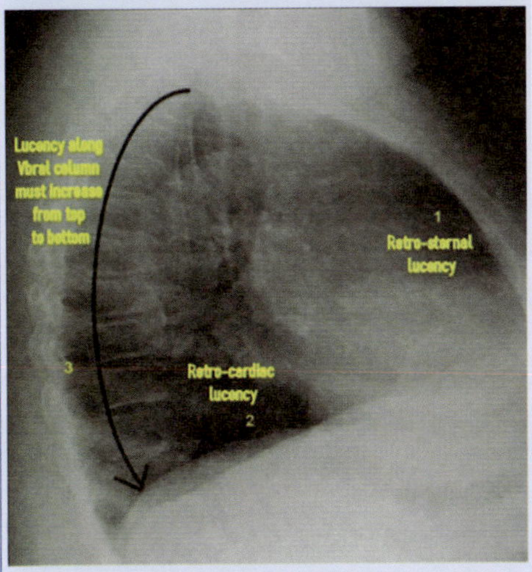

"3 Normal Findings on a Lateral CXR"[Q]

Retrosternal Lucency:

- Lucency/blackness just behind the sternum, where the two lungs meet.
- Obliteration of this space occurs with Anterior mediastinal masses[Q], ascending aorta aneurysms[Q] and lymph nodal masses[Q] and occasionally with RA enlargement

Retrocardiac Lucency

- Similar area of blackness behind the heart
- Lost in lower lobe pathologies[Q], pleural effusion[Q], descending thoracic aortic aneurysm[Q]

Vertebral Translucency

- Normally, as you travel from the top to the bottom the density over the vertebral bodies become progressively translucent/black[Q]. This is known as the **Spine sign**[Q]
- This gradient may be lost in lower lobe/posterior basal consolidation[Q]—where the lower portion appears whiter/denser.

CXR–NORMAL VARIANTS

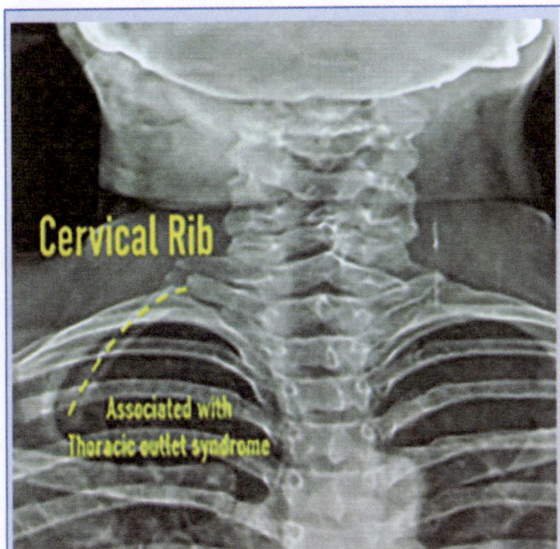

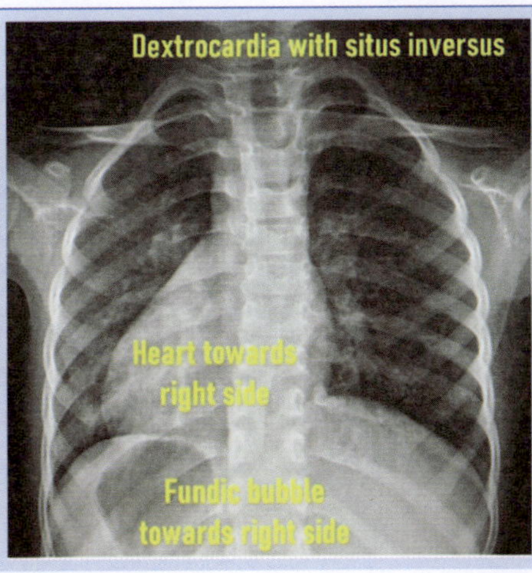

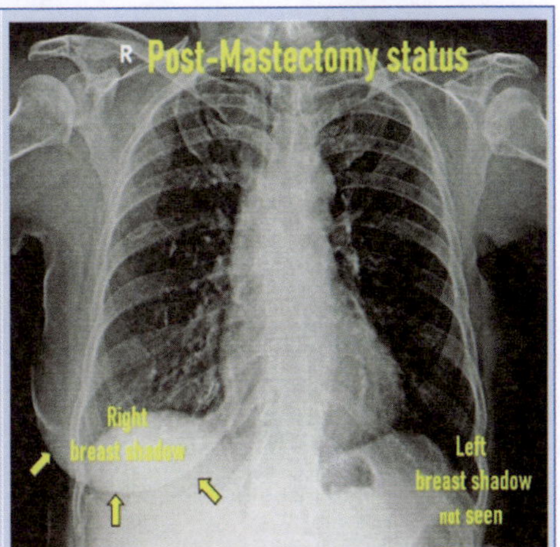

Contd...

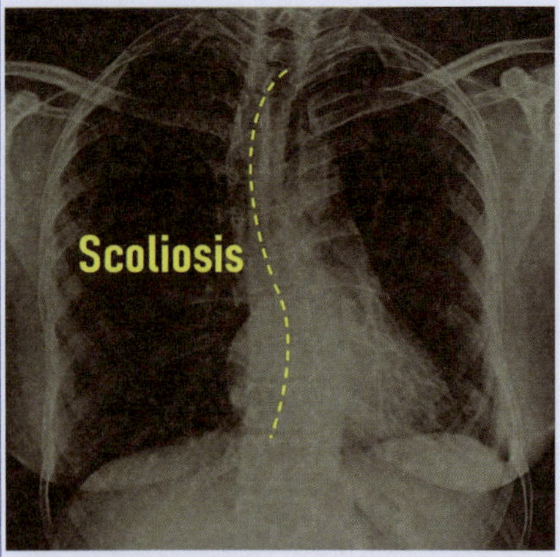

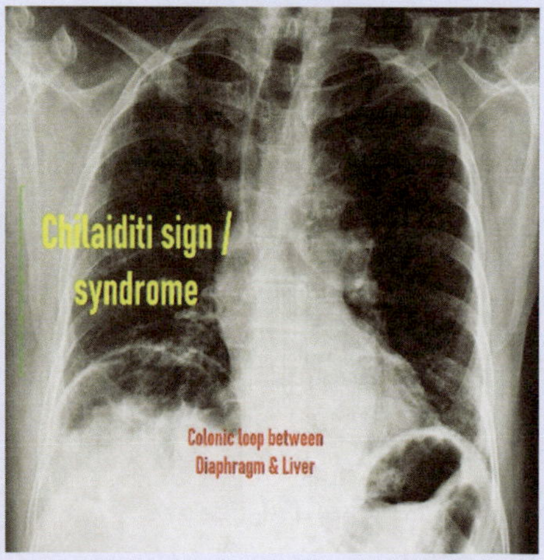

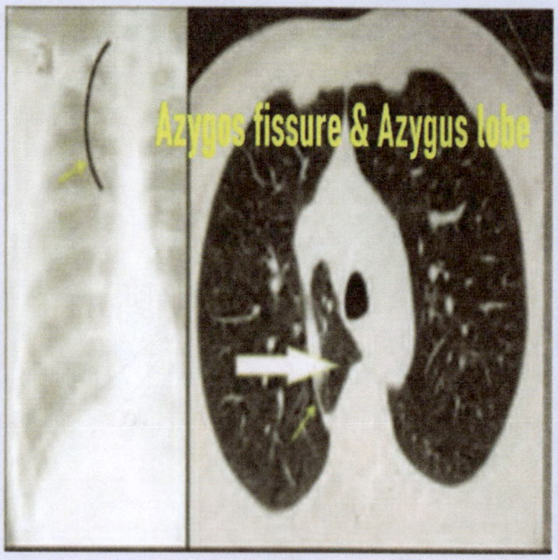

DIFFERENTIAL RADIOGRAPHIC DENSITY THEORY AND SILHOUETTE SIGN

- *Only five tissue densities are seen separately from each other on any CXR – Air – Fat – Water – Bone– Metal*
- *Whenever 2 tissues of DIFFERENT densities are located adjacent to each other – Sharp margin is seen between them. On a CXR – sharp margins of mediastinum, heart and diaphragm are seen because adjacent lung is normal and air-filled (this of different density)*
- *When 2 tissues of same density come to lie adjacent to each other – the intervening sharp margin is LOST. If any lung becomes consolidated(water density) the adjacent tissue (mediastinum/heart/ diaphragm) is also water density – thus the intervening sharp margin is lost.*
- *This is called positive silhouette sign.*

Obscured margins on CXR

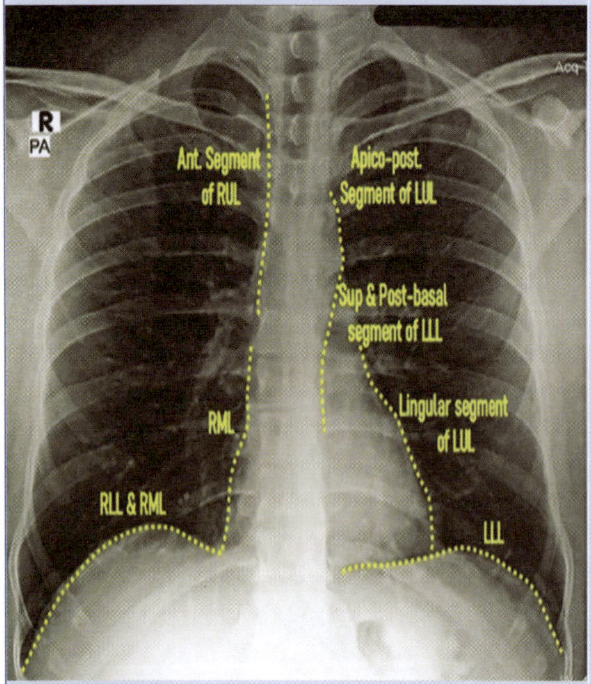

Silhouette Lost/ Obliterated	Lung Lobe/Segment Involved
Right upper mediastinal margin	Anterior segment of right upper lobe[Q]
Right heart border	Right middle lobe (medial segment)[Q]
Right dome of diaphragm	Right lower lobe, most commonly[Q] Right middle lobe, occasionally[Q]
Aortic knuckle	Left upper lobe (Apicoposterior segment)[Q]
Lateral margin of descending thoracic aorta	Left lower lobe (superior and posterior basal segment)[Q]
Left heart border	Left upper lobe (lingular segment)[Q]
Left dome of diaphragm	Left lower lobe[Q]

RUL consolidation

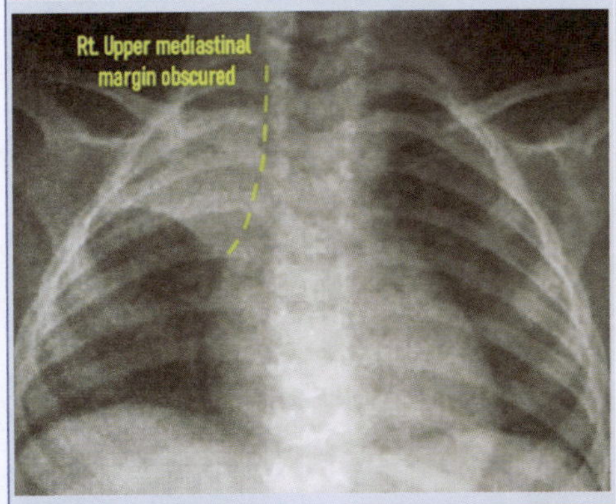

RML consolidation

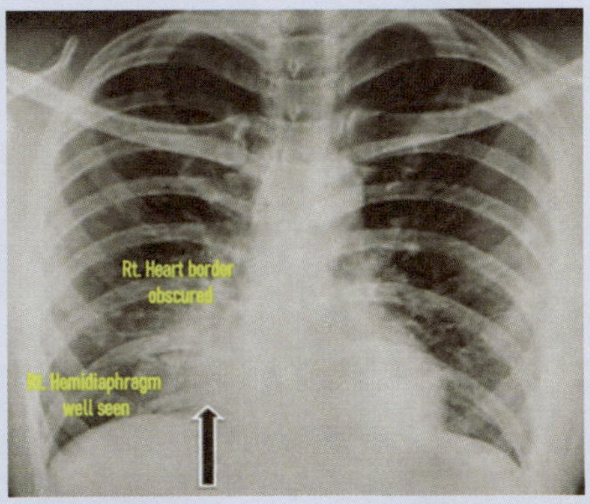

RLL consolidation

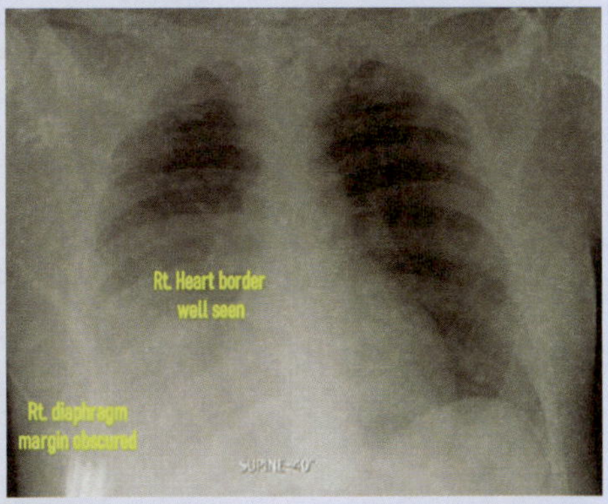

Lingular consolidation

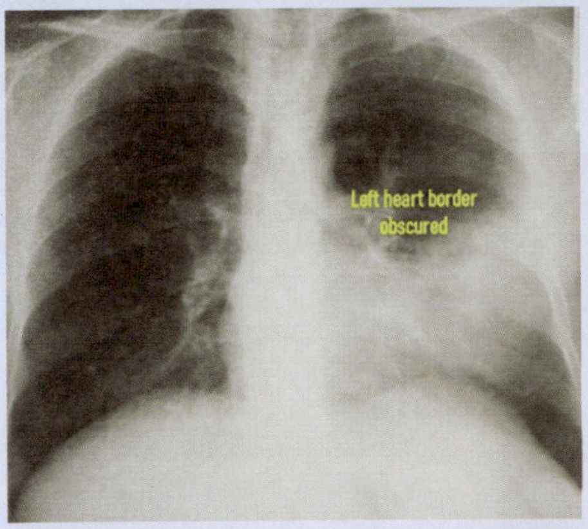

LLL consolidation

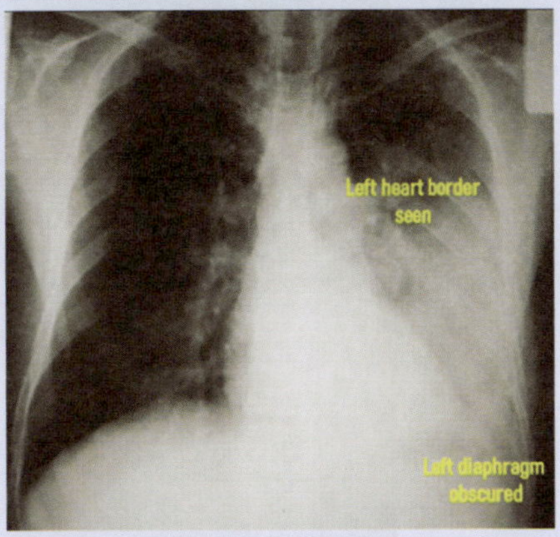

Air-bronchogram sign

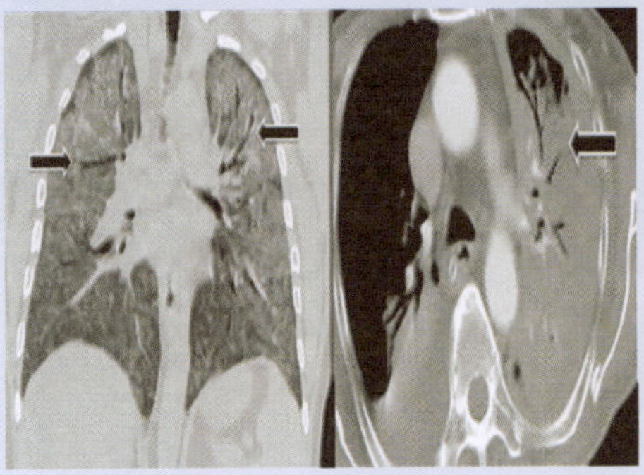

Air-bronchogram sign:

Seen in:

- Infective consolidation
- Pulmonary edema
- Hyaline membrane disease
- Expiratory film
- Lymphoma
- Alv. Proteinosis
- ARDS
- Sarcoidosis
- Alv. Cell carcinoma
- Radiation fibrosis
- Fibrosing alveolitis

Clinical integrated approach to respiratory tract infections

Let's integrate the clinical and radiological aspects of various infections and have some fun!!

Clinical history	Imaging findings	Diagnosis
• 12 years male • Fever and cough with expectoration • On Rx with antibiotics	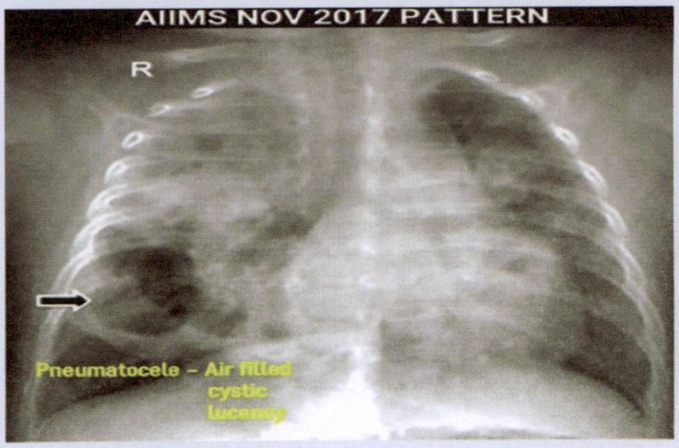	**Staphylococcal pneumonia**[Q]

Contd...

Clinical history	Imaging findings	Diagnosis
• Chronic alcoholic/ Debilitated patient • Fever and cough with expectoration and breathlessness	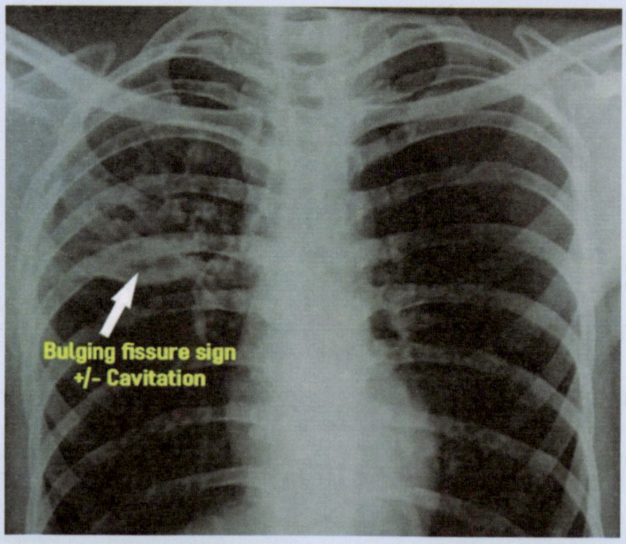	**Klebsiella pneumonia[Q]**
• Low grade fever, dry cough • More constitutional symptoms – Headache, Myalgia	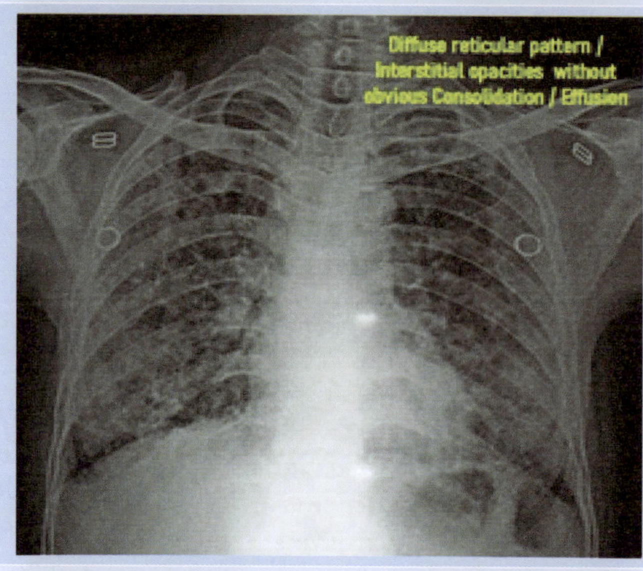	**Atypical/Mycoplasma pneumonia[Q]**
• Acute onset Respiratory illness after an indoor gathering with LRTI signs • GIT signs – Nausea, Vomiting, Diarrhea • CNS signs – Headache, Confusion, Lethargy • Infection spread through contaminated water in air coolers/ACs	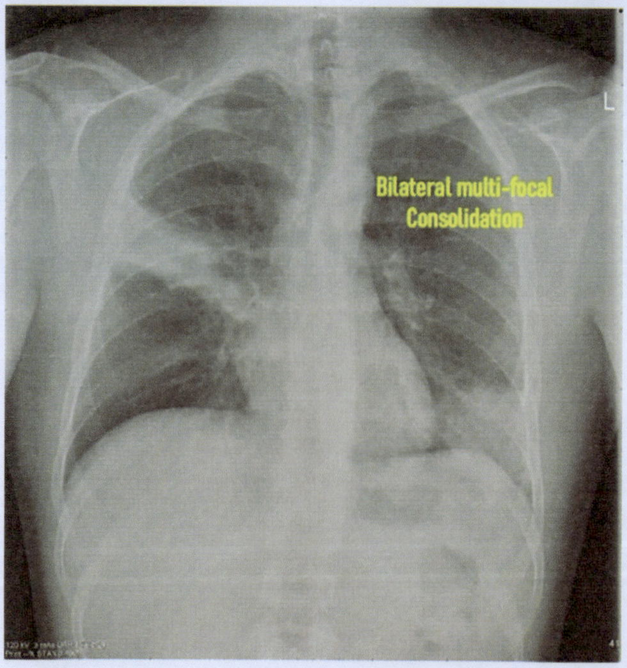	**Legionella pneumonia[Q]**

Contd...

<table>
<tr><th>Clinical history</th><th>Imaging findings</th><th>Diagnosis</th></tr>
<tr><td>

- K/c/o HIV with CD4 <200
- Gradual dyspnea and Nonproductive cough

</td><td>
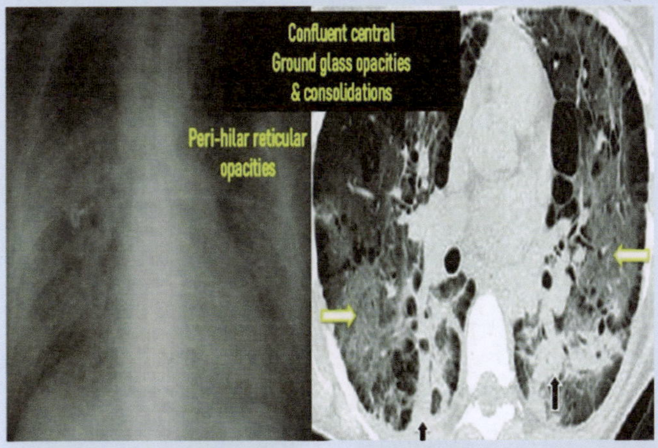

</td><td>Pneumocystis pneumonia[Q]</td></tr>
<tr><td>

- Chronic alcoholic, found unconscious
- Later develops high grade fever, cough with expectoration

</td><td>
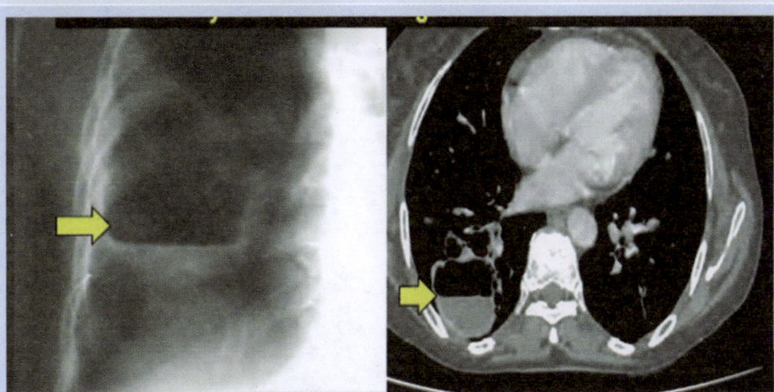
Cavitatory lesion in the lung with an Air-fluid level
</td><td>Lung abscess[Q]</td></tr>
<tr><td>

- Old treated case of TB
- Asymptomatic/ Occasional cough with hemoptysis

</td><td>
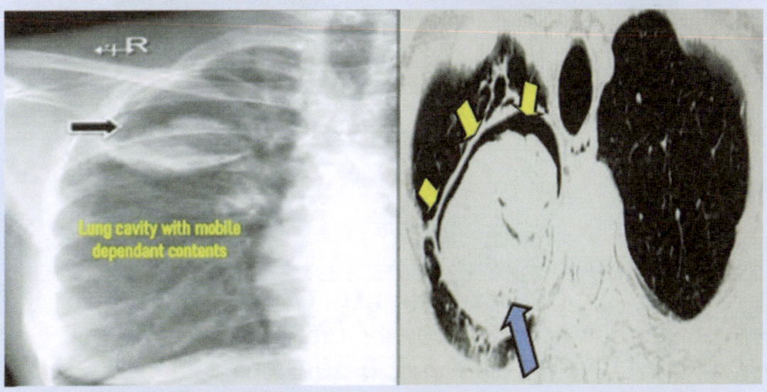

Monod signQ/Air crescent sign[Q]
</td><td>Aspergilloma[Q]</td></tr>
<tr><td>

- Child with persistent rhinorrhea and nasal congestion
- Repeated episode of Otitis media

</td><td>
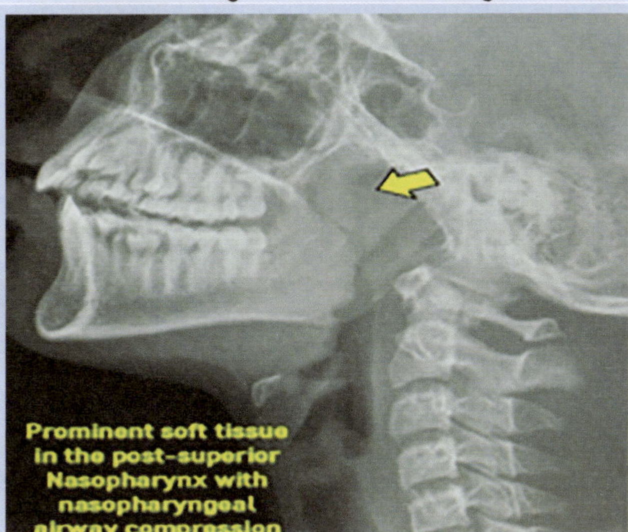

</td><td>Adenoid hypertrophy[Q]</td></tr>
</table>

Contd...

Clinical history	Imaging findings	Diagnosis
• Child with recent H. influenza B infection • C/o Fever with change in voice and difficulty in speaking • Inspiratory stridor	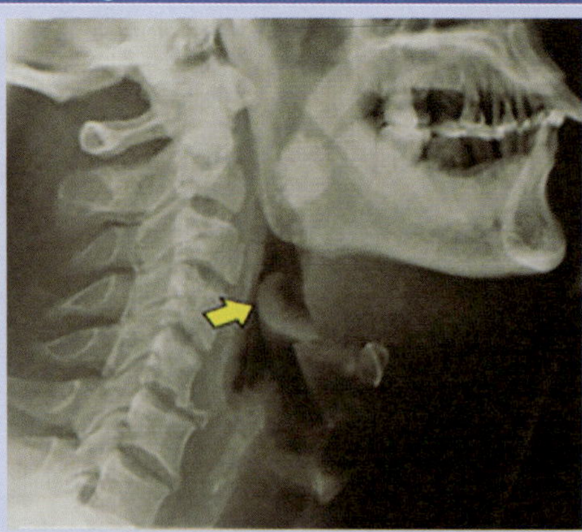 Thick epiglottis–Thumb sign[Q]	**Acute epiglottitis[Q]**
• Child with protracted barking cough • Inspiratory stridor	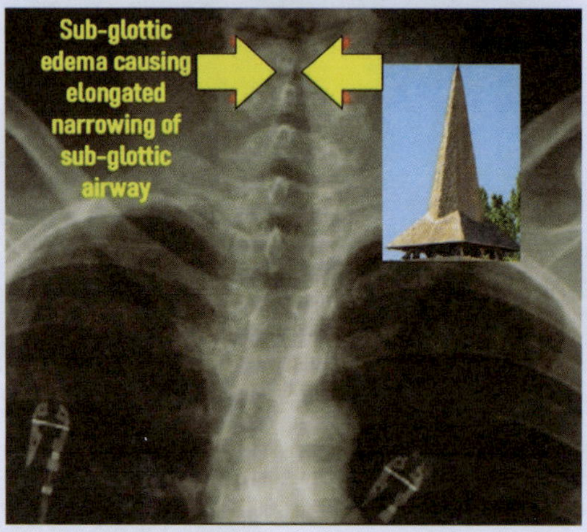 Steeple/Wine bottle sign[Q]	**Acute laryngo-tracheo-bronchitis[Q]/Croup[Q]**

TUBERCULOSIS

TB

Post-primary TB
- Endogenous reactivation of latent infection
- **CAVITATION is Hallmark finding[Q]**
- MC involves apical and posterior segments of the lobes and superior segments of the lower lobes[Q]
- Progressive involvement and lung fibrosis[Q]

Primary TB
- 1st infection/exposure
- Most common in <5 years age
- MC site – **lungs**
- Cavitation is never seen[Q]

Primary progressive TB
- Inadequate immunity hence, primary infection continues to progress instead of becoming latent
- No recovery from primary infection

Miliary TB
- Due to hematogenous dissemination of bacillus
- Diffuse tiny discrete nodules scattered in both lobes of lungs – resemble Millet seeds hence, the name

Contd...

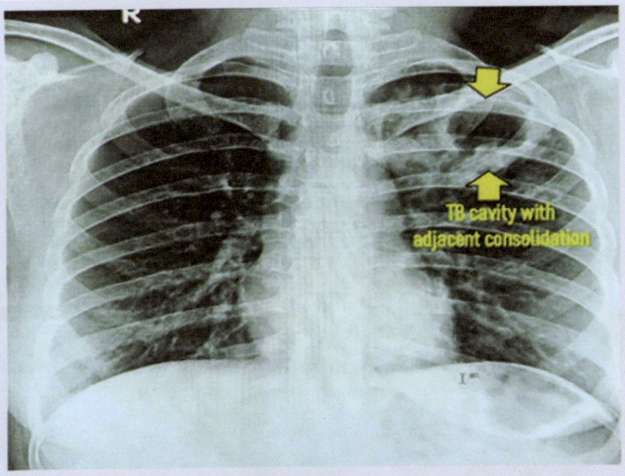

Post-primary TB

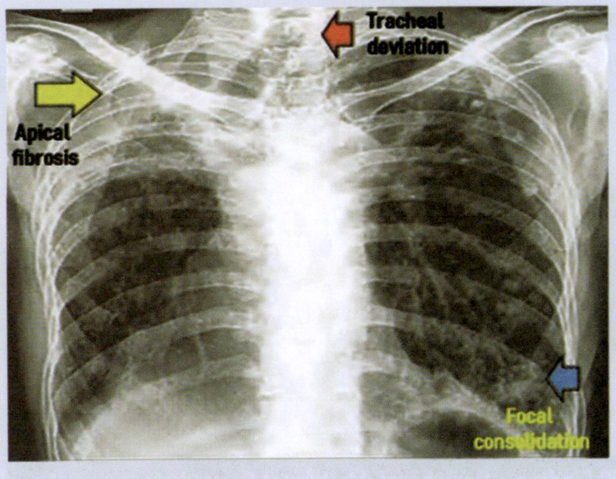

Post-primary TB

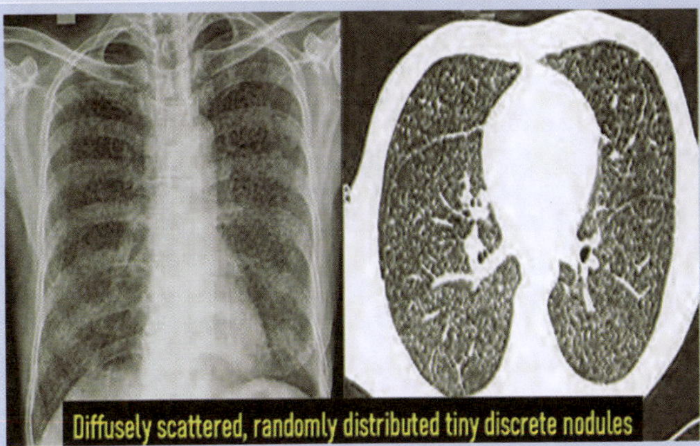

Miliary TB

Miliary Shadows on CXR

- **Infections:** TB, varicella, histoplasmosis, bronchopneumonia, brucellosis, coccidioidomycosis, cryptococcosis, blastomycosis
- **Cardiac causes:** Mitral stenosis, pulmonary edema
- **Neoplastic:** Lymphangitic carcinomatosis, metastasis, leukemia, lymphoma, alveolar cell carcinoma
- **Pneumoconiosis:** Silicosis, coal worker's pneumoconiosis
- **Allergic:** Löffler's syndrome
- **Others:** Interstitial pulmonary fibrosis, sarcoidosis, right arthritis, histiocytosis X, alveolar microlithiasis

Eponyms in Tuberculosis—All Potential MCQs

Ghon's focus/lesion	Lung parenchymal evidence of primary TB infection.
Ghon's Complex	Ghon's focus with involvement of hilar lymph nodes and the intervening lymphatics
Ranke's complex	Calcified Ghon's focus is Ranke's complex
Simon's focus	Apical lung nodule due to hematogenous spread from an extrapulmonary Primary TB — Heals by scarring

Puhl's lesion/nodule or Aschoff-Puhl reinfection/exogenous reinfection	Isolated lesion of chronic pulmonary TB—located in lung apex
Assman's foci	Reactivation of Simon's focus Typical infraclavicular location
Weigert focus	Caseating focus in the wall of a pulmonary vein Subintimal location
Rasmussen's aneurysm	Pulmonary artery aneurysm within/adjacent to a TB cavity May rupture and cause hemoptysis
Rich's focus	TB granuloma in cerebral cortex Ruptures into the subarachnoid space causing TB meningitis
Simmond's focus	TB focus in liver
Pott's disease, Pott's caries Pott's curvature, Pott's syndrome David's disease	TB involvement of Spine

IMAGING IN COVID-19

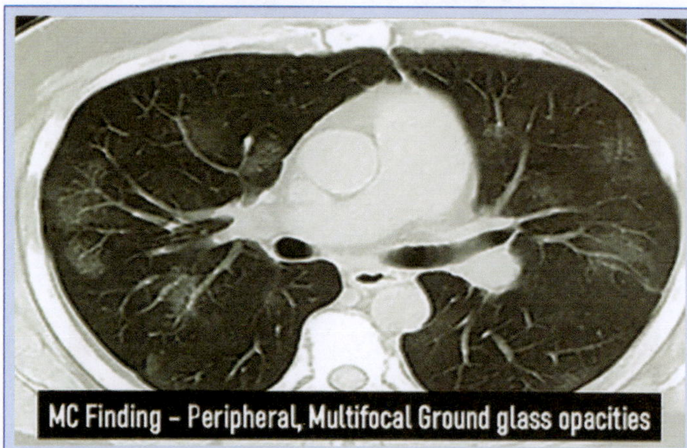

HRCT–IOC for COVID-19 Imaging

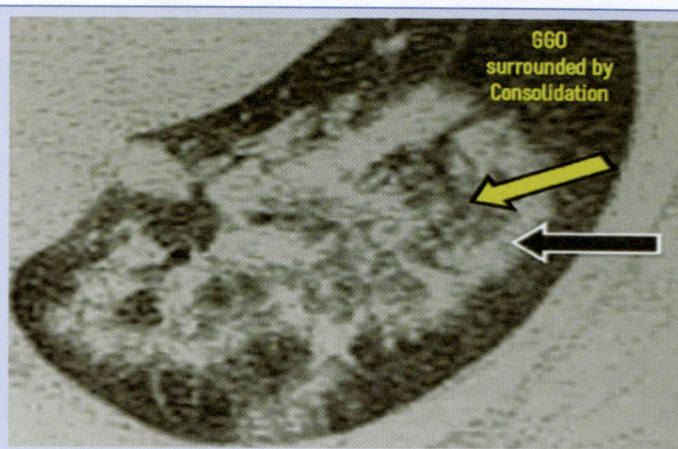

Reverse HALO sign/Atoll sign: COVID and cryptogenic organizing pneumonia (COP)

CO-RADS – COVID-19 Reporting and Data System to Predict the Probability of COVID based on CT findings		
CO-RADS 1	Highly unlikely	Normal CT
CO-RADS 2	Unlikely	Abnormalities other than COVID-19 (Effusion/Lnpathy)
CO-RADS 3	Equivocal	Unclear – single central GGO
CO-RADS 4	Probable	Few GGO
CO-RADS 5	Highly likely	Multifocal, Peripheral/ Subpleural GGO
CO-RADS 6	RT-PCR Proven	Irrespective of CT findings

CT involvement score in COVID-19

Assess the % of Each Lung Lobe Involved	
Lung lobe	Score
RUL	
RML	
RLL	
LUL	
LL	
TOTAL SCORE	0–25

Scoring Scale::

- No involvement = 0
- <5% = 1
- 5–25% = 2
- 25–50% = 3
- 50–75% = 4
- >75% = 5

PLEURAL EFFUSION IMAGING

Typical findings

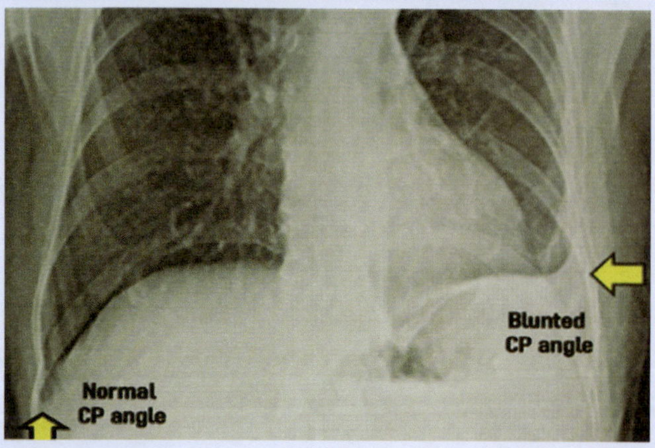

Blunting of CP angle[Q] (Earliest sign on CXR PA view)

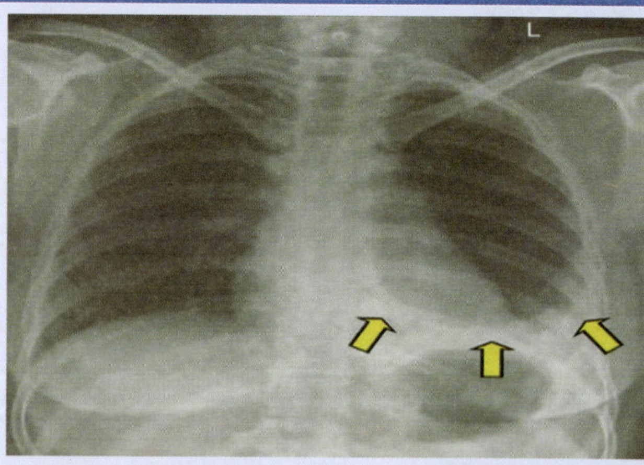

Meniscus sign[Q] (Concave-upward meniscus like opacity)

Contd...

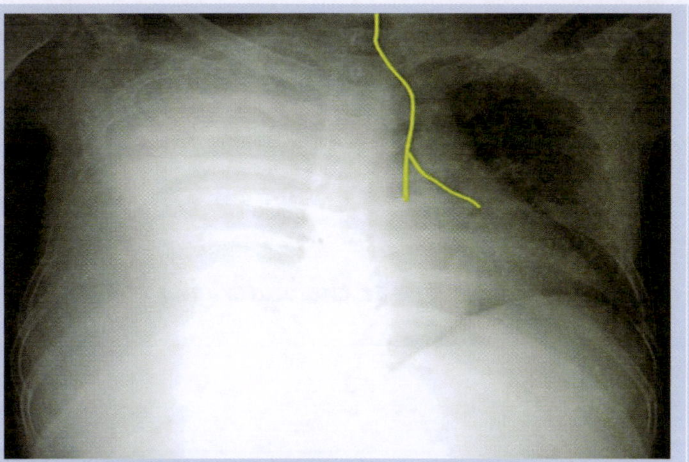

White-out lung[Q]/Opaque hemithorax[Q]

(Trachea/mediastinum pushed to apposite side)

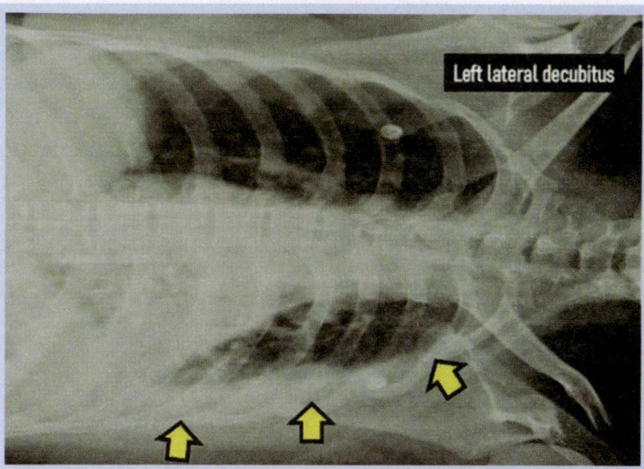

Lateral decubitus view

(Best X-ray projection for minimal pleural effusion[Q])

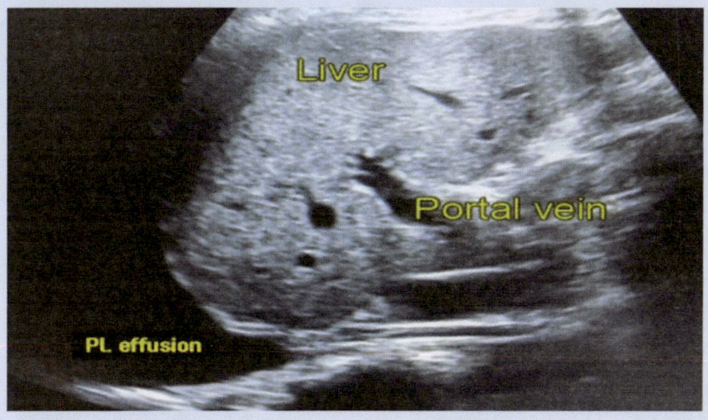

USG-IOC for pleural effusion[Q]

(Appears nechoic/hypoechoic)

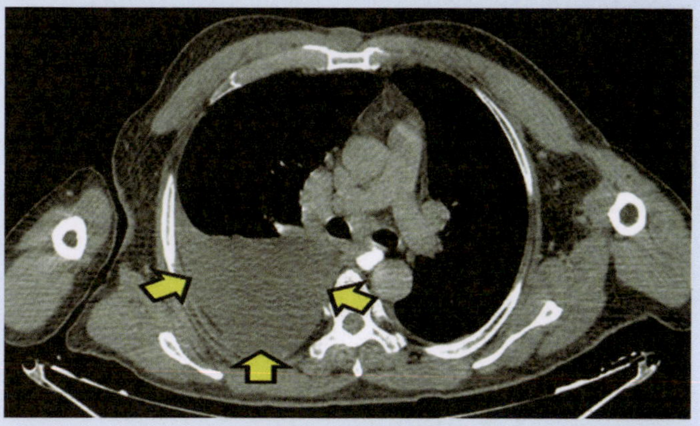

CT-pleural effusion

(Hypodensity in dependent part of right hemithorax)

Atypical findings

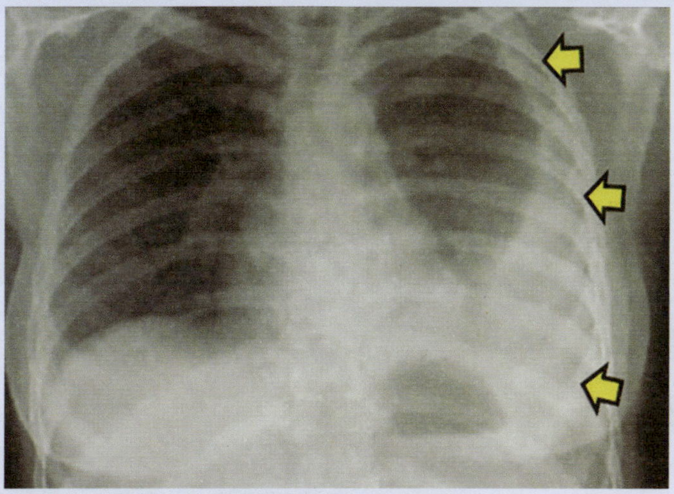

Lamellar effusion

(Band/layer like opacity parallel to lateral chest wall)

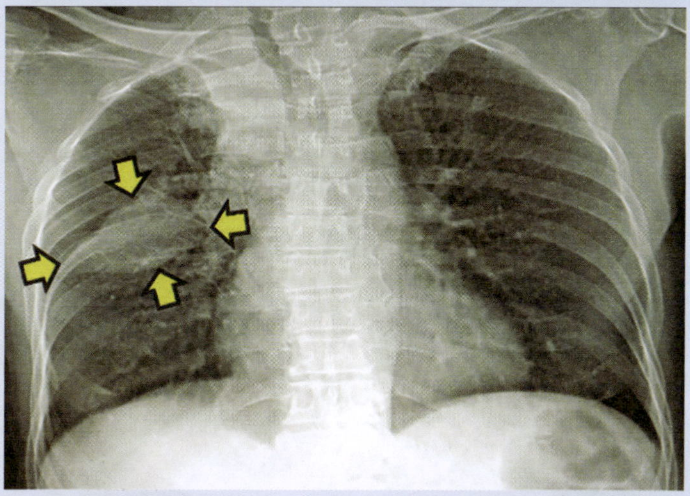

Loculated/fissural effusion

(Well-defined oval opacity with its long-axis along Horizontal fissure)

Contd...

Vanishing lung tumor/Phantom lung tumor

CLINICAL CLINCHER

- Elderly patient with Congestive heart failure
- Mass like opacity on CXR—reported as a Lung tumor
- Rx for CHF with Diuretics and Inotropes
- CXR tumor disappears in a few days!!

Loculated effusion in the fissures secondary to CHF—resolves completely once the underlying cause is treated.

PNEUMOTHORAX AIR IN PLEURAL CAVITY

Imaging Investigations for Pneumothorax

- CXR is the initial examination of choice[Q].
- An expiratory chest X-ray[Q] is much better for detection of minimal pneumothorax
- Overall, IOC for Pneumothorax – CT
- USG is used in the Emergency room setup.

Treatment of Tension Pneumothorax

- **Needle Thoracotomy: 1st step in treatment[Q]**
  - In adults—5th intercostal space slightly anterior to mid axillary line
  - In Children—2nd intercostal space in the midclavicular line
- **ICD Insertion: 2nd step after the tension component is relieved**

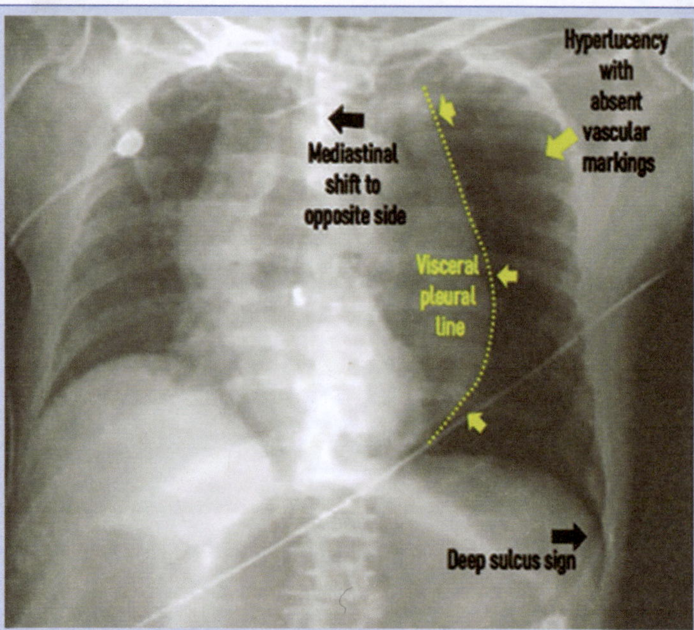

Tension pneumothorax

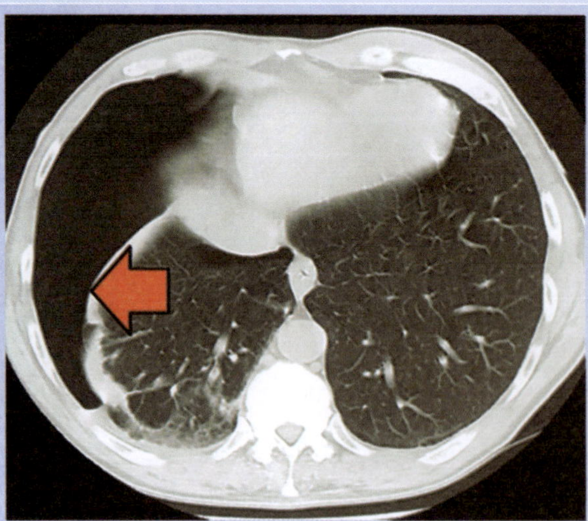

Pneumothorax-CT

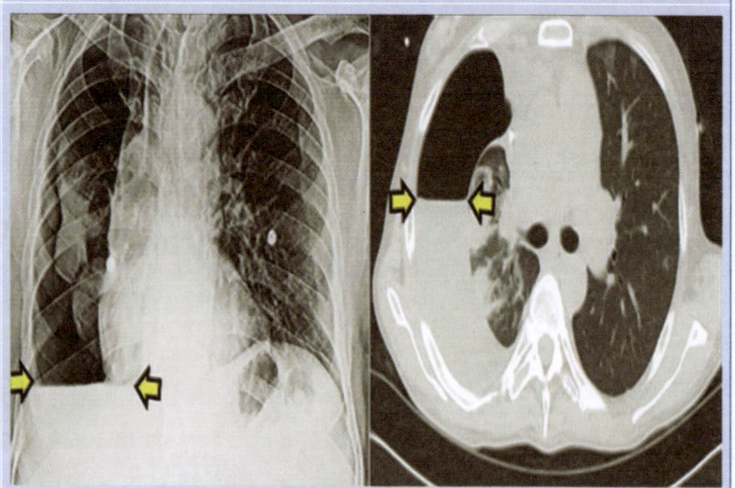

Hydro-Pneumothorax
(Air-fluid level in the pleural cavity)

Contd...

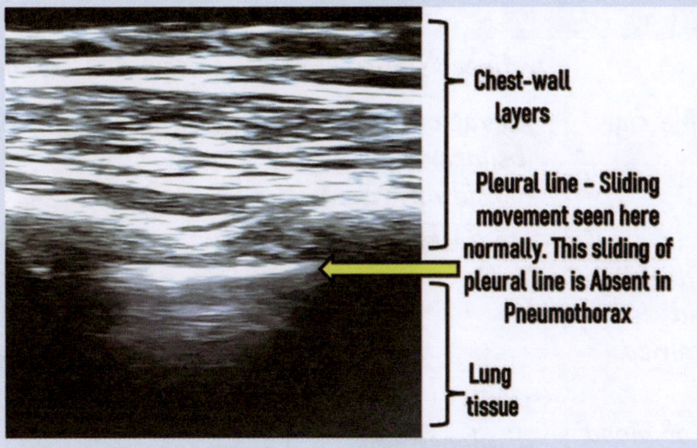

Normal USG thorax

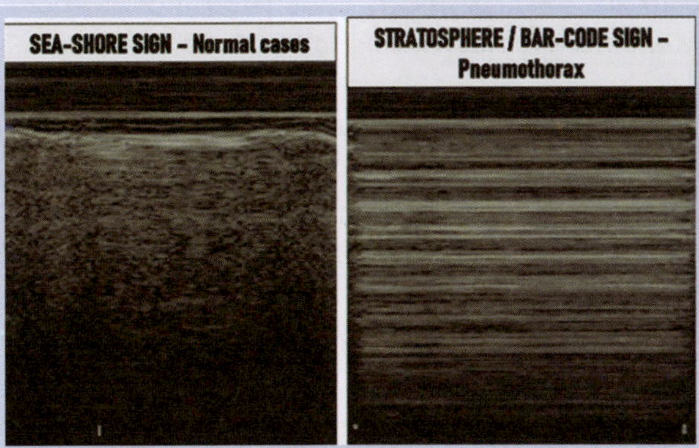

M-mode USG thorax

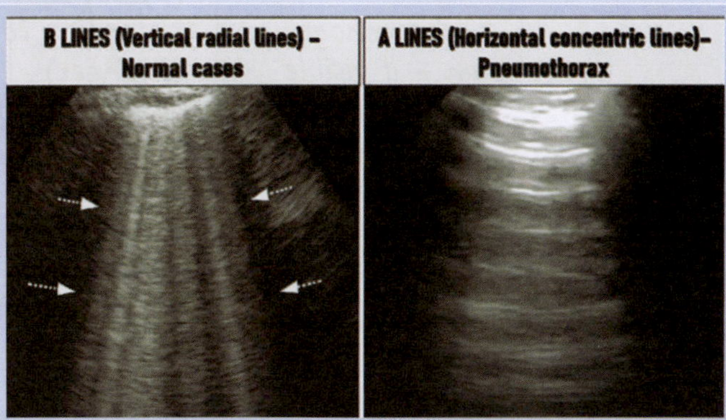

B-mode USG thorax

AIRWAY DISORDERS AND MISCELLANEOUS CONDITIONS

Bronchiectasis—chronic local, irreversible dilatation of bronchi, associated with inflammation.

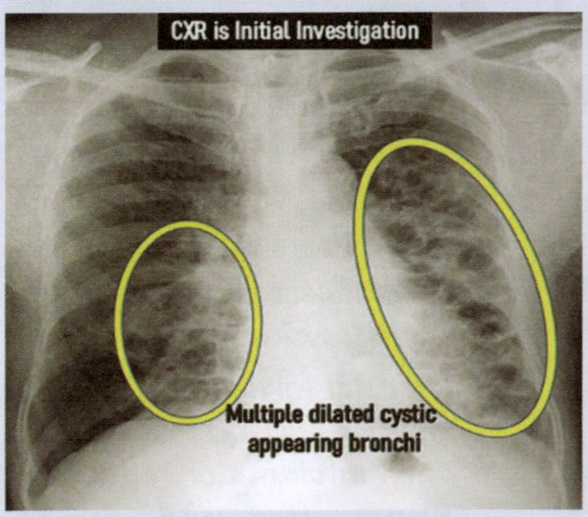

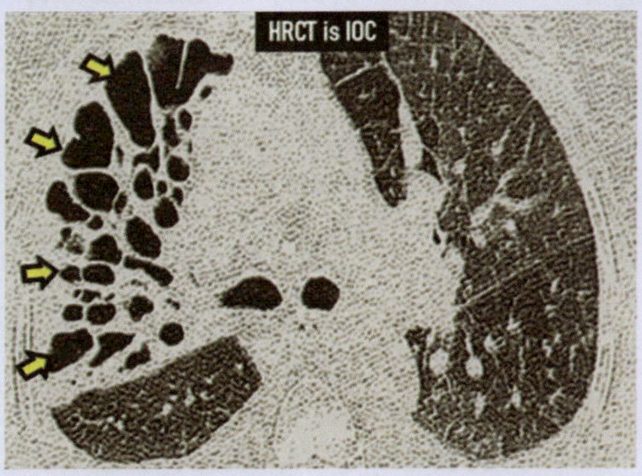

Bronchiectasis (Cluster of Grapes sign[Q])

HRCT signs:

- **Bronchial dilatation: Cardinal sign of bronchiectasis.**
- Increased bronchoarterial ratio: Diameter of a bronchus should measure approximately 0.65-1.0 times that of the adjacent pulmonary artery branch greater than 1.5 indicates bronchiectasis
- **Signet ring sign**
- **String of pearl sign**
- **Cluster of grapes sign**

Lobulated gloved finger, V or Y-shaped densities – seen due to mucus-filled bronchi. Often seen in ABPA.

Contd...

LOBAR COLLAPSE - CT is IOC/Best Investigation for Lobar Collapse

Direct signs

Displacement of interlobar fissures	Most reliable sign
Loss of aeration	Will result in increased density of lung field, is due to retained secretions
Vascular and Bronchial signs	Crowding of blood vessels Air bronchogram sign – if visible will reveal crowding of vessels

Indirect signs: These are seen due to compensatory changes

Elevation of ipsilateral hemidiaphragm	Juxtaphrenic peak sign[Q]:
Mediastinal shift	Lower lobe collapse – Heart may be displaced Least mediastinal shift is seen in RML collapse[Q] maximum mediastinal shift is seen in right/ left lower lobe collapse[Q]
Hilar displacement (Direct sign according to Grainger)	Upper lobe collapse – Hilum is elevated Lower lobe collapse – Hilum is depressed. More accurate description is that the hilum appears smaller than normal in lower lobe collapse.
Compensatory hyperinflation	Normal lung may appear hypertranslucent (black) with widely-spaced vessels **Shifting granuloma sign:** Hyperexpansion may result in a change in position of lung lesions previously documented Luftsichel sign (meaning air crescent)[Q]– seen in LUL collapse

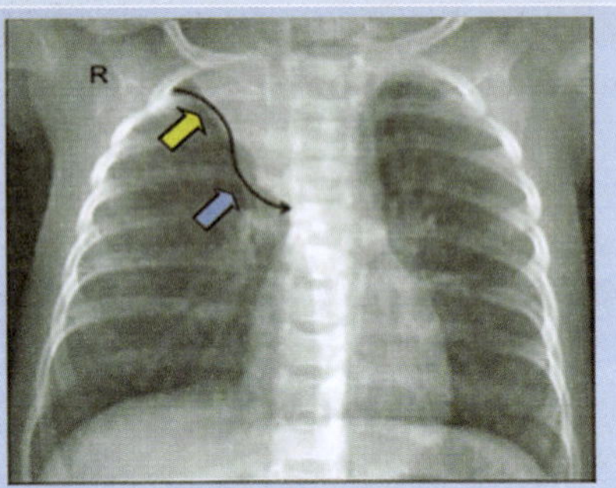

Golden S sign[Q]

(Right upper lobe collapse due to a central mass lesion)

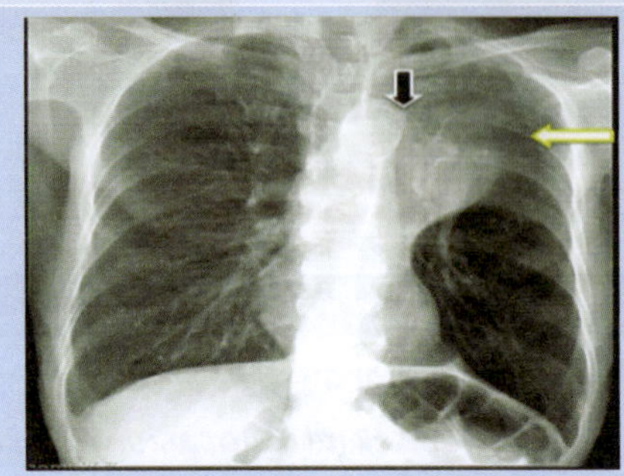

Luftsichel sing[Q]

(Left upper lobe collapse with resultant overinflation of LLL)

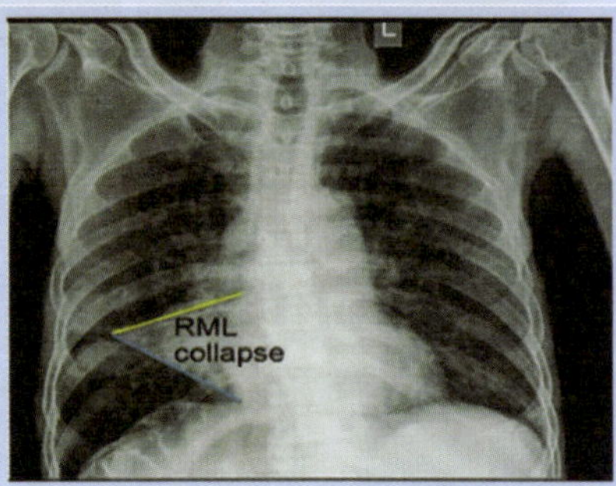

RML collapse

(Lordotic AP view - is better for diagnosis)

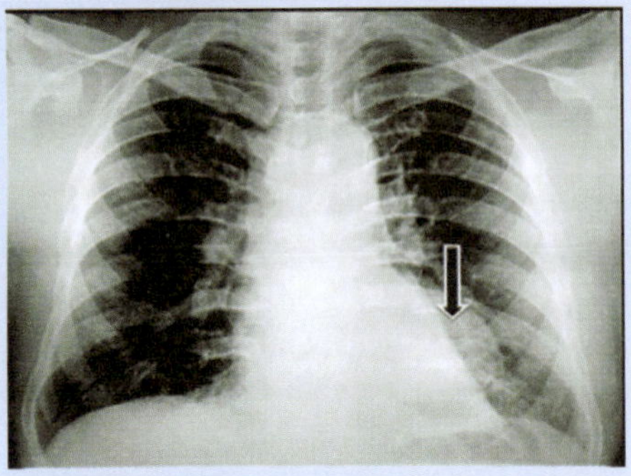

LLL collapse

(Triangular para-spinal wedge shaped opacity)

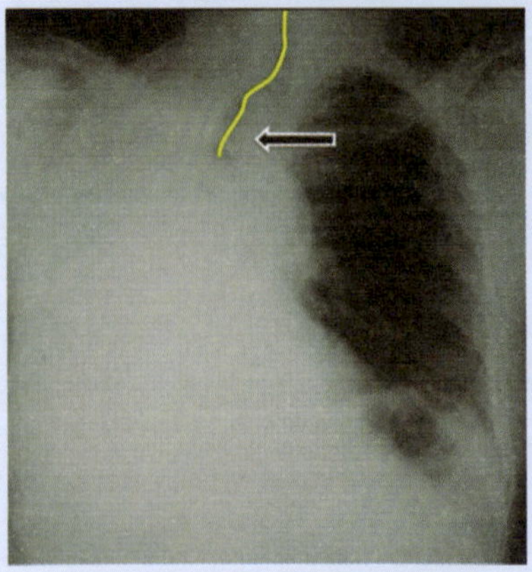

Complete lung collapse

(Right opaque hemithorax with ipsilateral mediastinal shift)

Round Atelectasis/Folded Lung/Blesovsky's Syndrome

- Unusual form of collapse related to asbestos exposure with infolding of redundant pleura, often misdiagnosed as a mass lesion.
- IOC - CT[Q]
- On CXR appears as a homogenous mass, up to 5 cm diameter, with ill-defined edges. It is always pleural based and is associated with pleural thickening.
- **Comet tail sign[Q] and Crow feet sign[Q]:** Vascular shadows radiating from the opacity

Contd...

Diaphragmatic hernia

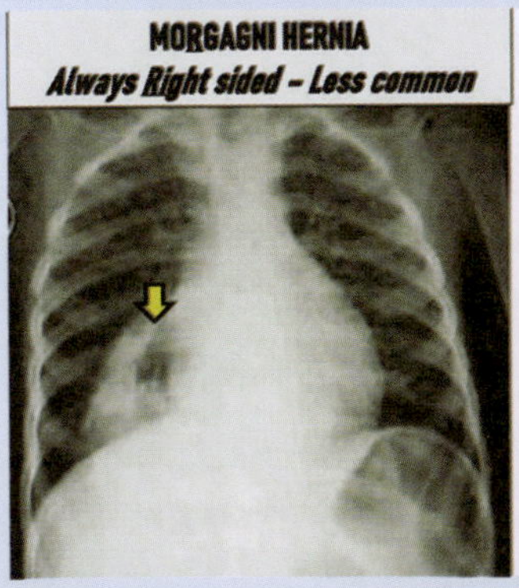

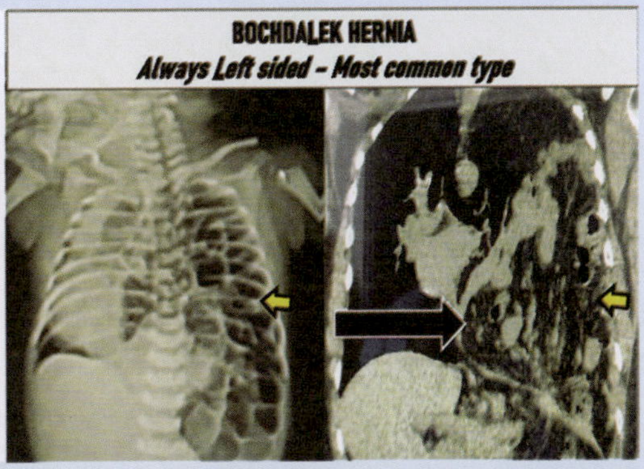

Sarcoidosis

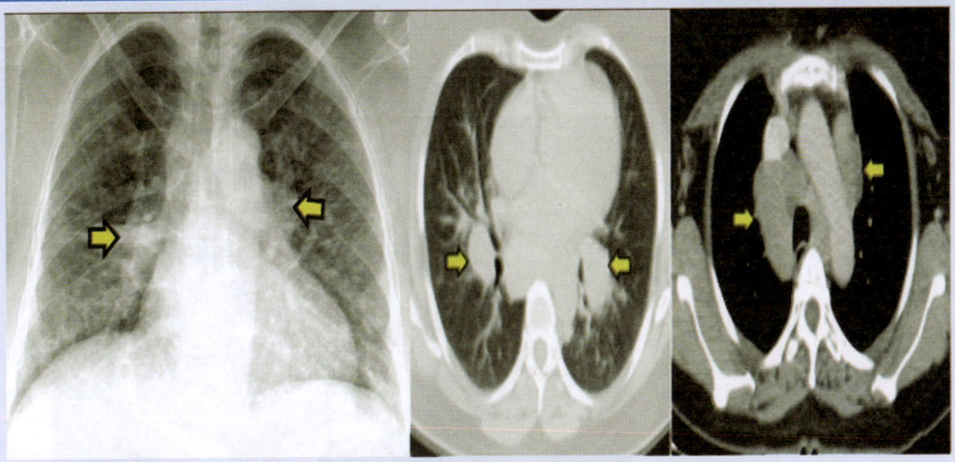

Sarcoidosis – bilateral hilar lymphadenopathy

- A middle-aged female patient with bilateral hilar lymphadenopathy and few clinical complaints like cough, dyspnea – suggests Sarcoidosis.
- On CT scan – **Lambda sign**[Q] **or 1-2-3 sign**[Q]
- **On Gallium scan**[Q] **Lambda sign and Panda sign**[Q]
- In lung, **perilymphatic and subpleural nodules** are seen.
- In later stages, coalescent nodules surrounded by multiple satellite nodules – **Galaxy sign**[Q] can be seen.

Most common radiologic finding at presentation

- **In Indian patients:** Bilateral adenopathy with parenchymal infiltrates
- **In Western patients:** Bilateral adenopathy

Lung tumors

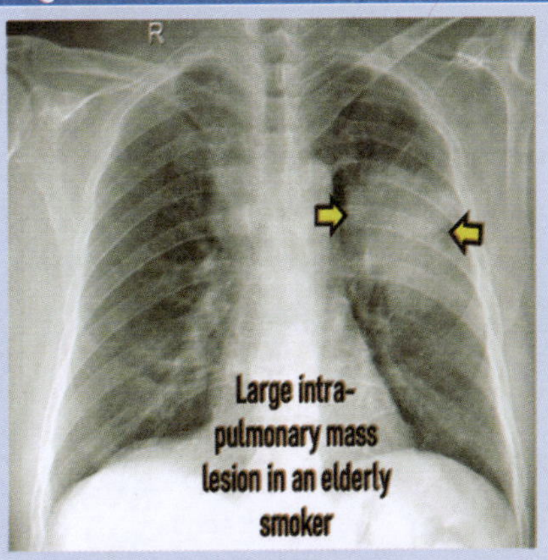

Lung cancer

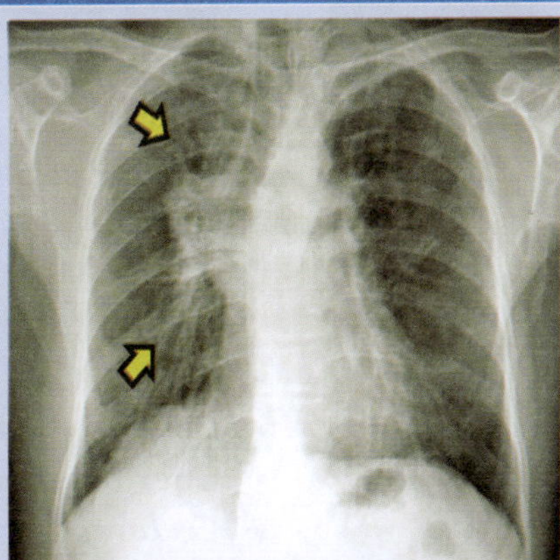

Lung cancer (Corona radiata appearance)

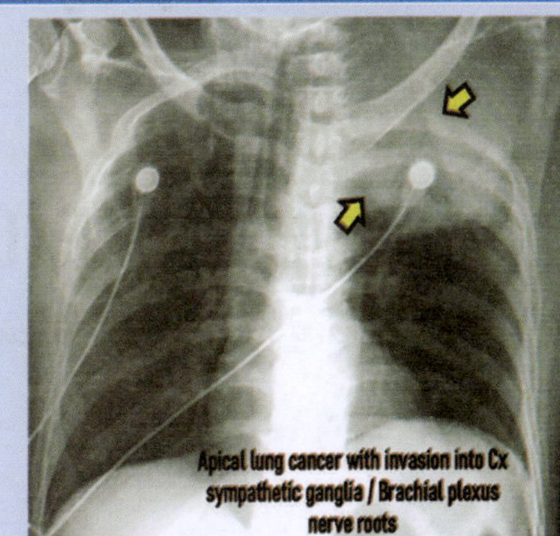

Pancoast tumor

Contd...

Lung tumors

CLINICAL CLINCHER—PANCOAST TUMOR

- An elderly male, chronic smoker – predisposition to malignancy
- Cough with hemoptysis and mass lesion on CXR – suggests malignancy
- Ipsilateral upper limb pain, paresthesia and weakness and Ptosis – suggests neural extension into brachial plexus nerve roots and cervical sympathetic ganglia.

- Lung cancer – located in the apex of the lung.
- Invades into adjacent vital neural structures such as cervical sympathetic ganglia (resulting in Horner's syndrome) and into brachial plexus nerve roots (resulting in upper limb pain, paraesthesis and weakness).
- IOC for all lung tumors is CE-CT, except for Pancoast tumor – it is MRI. Pancoast tumor is known to infiltrate into the brachial plexus nerve roots/cervical sympathetic ganglia—hence, MRI is IOC.

Miscellaneous lung tumors

Lung hamartoma

Carney's Triad[Q]–Seen in cases of Pulmonary hamartomas/chondromas. Consists of:

- Multiple pulmonary chondromas[Q]
- Gastric epithelioid leiomyosarcoma/GISTs[Q]
- Functioning extra-adrenal paragangliomas[Q]

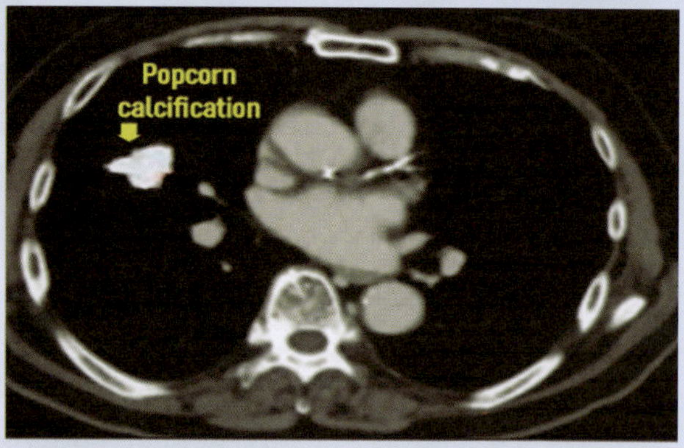

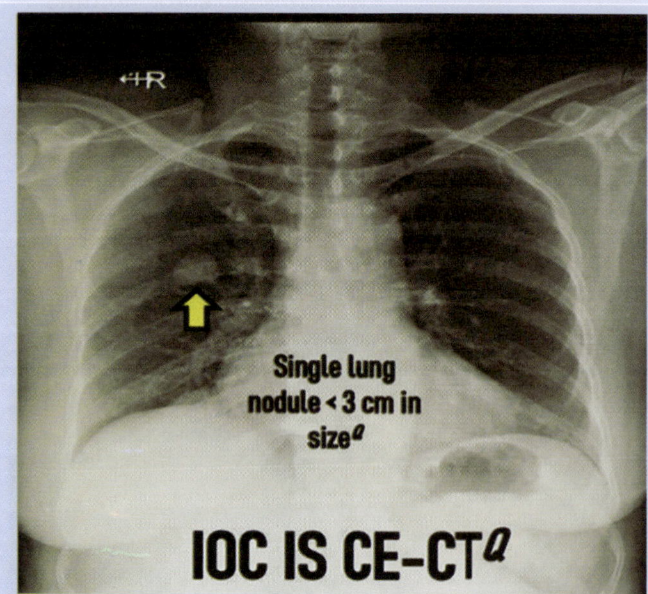

Solitary pulmonary nodule (SPN)

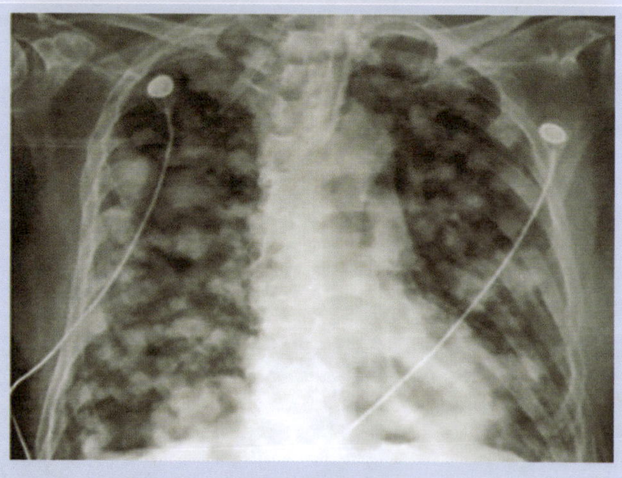

Cannon-ball lung metastases

Multiple large round well-defined lesions in both lungs–as the rich vascular bed of the lungs is hospitable to tumor emboli.

Causes:

- Renal cell carcinoma–most common[Q]
- Choriocarcinoma
- Endometrial carcinoma
- Germ cell tumors
- Synovial sarcoma
- Prostate carcinoma

Mediastinal Abnormalities

Mediastinal tumors

CLINICAL CLINCHER

Most common in Mediastinal lesions:

- Overall most common mediastinal mass – Thymoma[Q]
- Most common anterior mediastinal mass – Thymoma[Q]
- Most common middle mediastinal mass – Lymph nodal mass[Q]
- Most common middle mediastinal mass in children – Duplication cysts[Q]
- Most common posterior mediastinal mass – Neurogenic tumors[Q]

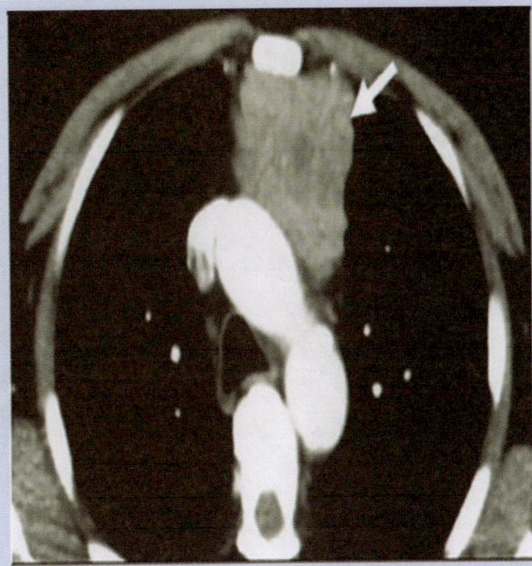

Thymoma

- MC mediastinal tumor overall[Q]
- MC anterior anterior mediastinal tumor[Q]
- MC tumor of thymus in adults[Q]
- Associated with Myasthenia gravis[Q]/ Hypogammadlobulinemia[Q]/Goods' syndrome[Q]

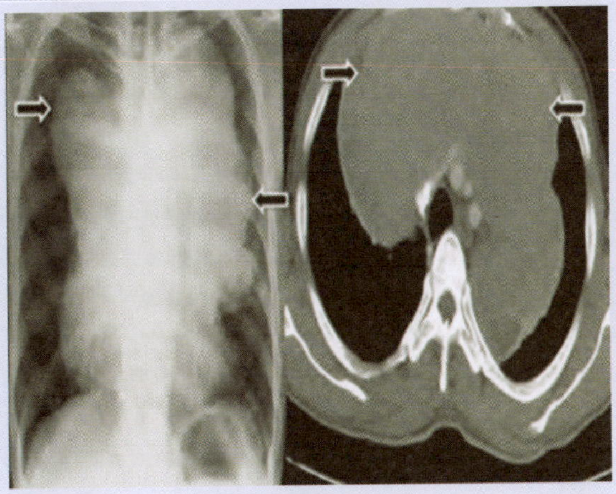

Lymphoma

(Large uniformly enhancing solid mass lesion – so large that it extends to all mediastinal compartments)

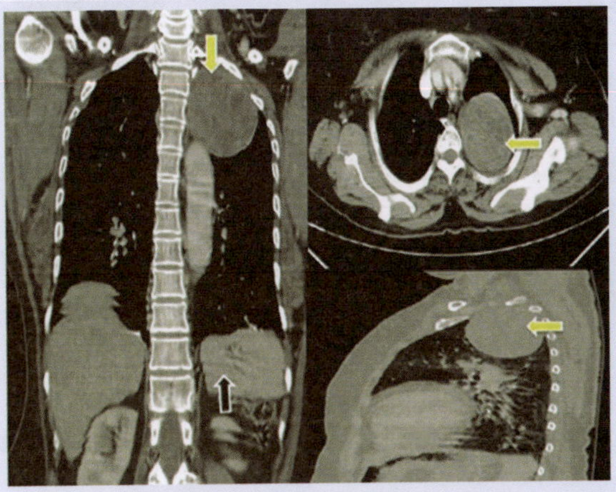

Posterior mediastinal mass

(MC - neurogenic tumor)

Egg-shell calcification of lymph nodes:

- Silicosis
- **Treated lymphoma:** (Post-irradiation Hodgkin disease)
- Coal workers pneumoconiosis
- TB
- Sarcoidosis
- Scleroderma
- **Amyloidosis:** Rare
- Blastomycosis
- Histoplasmosis

CLINICAL CLINCHER

IOC for all Mediastinal tumors is CE-CT, except for Posterior mediastinal masses—it is CE-MRI.

This is because most of the posterior mediastinal masses are neurogenic in origin. Hence, may have an intraspinal component. For better delineation of this neurological extension/intraspinal component, MRI is IOC (as CT fails to image this extent well).

Pneumomediastinum

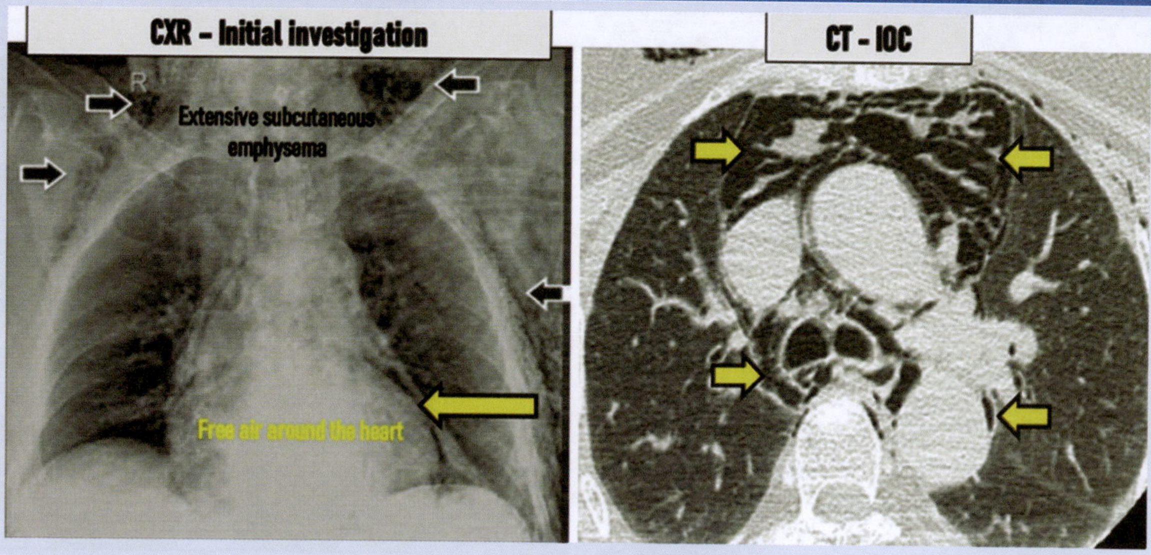

Pneumomediastinum

Various named signs are seen in Pneumomediastinum on a CXR:

Ring around the artery[Q]:	A radiolucent area is observed surrounding the right pulmonary artery.
Tubular artery sign[Q]:	Air around the major aortic branches.
Double bronchial wall sign[Q]:	Clear depiction of bronchial walls due to air both on inside and outside, Silhouette sign.
Thymic sail sign[Q]/ Spinnaker sail sign[Q]/Angel wing sign[Q]:	In infants with pneumomediastinum, the thymic lobes are shifted upward resembling a full sail.
Continuous diaphragm sign[Q]:	Free air is present between the pericardium and diaphragm, causing the central parts of the diaphragm to become apparent as a sharp margin, Silhouette sign.
Naclerio's V sign[Q]:	Free air outlines the lateral margin of descending aorta and laterally between the parietal pleura and medial left hemidiaphragm. Seen in pneumomediastinum secondary to esophageal rupture – not specific for this cause.

3. CARDIOVASCULAR SYSTEM IMAGING

Congenital heart diseases

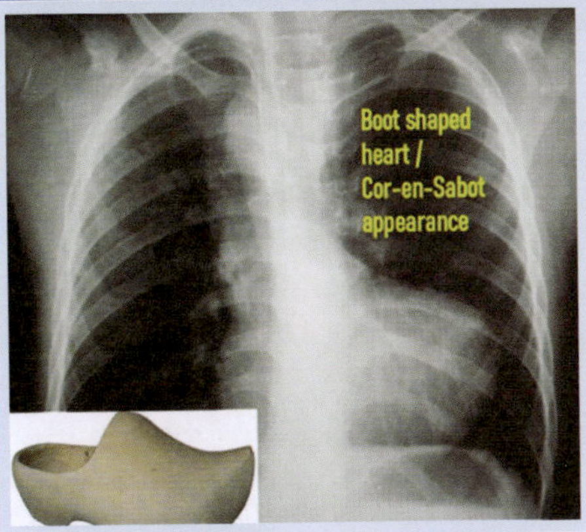

Tetralogy of Fallot:

- Only cyanotic heart disease that may present in adulthood[Q].
- Four components:
  1. Ventricular septal defect
  2. Over-riding of aorta
  3. Right ventricular hypertrophy
  4. Right ventricular outflow tract obstruction/Pulmonic stenosis.
- Boot-shaped heart[Q]/Cor en Sabot[Q]—mainly due to RVH[Q]

Trilogy of Fallot

Consists of ASD, Right ventricular hypertrophy and Pulmonary stenosis.

Pentalogy of Fallot

- Has additional ASD[Q] along with other tetralogy features.

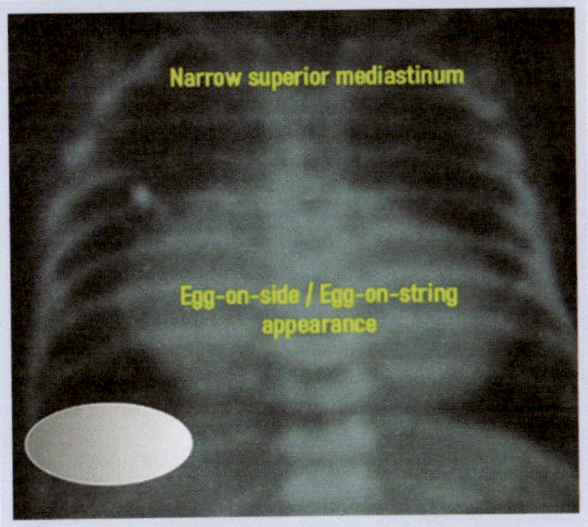

Transposition of Great Arteries (TGA):

- Narrowing of superior mediastinum[Q]—most consistent CXR finding
- Egg-on-side/Egg-on-string appearance—due to mild biventricular hypertrophy—starts after ductus arteriosus closure—around 2 weeks of age

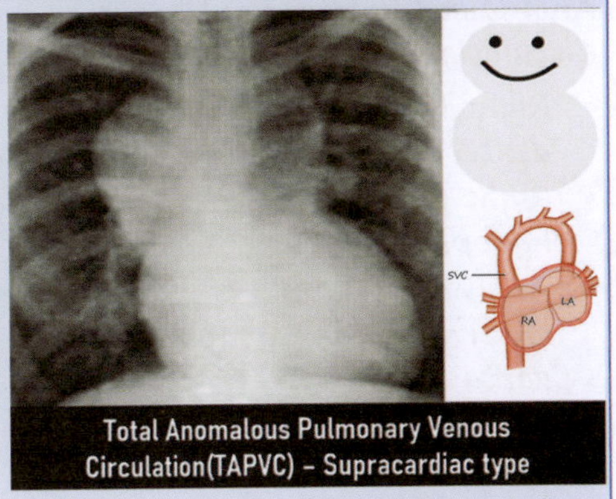

Figure- of-8/Snowman heart

Total Anomalous Pulmonary Venous Connection(TAPVC):

- MC type – Supracardiac type[Q] – Snowman's heart[Q]/Figure of -8 heart seen[Q]
- MC type associated with venous obstruction/MC type associated with cyanosis—Infracardiac type[Q]

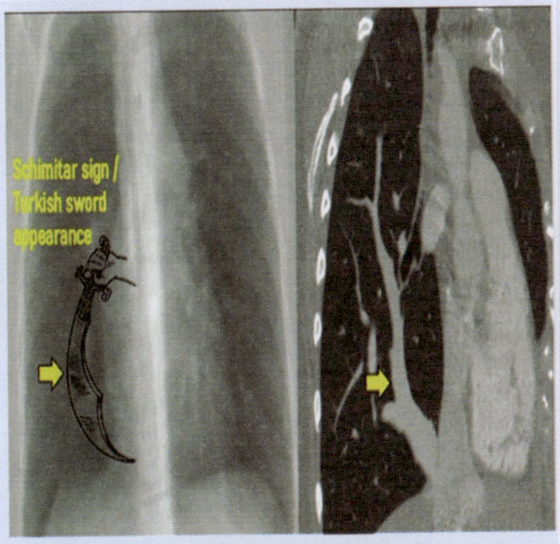

Scimitar syndrome

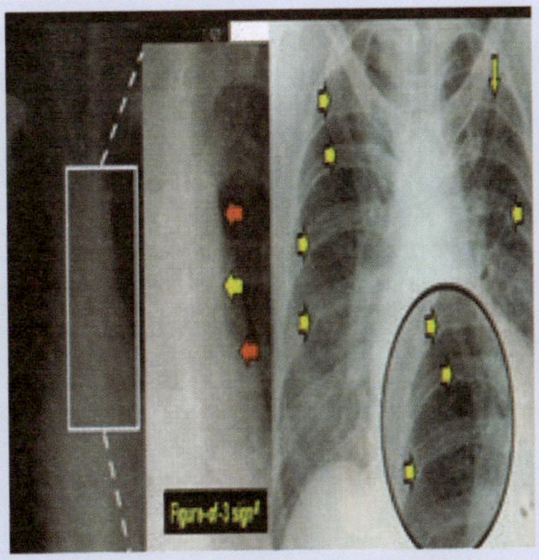

Coarctation of aorta

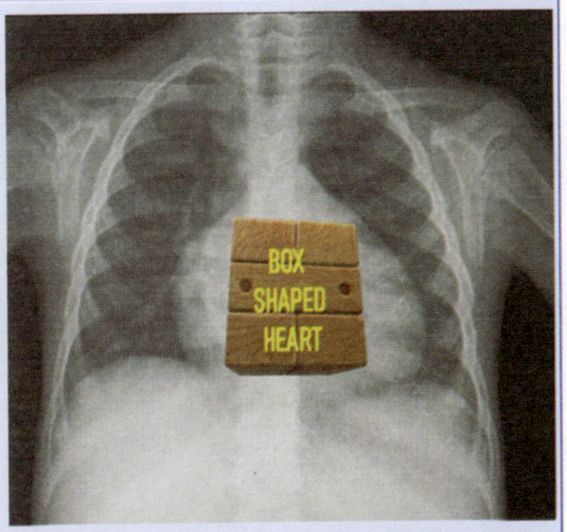

Ebstein anomaly

Contd...

Congenital heart diseases

Scimitar syndrome/Hypogenetic lung syndrome/Partial Anomalous Pulmonary Venous Circulation (PAPVC):

- Right lung hypoplasia with dextroposition of heart[Q]
- Right pulmonary artery hypoplasia
- Anomalous supply of right lower lobe from abdominal aorta
- Anomalous drainage by Scimitar vein[Q] into IVC[Q] – this vein travels downward and creates a Turkish sword[Q] like appearance

Coarctation of aorta:

- Congenital narrowing of aorta
- MC site – just distal to origin of left subclavian artery[Q]
- Figure-of-3 sign[Q] on CXR – Constriction at coarctation site with proximal subclavian and distal aortic dilatation
- Reverse-figure-of-3 sign[Q] – exact reverse impression on esophagus seen on Barium swallow
- Inferior rib notching[Q]/ Roesler's sign[Q] –
    - Involves 3rd/4th to 8th rib bilaterally[Q]
    - Due to collaterals from Intercostal arteries[Q]
    - 1st and 2nd ribs always spared[Q]

Other named appearances:

Appearance/sign	Seen in
Tear drop heart	Chronic emphysema
Egg in cup heart	Constrictive pericarditis
Triangular-shaped heart	Constrictive pericarditis
Tubular heart	Emphysema/ Addison's disease
Pentagon-shaped heart	Mitral incompetence
Ground glass appearance of lung	Obstructive type of TAPVC
Sitting duck heart	Persistent truncus arteriosus
Jug handle appearance	Primary pulmonary hypertension
Cortriatriatum	Pulmonary vein obstruction
Maladie-de-roger defect	Ventricular septal defect (VSD) – Most common heart defect
Swiss cheese appearance	VSD – on USG
Great hilar dance on fluoroscopy	Atrial septal defect (ASD)
Goose neck deformity	Endocardial cushion defect

ACQUIRED CARDIOVASCULAR DISORDERS

Mitral stenosis—IOC is echocardiography

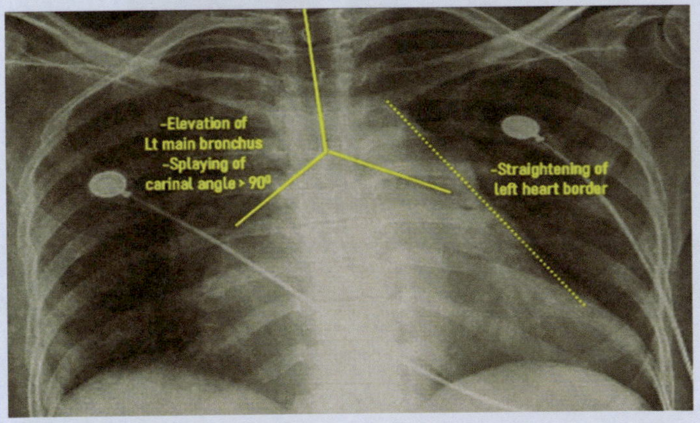

Mitral stenosis

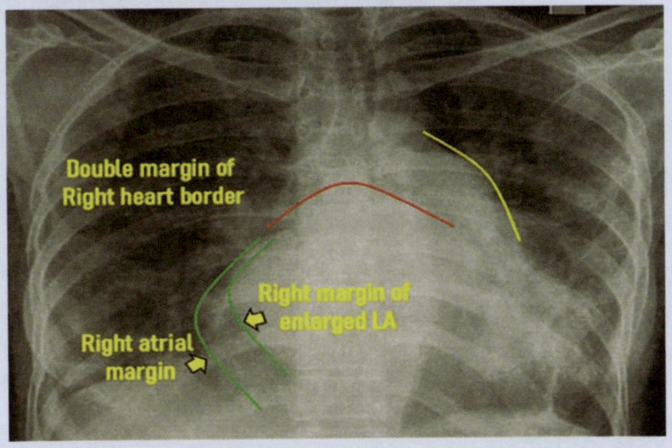

Mitral stenosis—double density sign

- IOC Echocardiography[Q]
- X-ray signs:
  - Fullness beneath the pulmonary artery shadow—earliest sign[Q]
  - Elevation of left main bronchus[Q]
  - Splaying/Widening of carinal angle >900[Q]
  - Straightening of left heart border[Q]
  - Third mogul sign[Q]
  - Double density sign[Q]–Double right heart border
  - Anterior esophageal impression[Q] on Barium swallow
  - Walking man sign[Q]–On Lateral CXR – posterior displacement of left main bronchus due to LA enlargement

Congestive heart failure—CXR staging

PCWP 13 – 18 mm Hg
Stage 1 : Redistribution of blood flow

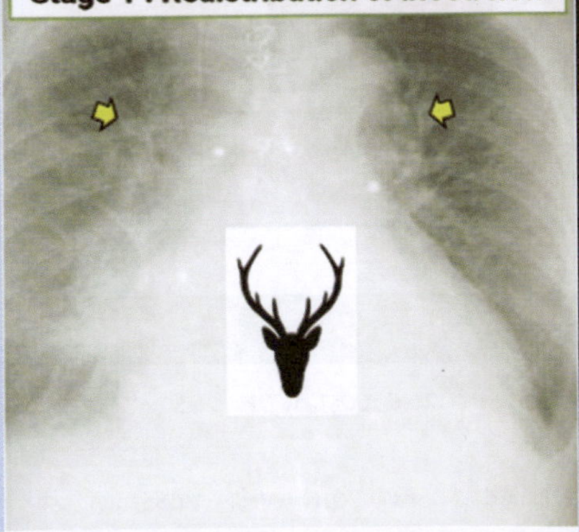

- Prominent upper lobe vessels-cephalization of blood flow[Q]-stag antler sign[Q]/inverted moustache sign[Q]/hands up sign[Q]
- Cardiomegaly[Q]
- Broad vascular pedicle

PCWP 18 – 25 mm Hg
Stage 2 : Interstitial edema

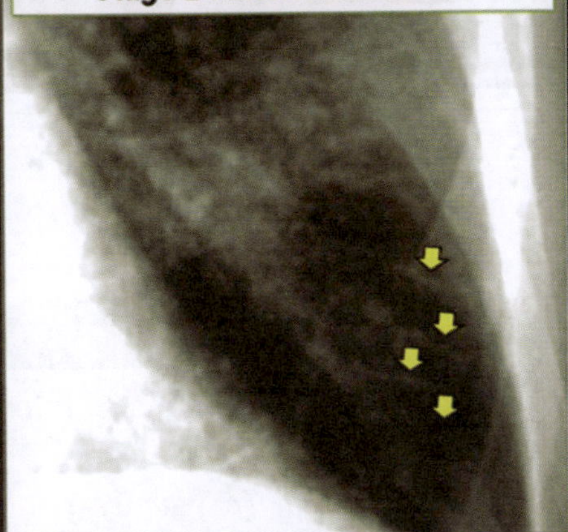

- Kerley B lines[Q]-due to thickening of deep interlobular septae-as fluid leaks along these septae
- Peri-bronchial cuffing

PCWP > 25 mm Hg
Stage 3 : Alveolar edema

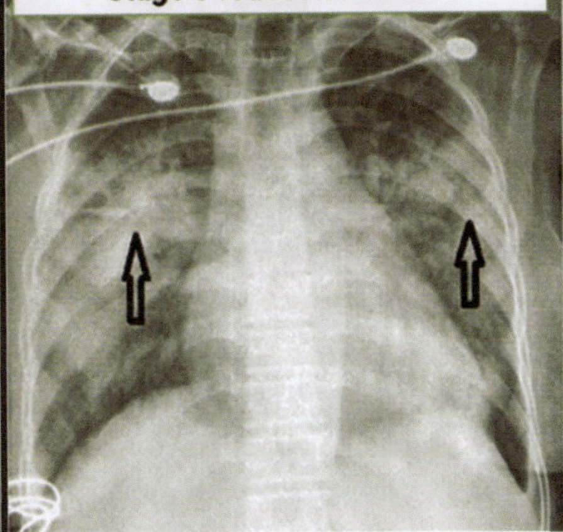

- Bat-wing[Q]/angle-wing[Q]/central peri-hilar opacities[Q]
- Consolidation
- Cotton-wool spots

Contd...

Pericardial effusion—IOC is USG/Echocardiography

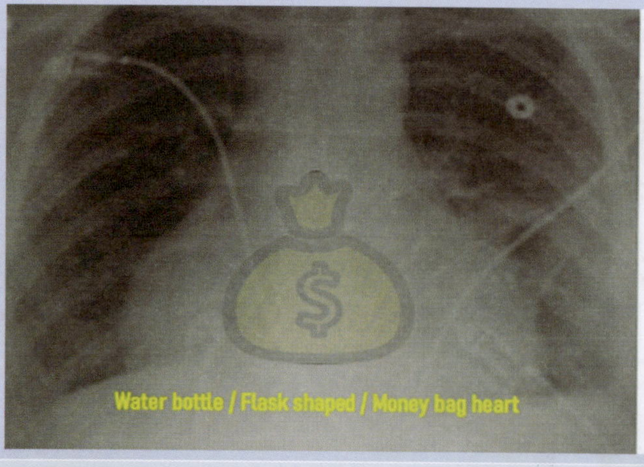

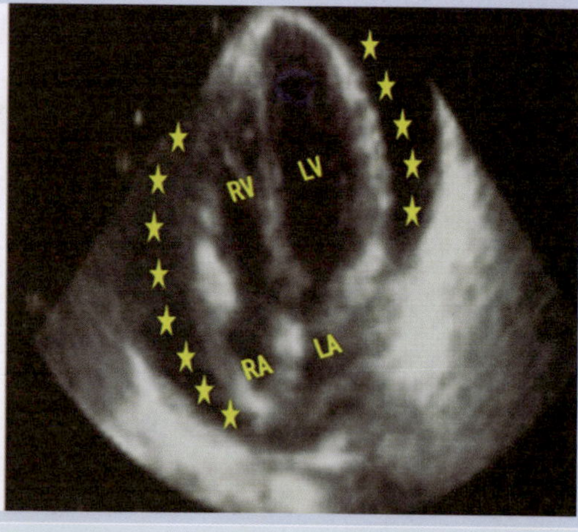

PYQ ALERT "FMGE JAN 2023 PATTERN"

Pulmonary Embolism

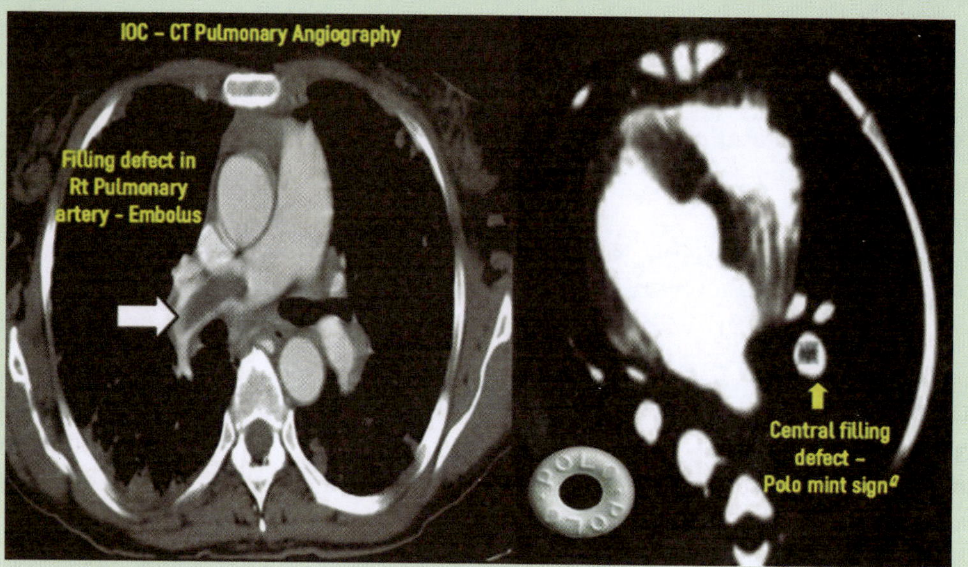

Pulmonary Embolism:

CXR – Poor sensitivity: Normal in early cases

CT Pulmonary Angiography: Investigation of Choice[Q]

PYQ ALERT

- **Acute emboli: Show Polo mint sign[Q]**—Central nonenhancing filling defect due to thrombus with the contrast flowing peripherally.
- **Chronic emboli:** The thrombus forms obtuse angle (c/f acute angle in acute emboli) with vessel walls + calcification
- **Ultrasound/echocardiography:** Right ventricular hypokinesia (**McConnell sign**[Q]), right ventricular dilatation and pulmonary arterial hypertension can be identified.
- **Nuclear/radionuclide scans: Second Line Test for PTE**, also known as Ventilation-Perfusion (V/Q) scan.
- **Mismatched defects[Q] on V/Q scan—suggestive of pulmonary embolism** present ventilation—absent perfusion in the same segment of lung
- **Invasive pulmonary angiography: Gold Standard/Most Accurate Method**—Invasive hence, CT angiography is preferred for diagnosis.

Contd...

CONCEPT

Vascular abnormalities is an absolute favorite topic of your examiners! Remember, whenever you are asked about the gold standard investigation for any vascular abnormality, the Answer is Invasive catheter angiography[Q]. See the following table.

Condition	Gold standard investigation
Berry aneurysm	Cerebral digital subtraction angiography (DSA)
Brain AV malformation	Cerebral digital subtraction angiography (DSA)
Renal artery stenosis	Invasive catheter angiography
Varicose veins/DVT	Invasive catheter venography
Aortic dissection	Invasive catheter venography
Pulmonary embolism	Invasive pulmonary angiography
Mesenteric artery thrombosis	Invasive abdominal/mesenteric angiography

Aortic dissection

PYQ ALERT "FMGE JAN 2023 PATTERN"

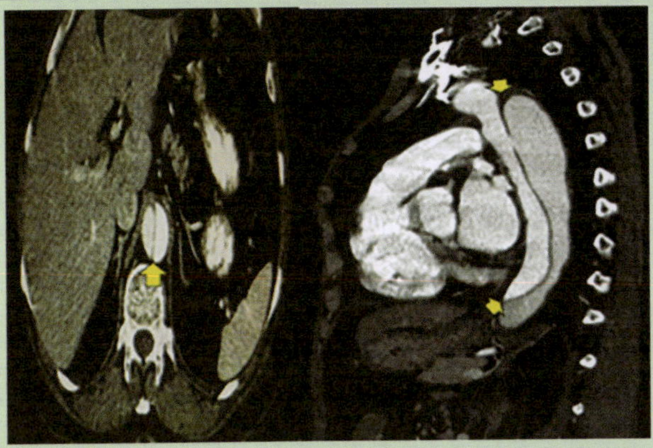

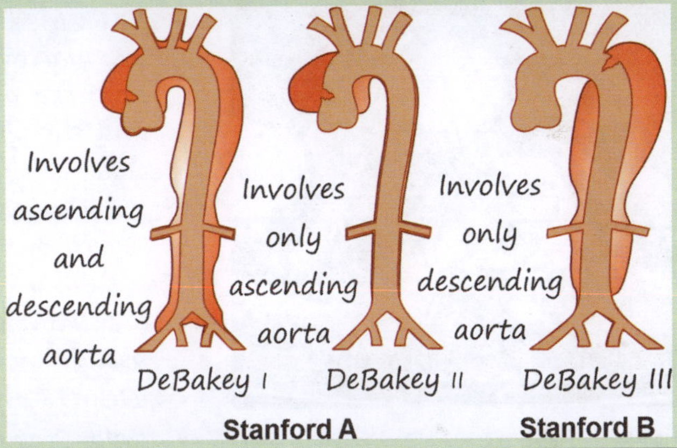

- Hypertension[Q] is the most common underlying cause.
- **IOC—CE-CT/CT Angiography**
- **Transesophageal Echocardiography used in emergency conditions**
- Gold standard invasive catheter angiograpjhy
  - On CT angiography—intimal flap seen in aortic lumen separating it into true and false lumen
  - Mercedes Benz sign[Q]—in triple dissection,
  - Windsock sign[Q]—associated hematoma or thrombus.
  - Cobweb sign[Q]—is seen along the false lumen due to shreds of media seen along the wall.
  - Beak sign[Q] is seen at the terminal end of the dissection.

CLINICAL CLINCHER

Treatment of Aortic dissection:

- Whenever ascending aorta is involved (DeBakey I and II and Stanford Type A) – Rx is usually surgical by Dacron graft reconstruction
- DeBakey III/Stanford B can be treated conservatively

Aortic aneurysm

Focal dilatation of aortic lumen. Diagnosed as aneurysm if diameter is more than:	• Ascending aorta diameter >5 cm • Descending aorta diameter >4 cm • Abdominal aortic diameter >3 cm

Contd...

Aortic aneurysm

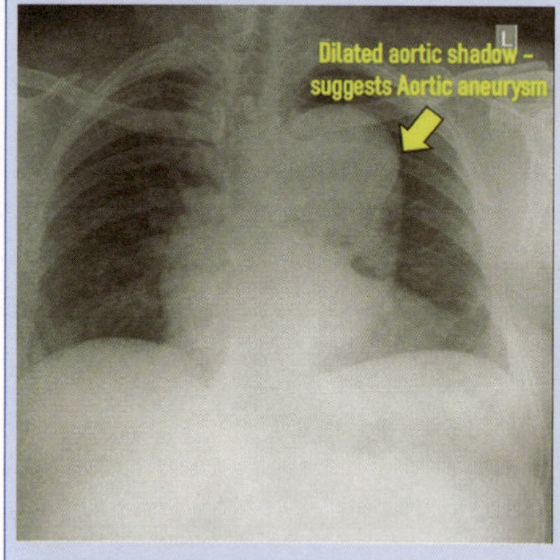

Aortic aneurysm

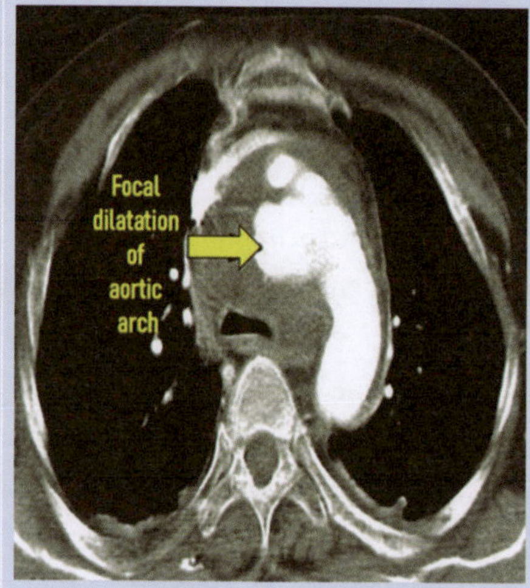

Aortic aneurysm

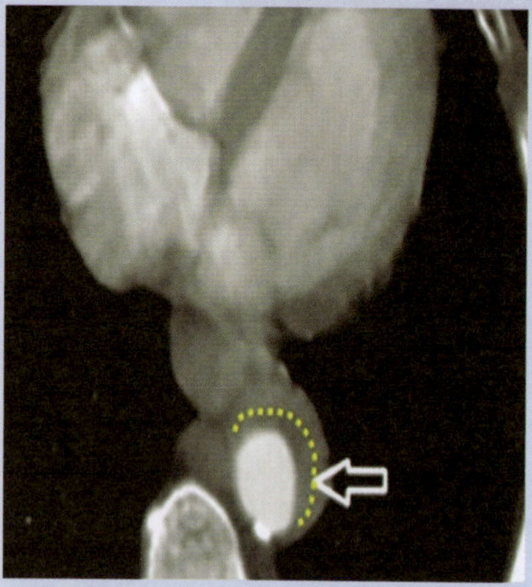

Aortic aneurysm—Crescent sign[Q]

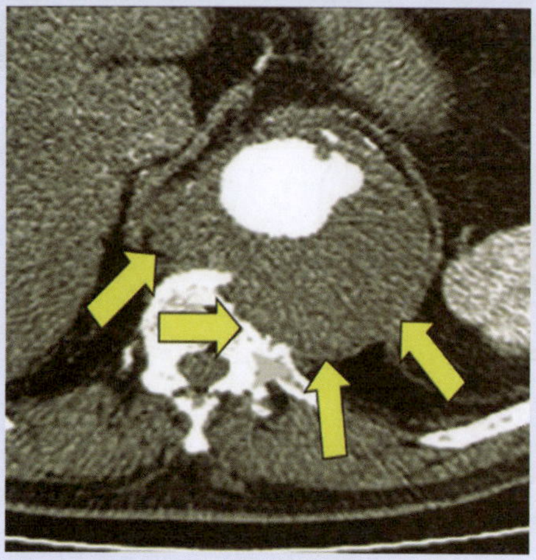

Aortic aneurysm—Draped aorta sign[Q]

- **Atherosclerosis**[Q]: Most common cause
- **CXR**: Mediastinal widening, an opacity with long axis oriented along the aorta and showing curvilinear wall calcification.
- **Yin-Yang sign**[Q]: Traditionally described in pseudoaneurysms – but is seen in both true and pseudoaneurysms
- **IOC**: CT angiography[Q]
- **Gold Standard**: Invasive catheter angiography[Q]

CLINICAL CLINCHER

Impending rupture of aneurysm is indicated by the following features and requires emergency surgical treatment:

- Rapid increase in size[Q]
- Crescent sign[Q]—hyper-attenuation peripheral cresent-shaped thrombus around the aneurysm
- Draped aorta sign[Q]—aorta loses its round shape and drapes over the surface of adjacent vertebra
- Periaortic fat stranding[Q]
- Extravasation of contrast[Q]
- Missing calcium sign[Q]
- Tangential calcium sign[Q]

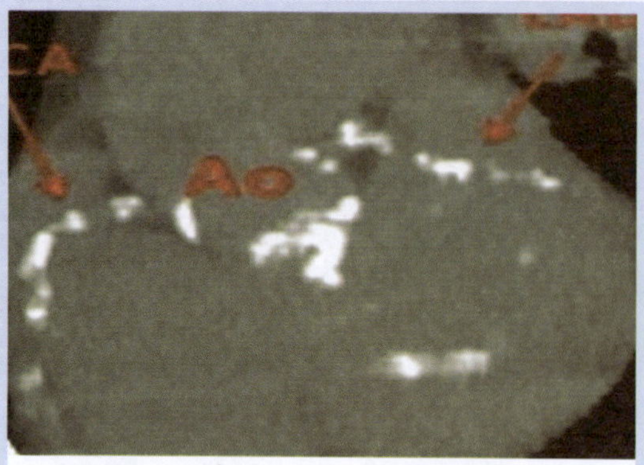

- Measured on non-contrast CT
- Moderate score 101–400
- Higher score–poor prognosis

Agatston score

Semi-quantitative estimation of calcium burden on coronary arteries

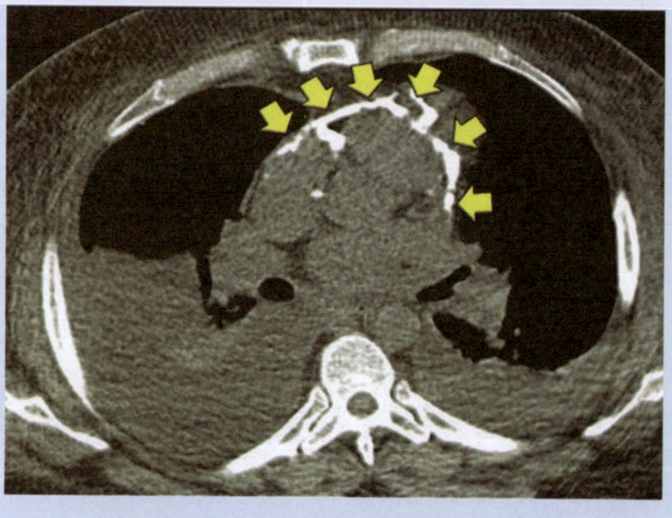

Constrictive pericarditis pericardial calcification

4. GASTROINTESTINAL TRACT IMAGING

PNEUMOPERITONEUM CLINCHERS

- **MC cause in adults**—bowel perforation[Q]
- MC cause in neonates—necrotizing enterocolitis[Q]
- Best X-ray projection — X-ray chest erect[Q]
- IOC overall — CT abdomen[Q]

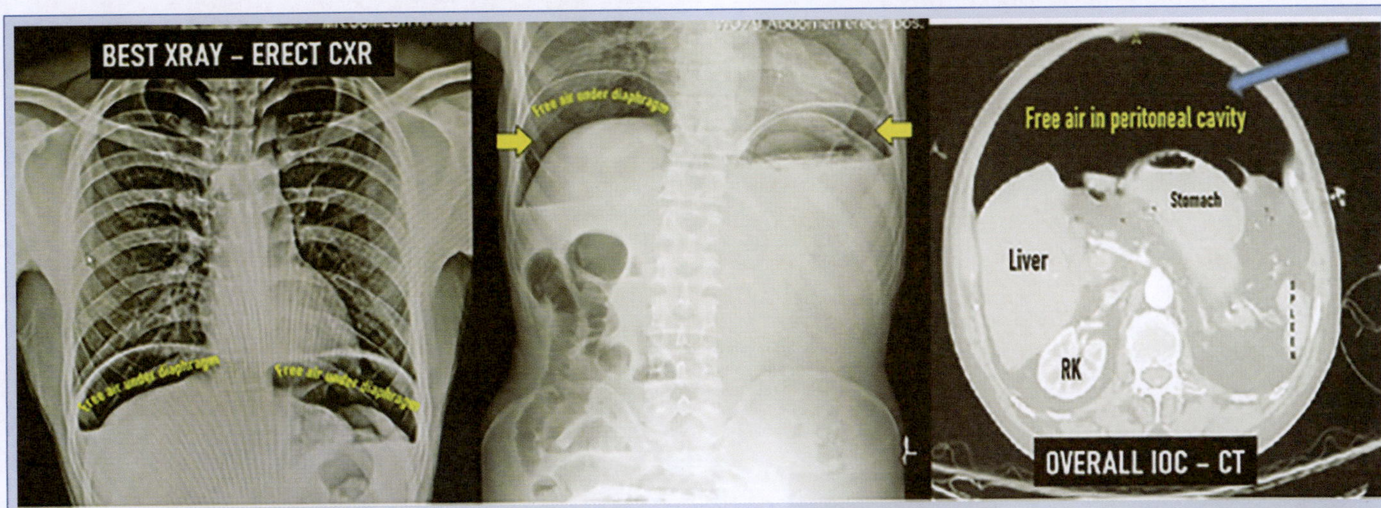

Supine abdomen X-ray—Multiple Named signs

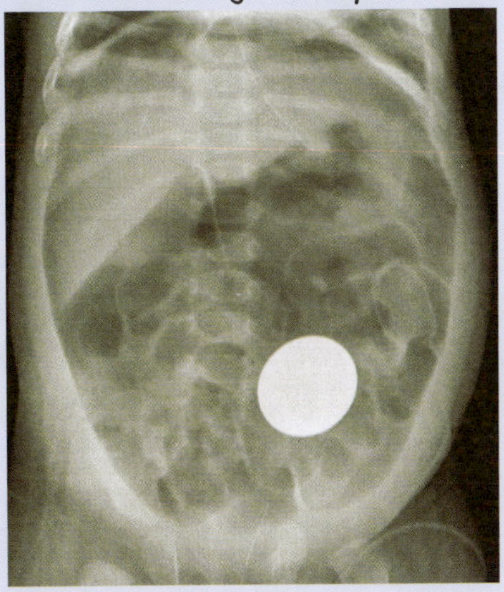

Football sign[Q]/Rigler's double wall sign[Q]/Doge's cap sign[Q]/ Leaping dolphin sign[Q]/Cupola sign[Q]/Inverted V sign[Q]

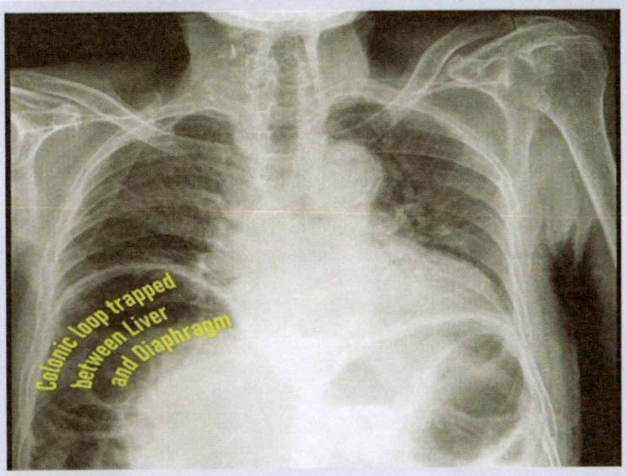

Pseudopneumoperitoneum

Conditions simulating pneumoperitoneum on an abdominal radiograph

- **Chilaiditi sign[Q]**: Colon trapped between liver and right hemidiaphragm
- **Chilaiditi syndrome[Q]**: Chilaiditi sign + Right upper quadrant pain

Ascites Imaging

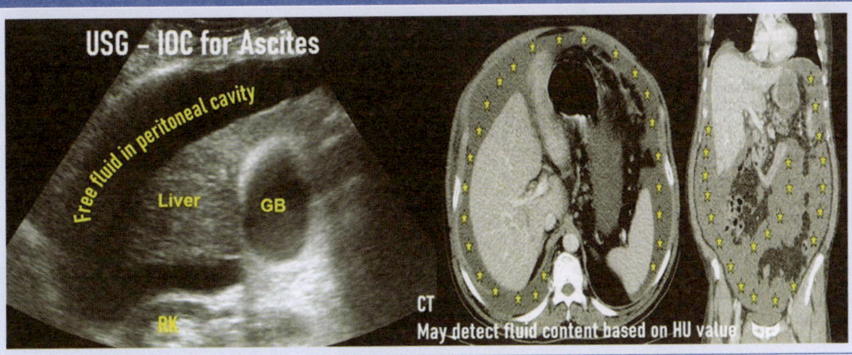

FOCUSSED ASSESSMENT WITH SONOGRAPHY IN TRAUMA (FAST)

- Longitudinal Right Upper Quadrant (RUQ) – Most sensitive quadrant for detection of hemoperitoneum
- Most commonly used probe for FAST – Convex/curvilinear probe with a frequency of 3.5–5 MHz
- Extended FAST (e-FAST):
  - Bilateral anterior thoracic region assessment to rule out Pneumothorax
  - Bilateral lower thorax assessment to rule out pleural effusion/hemothorax

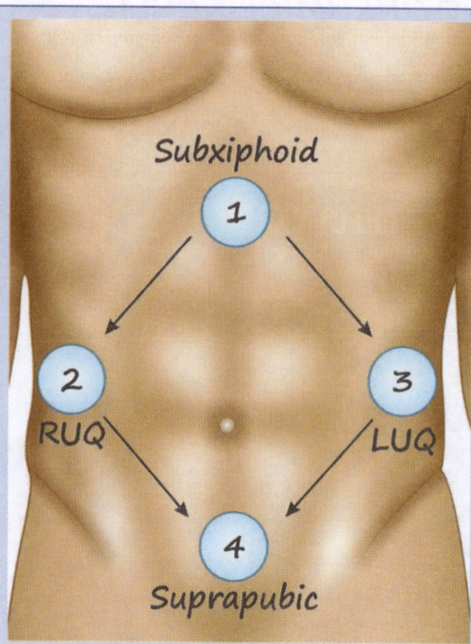

Standard fast protocol

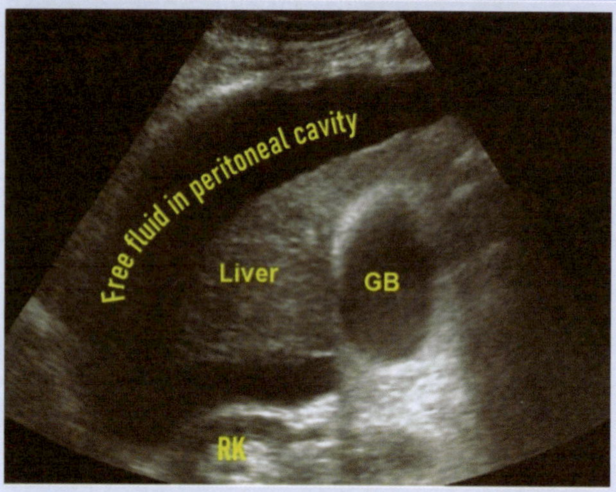

A FAST image showing hypoechoic free fluid around the liver and in the Morrison's pouch (Hepatorenal pouch) in a case of abdominal trauma—FAST positive

H/o trauma
→ Fast-free fluid +ve
→ Suggests hemoperitoneum due to solid organ injury
- Patient hemodynamically Stable → CE-CT: Modality of choice for solid organ injury
- Patient hemodynamically Unstable → Operative management

CLINICAL CLINCHER

Child presents with vomiting
- Newborn – at birth → Bilious vomiting → Duodenal atresia
- Presents at 6-12 weeks age → Nonbilious vomiting → Pyloric stenosis

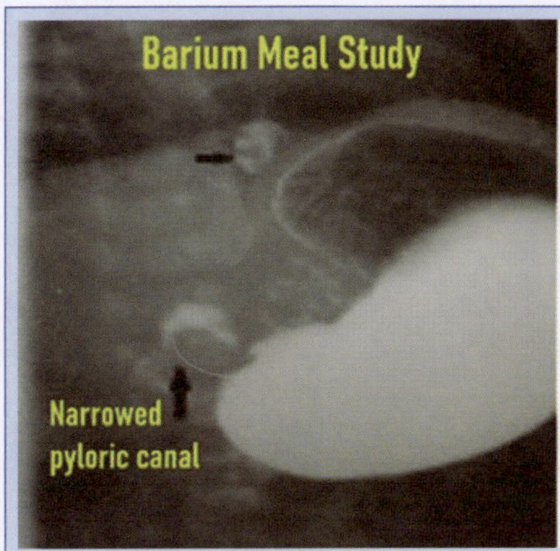

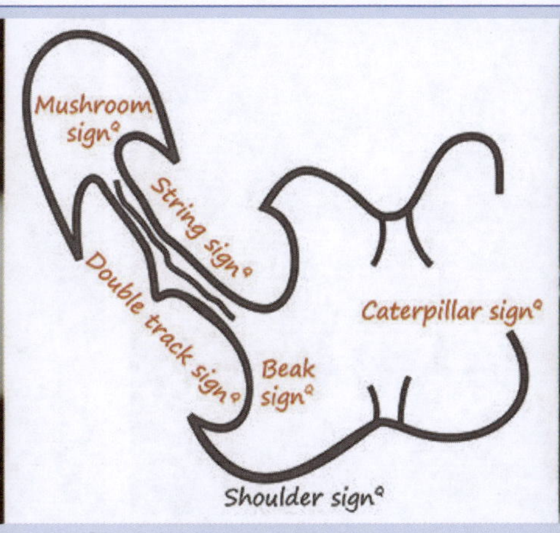

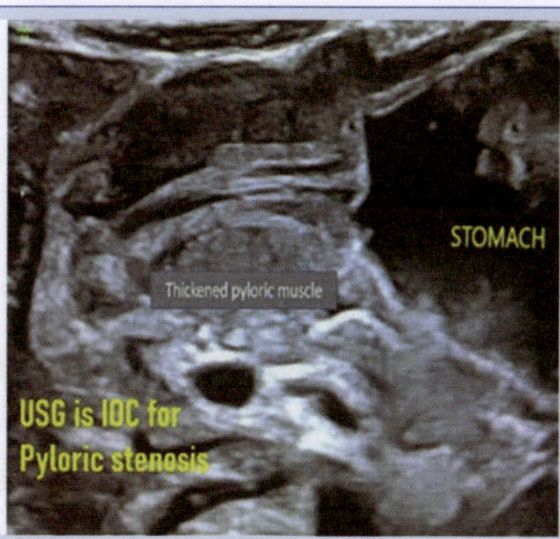

- On USG—Longitudinal pyloric length >16 mm[Q] (Cervix sign[Q]) and pyloric muscle thickness >3–4 mm[Q]
- Signs on barium meal:
  - Caterpillar sign[Q]: Stomach hyperperistalsis
  - Beak sign[Q]: Beak-shaped entrance of pylorus
  - Shoulder sign[Q]: Pylorus indenting the gastric antrum
  - String sign[Q]: Elongated pylorus with narrowed lumen
  - Double tract sign[Q]: Puckering of mucosa with double lining of pyloric canal
  - Mushroom sign[Q]: Pylorus indenting the duodenal bulb

Duodenal Atresia

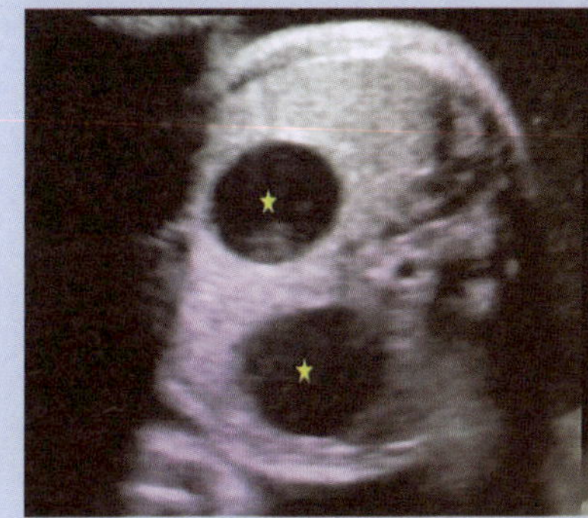

Double bubble sign—Antenatal USG

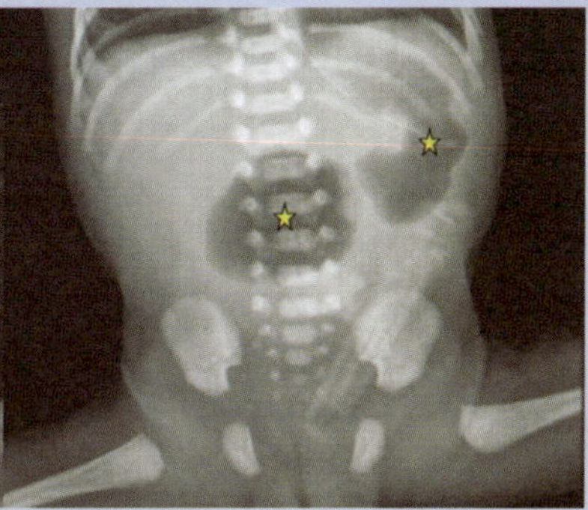

Double bubble sign—X-ray Abdomen

CLINICAL CLINCHER

Bubble signs on an infantogram/ Babygram

- **Single bubble sign:** Pyloric stenosis[Q] - due to dilated stomach
- **Double bubble sign:** Duodenal atresia[Q] (or any cause of duodenal obstruction) due to dilated stomach and duodenal cap
- **Triple bubble sign:** Jejunal atresia[Q] due to dilated stomach, duodenal cap and duodenal loop
- **Multiple bubble sign:** Ileal atresia[Q]

ESOPHAGEAL SPOTTERS

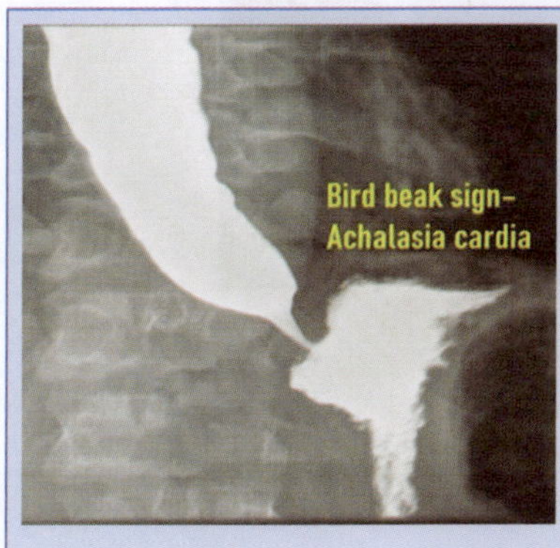

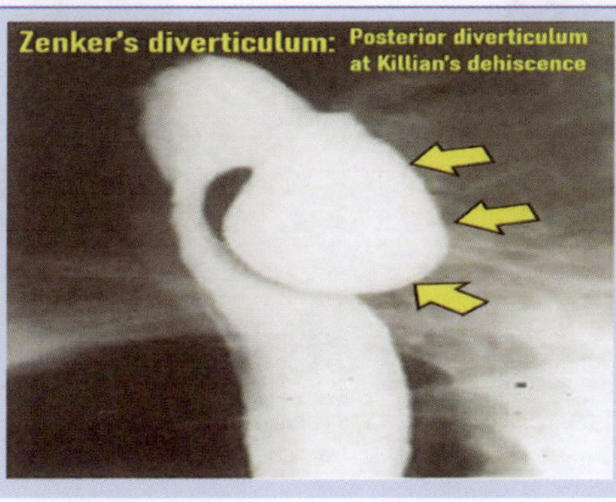

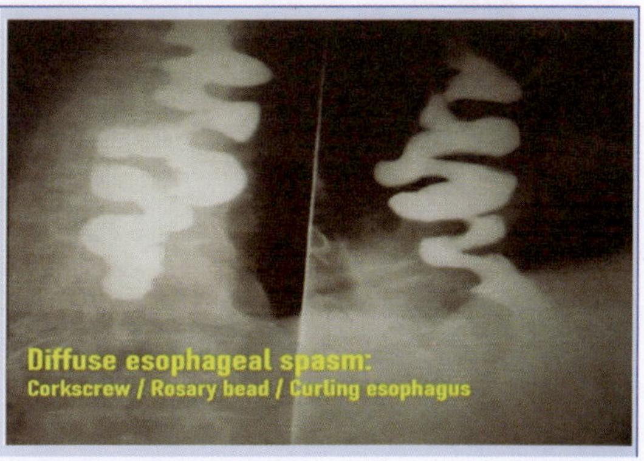

Contd...

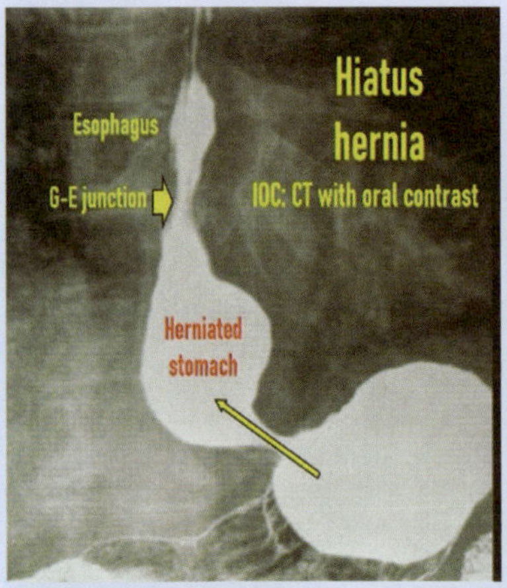

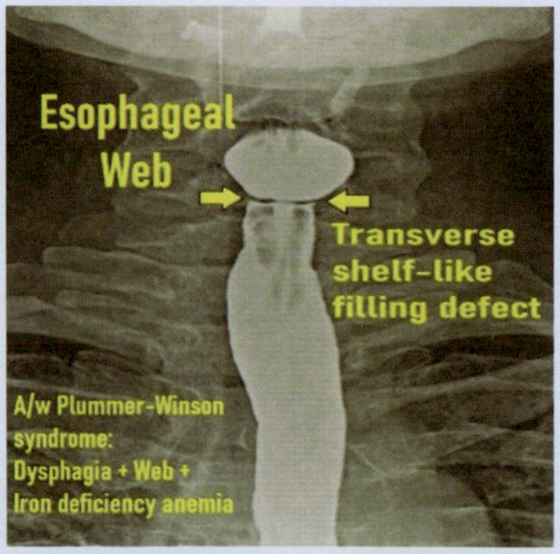

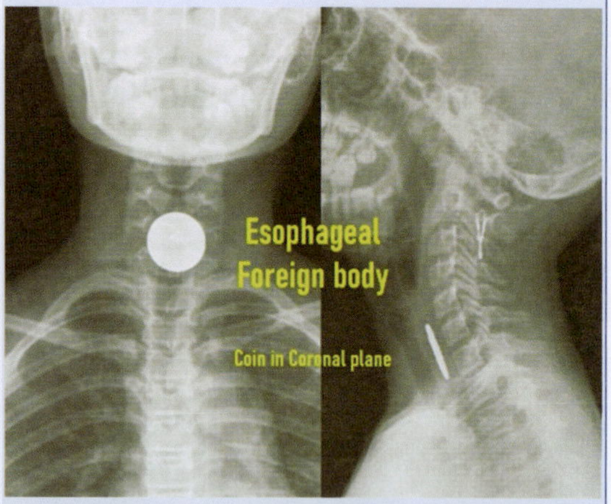

CLINICAL CLINCHER

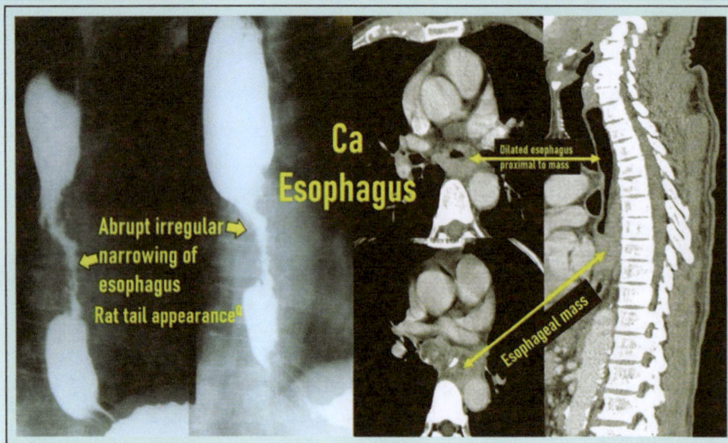

- Elderly patient with weight loss and dysphagia —equal for solids and liquids[Q]
- Barium swallow—Abrupt irregular narrowing—Rat tail appearance[Q]
- Ovarall IOC—Endoscopy + Biopsy[Q]
- Imaging IOC for staging—PET-CT[Q]
- Imaging IOC for TN staging—Endoscopic USG[Q]

BOWEL OBSTRUCTION

Small bowel obstruction	Large bowel obstruction
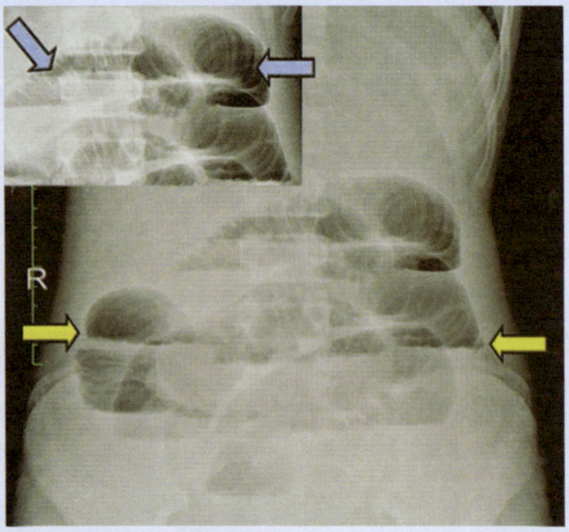	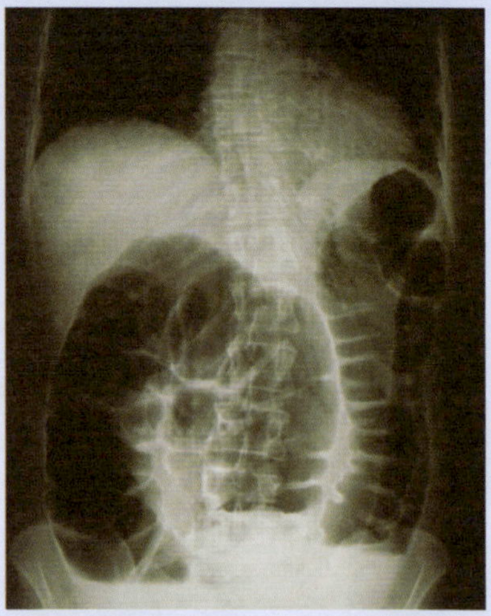
Multiple dilated small bowel loops—centrally located loops with multiple air-fluid levels and volvulae conniventes—Herring bone appearance/Concertina effect—suggests SBO	Dilated large bowel loops—Predominantly peripheral bowel loops with haustrations and few long air-fluid levels—suggests LBO

Contd...

	Small bowel obstruction (SBO)	Large bowel obstruction (LBO)
Bowel diameter	>3 cm to <5 cm	>5 cm (Cecum >9 cm)
Location of loops	Central	Peripheral
Bowel wall folds	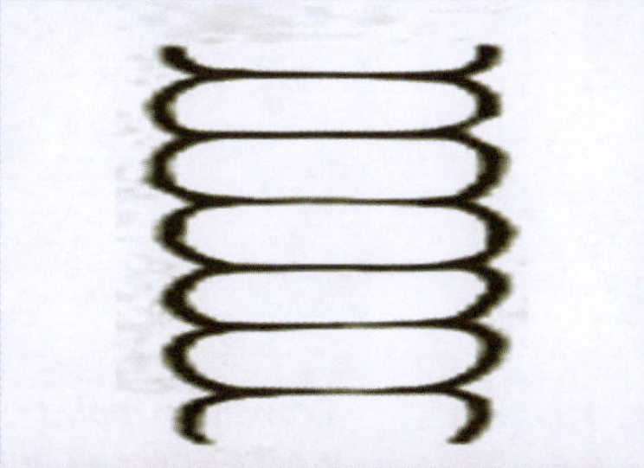 Volvulae conniventis / Kerckring folds/valves / plicae circulares – Complete transverse mucosal folds	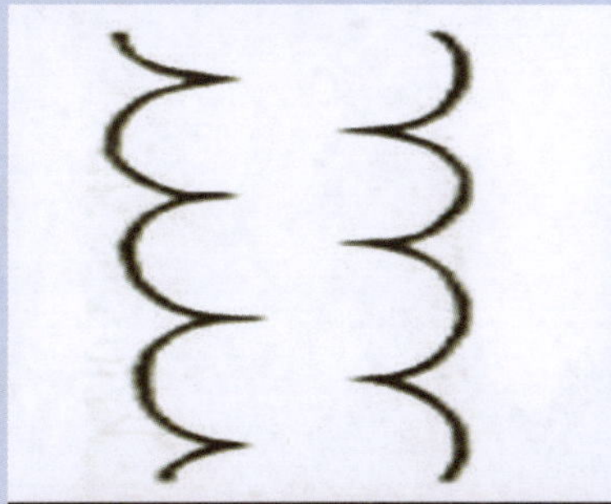 Haustrations – incomplete transverse wall folds
Number of dilated bowel loops	Multiple	Few
Air-fluid levels	Multiple short air-fluid levels	Few long air-fluid levels
Air in Large bowel	Not seen as nothing passes beyond obstruction site	Seen proximal to obstruction site
Named signs	• Step-ladder appearance • Small bowel feces sign • Transition point • Herring bone appearance/concertina effect • String of beads/pearls sign	Cut-off sign at obstruction site

Bowel obstruction spotters

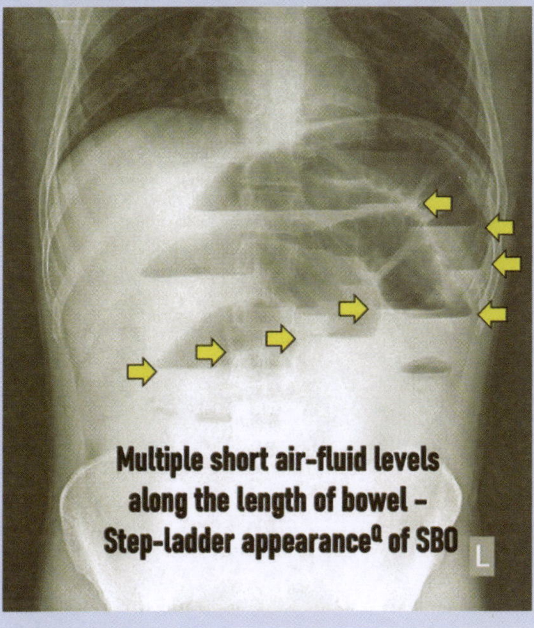

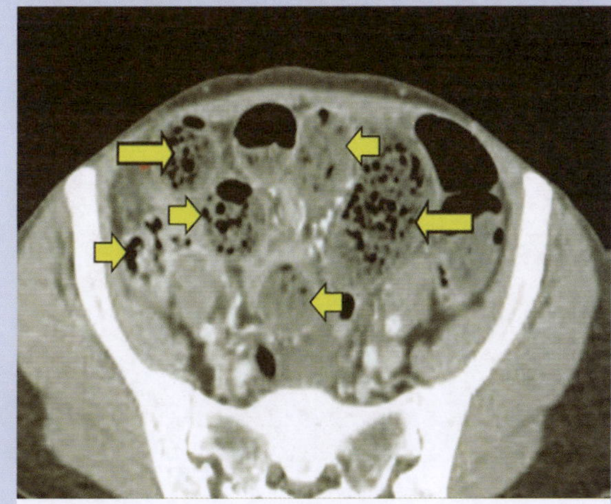

Axial CT–dilated small bowel loops filled with solid material with interspersed air–small bowel feces sign[Q]–small bowel obstruction

Contd...

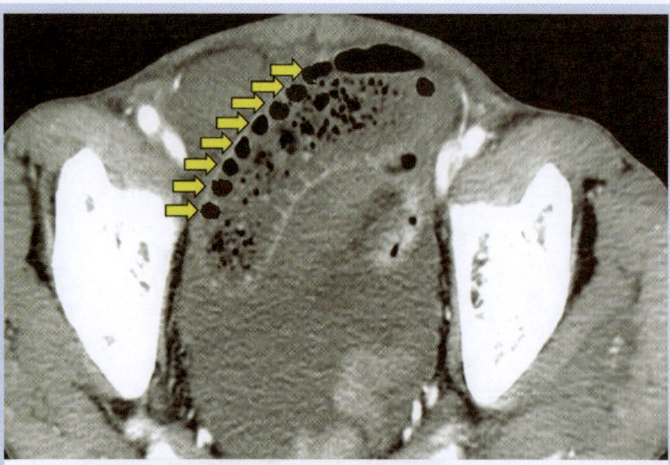

String of beads sign[Q]—axial CE-CT showing small linear gas bubbles trapped between the vulvulae conniventes in the non-dependent part of a fluid filled dilated bowel

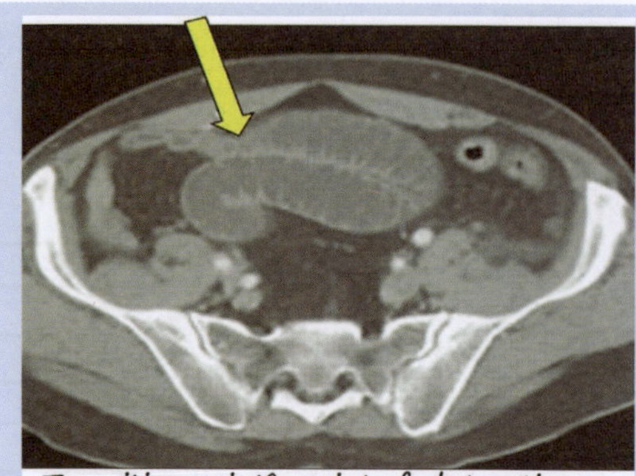

Transition point[Q]—point of obstruction where there is abrupt transition between dilated loops proximally and collapsed/ empty loops distally—most reliable CT criteria for diagnosis[Q]

CLINICAL CLINCHER

Air-fluid Levels

- May be seen on abdomen X-rays normally too.
- Considered abnormal when:
  - >2 in number
  - >2.5 cm in width
  - >2 cm away in height when within the same bowel loop

Gallstone Ileus

- Due to impaction of a large gallstone, following its passage into the bowel through a fistula between GB and small bowel usually the duodenum
- Most common site of impaction and mechanical obstruction— Terminal ileum[Q].
- Rigler's triad[Q]:
  - Pneumobilia
  - Small bowel obstruction
  - Ectopic gallstone—usually in the RIF

Inflammatory Bowel Disease—Spotters

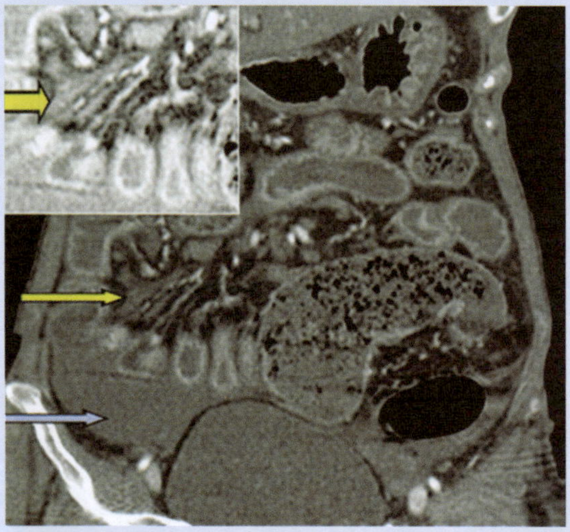

Coronal reconstructed image CE-CT — Prominent vasa recta resulting in Comb sign of Crohn's disease (yellow arrows). Ascites (blue arrow) is also seen due to the bowel inflammation

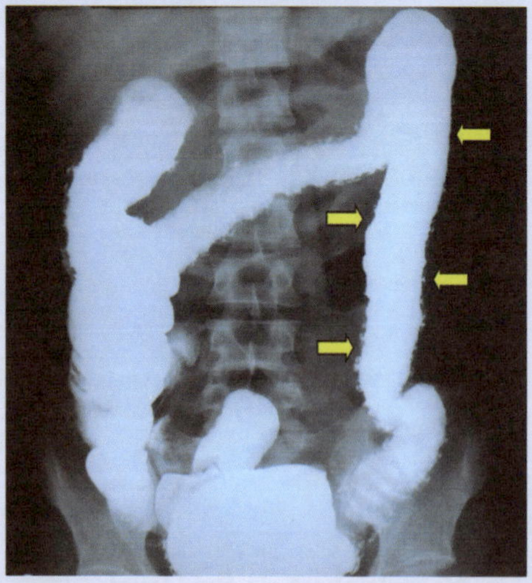

Lead pipe colon

Loss of haustral pattern of colon seen on barium enema – suggestive of Ulcerative colitis[Q]

Small Bowel Spotters

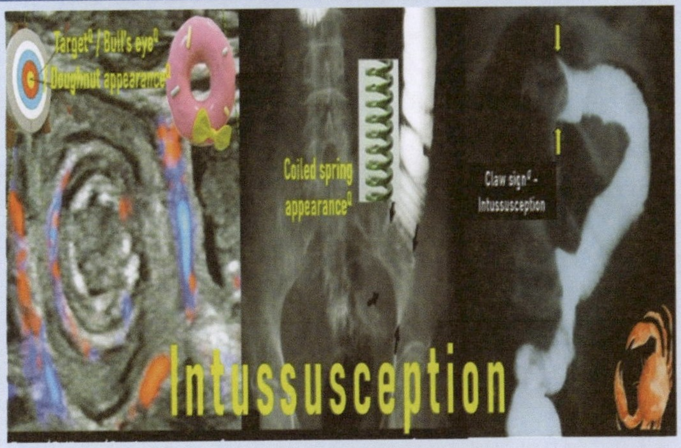

Intussusception

Intussusception:

CLINICAL CLINCHER

- Child 2 months – 2 years of age
- Pain in abdomen
- Red currant jelly stools

- Most common site in children — Ileocolic[Q]
- Most common site in adults — Colocolic[Q]
- IOC in pediatric age group — USG[Q]
- IOC in adults — CE-CT[Q]

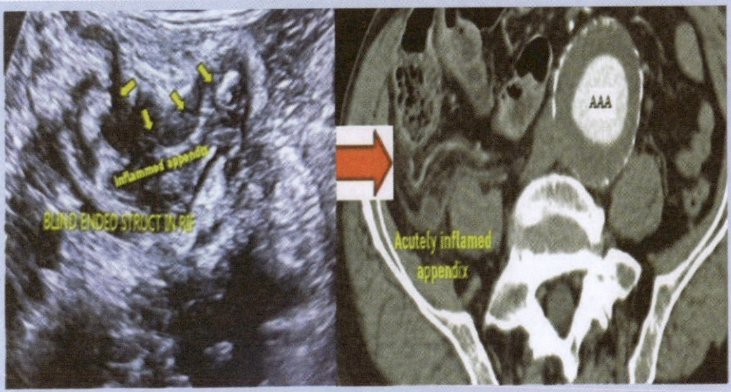

Acute appendicitis

Acute Appendicitis:

CLINICAL CLINCHER

- Child with fever
- Pain in abdomen, vomiting
- Pain at tenderness in RIF at McBurney's point

- IOC in children — USG[Q]
- IOC in adults — CE-CT[Q]
- Named signs on CE-CT
  - Cecal bar sign[Q]
  - Arrowhead sign[Q]
- Appendicular mucocele – Appendix distended with mucinous contents. Associated with mucinous cystadenoma of appendix[Q]

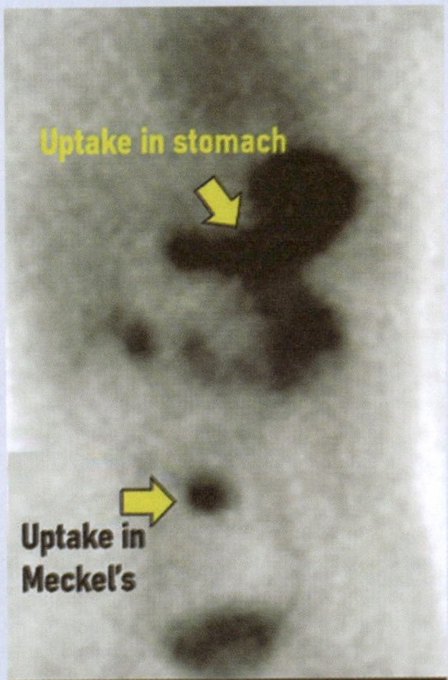

99m-Tc-pertechnate scan - showing focal uptake in the Meckel's diverticulum

Meckel's Diverticulitis:

CLINICAL CLINCHER

Meckel's Diverticulum Secifics

Rule of 2[Q]:

- 2 inches long
- 2 feet from Illeocecal junction
- 2% population affected
- 20% ectopic mucosa (gatric mucosa > pancreatic)
- GI bleeding — MC presentation in adults
- Littre's hernia[Q] — Meckel's diverticulum in the hernia sac

- Meckel's diverticulum has ectopic gastric mucosa in it – this secretes acid – hence, presents clinically as GI bleeding.
- IOC – 99mTc-pertechnetate scan. The radionuclide is concentrated in the gastric mucosa—that is in the stomach as well as that is in the Meckel's thus localizing it

Colonic Spotters

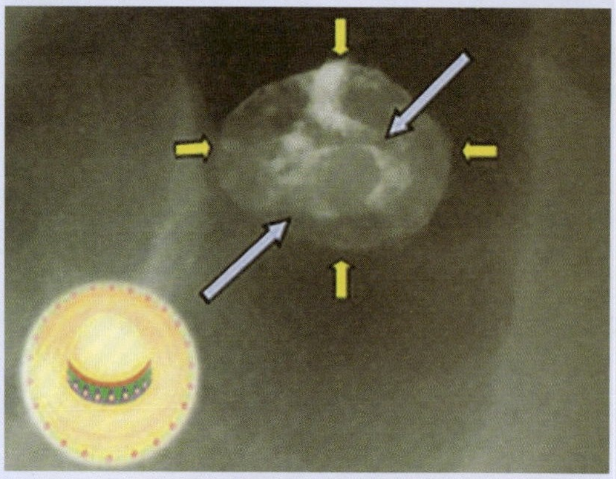

Mexican hat sign[Q]
Pedunculated colonic polyp

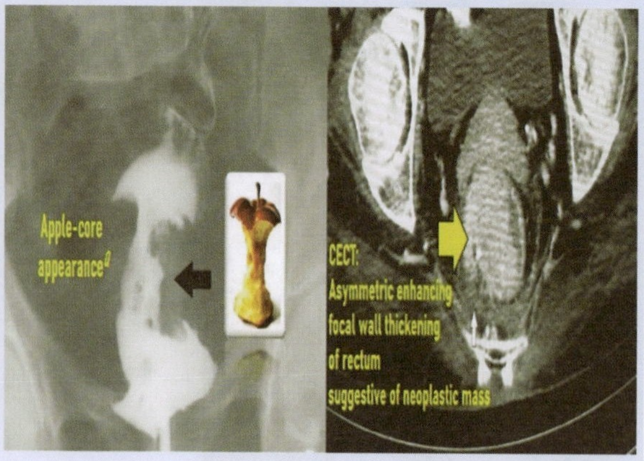

Ca Colon/Rectum

Ca Colon specifics:

- IOC for diagnosis – colonoscopy guided biopsy
- Overall IOC for staging – PET-CT
- Most common site for metastases – Liver

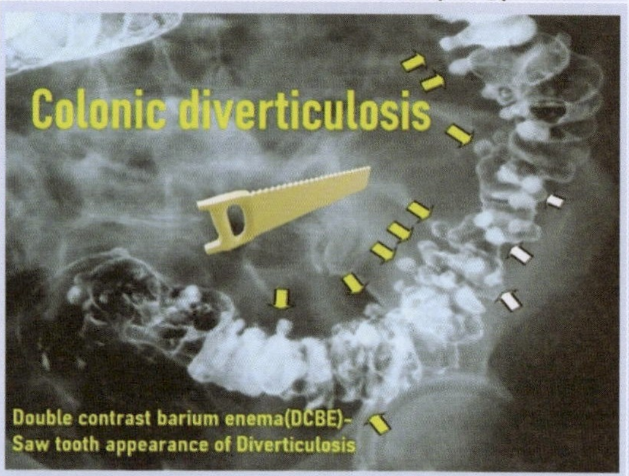

Colonic diverticulosis

Colonic diverticulosis:

- Most common site - Sigmoid colon[Q]
- Least common site - Rectum[Q]
- Saw tooth appearance of diverticulosis
- Bowler hat appearance[Q] is seen when viewed en-face
- CE-CT: IOC for diverticular disease

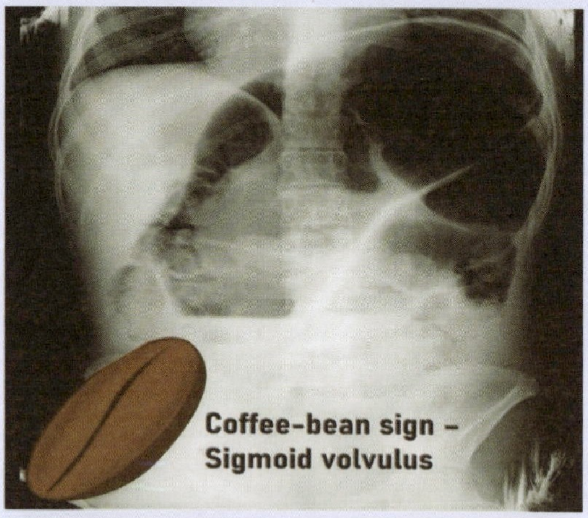

Sigmoid Volvulus – MC site of volvulus of bowel[Q]

CLINICAL CLINCHER

- Elderly female
- Known case of mental handicap/institutionalization
- Massive gaseous distension of abdomen

Named signs:

- Inverted U-shaped loop[Q]
- Kidney bean sign[Q]
- Omega sign[Q]
- Left flank overlap sign[Q]
- Frimann-Dahl sign[Q]
- Coffee bean sign[Q]
- Bent inner tube sign[Q]
- Liver overlap sign[Q]
- Pelvis overlap sign[Q]

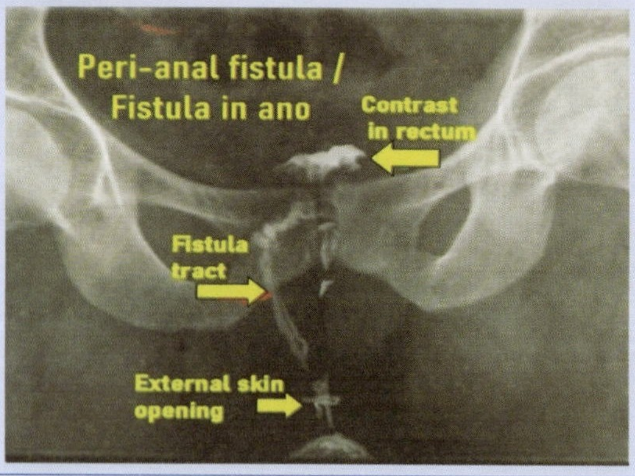

Perianal fistula/Fistula-in-ano

- IOC - MRI Fistulography
- Initial investigation – Conventional sinogram/fistulogram

FOCAL LIVER ABNORMALITIES

Liver abscess

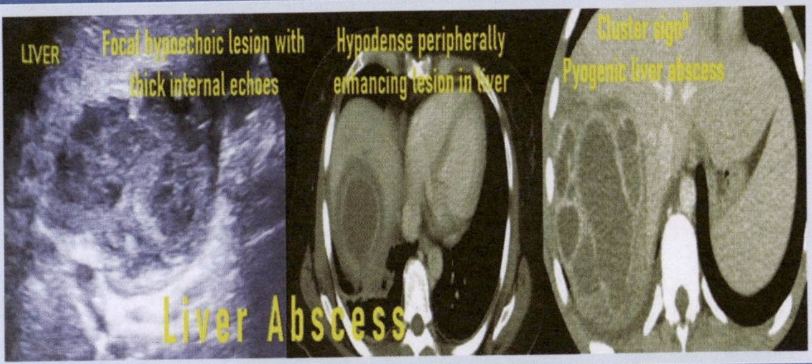

- Initial investigation—USG[Q]
- Imaging modality of choice for follow-up to assess liquefaction[Q]—USG[Q]
- Overall IOC — CE-CT[Q]—Double target sign[Q]
- Cluster sign[Q] of pyogenic abscess—Multiple smaller hypodense lesions coalesce together to form a larger abscess cavity.

Hepatocellular cancer (HCC)

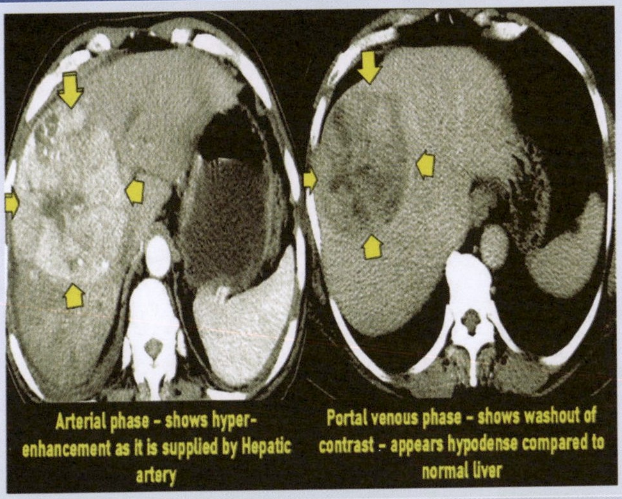

Most common malignant liver lesion[Q]

- On CE-CT
- Arterial phase—enhancement due to hepatic arterial supply[Q]
- Portal venous phase—Iso/hypodense liver due to wash-out of contrast
- Delayed phase—Capsule/fibrous components may enhance
- On angiography a streaks and threads like appearance[Q] is seen.
- LI-RADS[Q]: Liver imaging—reporting and data system is used.

CLINICAL CLINCHER

HCC Versus Fibrolamellar HCC

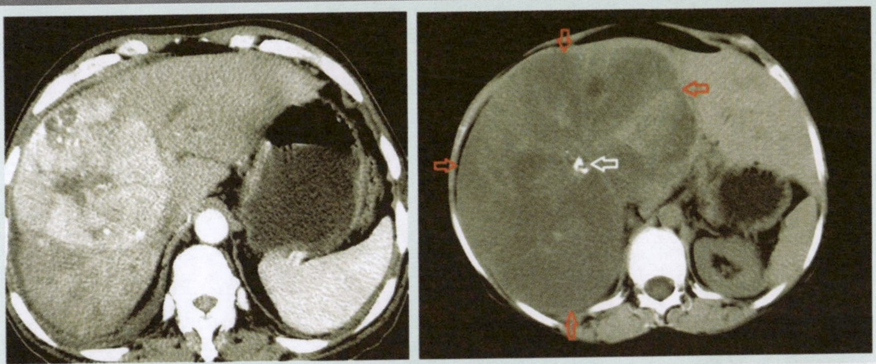

	HCC	Fibrolamellar HCC
Age	Middle age - Elderly	Young
Associated liver cirrhosis	Present	Absent
Sr. Alpha-fetoprotien (AFP)	Elevated	Normal
Sr. Neurotensin B	Normal	Elevated
Central fibrous scar with stellate calcification	Absent	Present
Overall prognosis	Poor	Good

Contd...

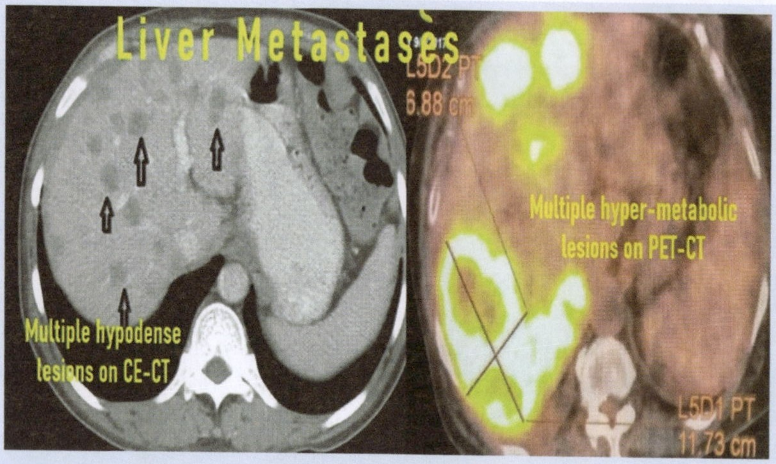

Liver Metastases

Liver metastases:

- IOC – PET-CT[Q] > Triphasic CE-CT[Q]
- Most common primary resulting in liver metastasis—Colon carcinoma[Q]
- Target/Bull's eye appearance[Q] on USG
- Calcified liver metastasis[Q] seen in—Mucinous metastasis from ovary/colon
- CT— Hypovascular mets[Q] are most common—appear hypodense to normal liver on portal venous phase
- Hypervascular liver metastasis[Q] occurs from:
  - RCC
  - Thyroid cancer
  - Neuroendocrine tumors (Carcinoid, Islet cell tumors)
  - Choriocarcinoma
  - Melanoma

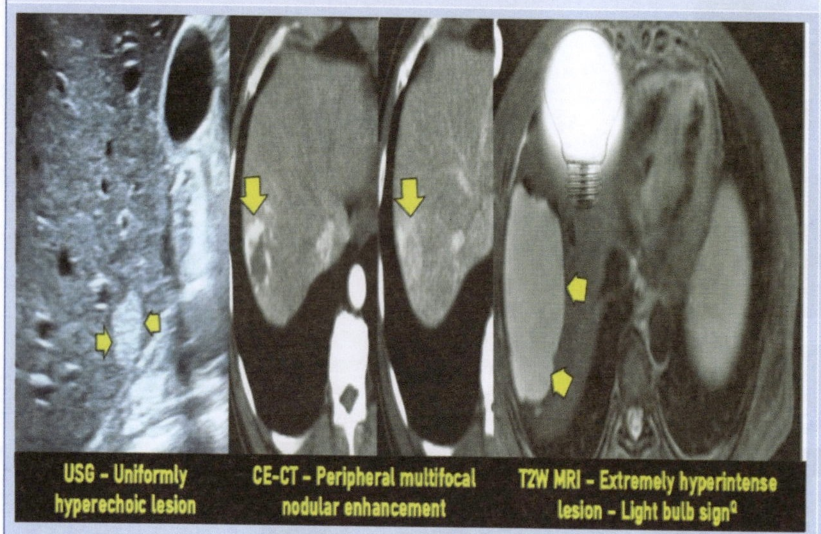

Liver hemangioma

Liver hemangioma:

- Most common benign neoplastic liver lesion
- IOC—Multiphasic CE-CT[Q]
- Bright dot sign[Q]—Bright dot seen within a hemangioma seen on arterial and portal venous phases of CT
- MRI—light bulb sign[Q]— on increasing T2 weighting of the images it appears progressively hyperintense (bright)

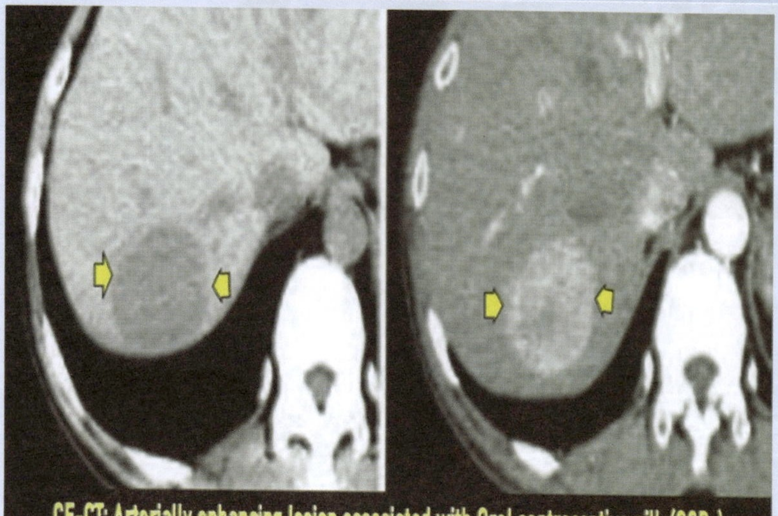

Hepatic Adenoma

Hepatic adenoma:

- Seen in young females on oral contraceptive pills[Q]
- Predilection for Intratumoral hemorrhage

BILIARY ABNORMALITIES

CLINICAL CLINCHER

Endoscopic retrograde cholangio-pancreatography (ERCP)	Magnetic resonance cholangio-pancreatography (MRCP)
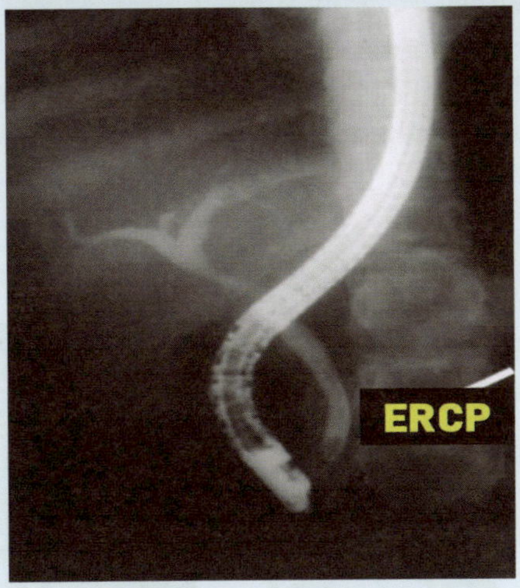	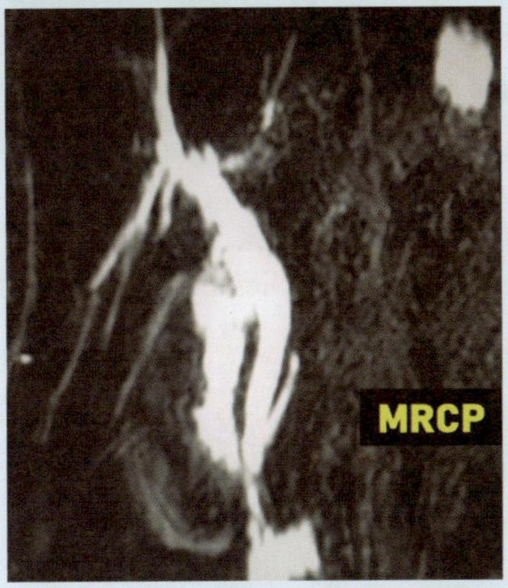
• Invasive technique • Two-Dimensional imaging technique • Involves cannulation of the ampulla endoscopically • Iodinated contrast injected into the biliary tree • Done under fluoroscopy guidance—so will have X-ray radiation exposure • Therapeutic use—can be used for stenting/ sphincterotomy/CBD stone removal	• Noninvasive technique • Three-Dimensional imaging technique • No endoscopy needed • No contrast needed • No radiation exposure • No therapeutic applications

BILIARY TREE SPOTTERS

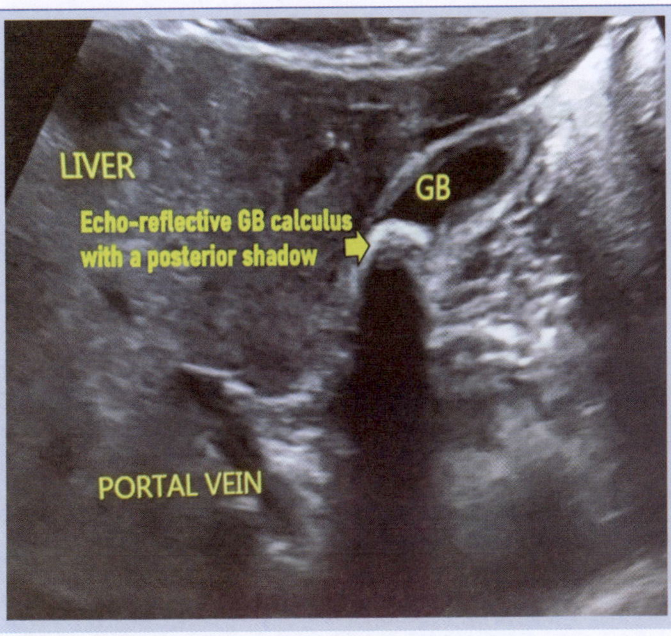

Cholelithiasis:

- Mixed stones[Q]—Most common type followed by cholesterol and pigment stones
- IOC for biliary calculi – USG[Q] – as they have poor calcium content – hence, not seen on X-ray/CT
- Mercedes-Benz sign[Q]—Star-shaped pattern of air fissuring within a gallstone, seen on a X-ray
- Rolling stone sign[Q]—Movement of stones, upon change in patient position

Contd...

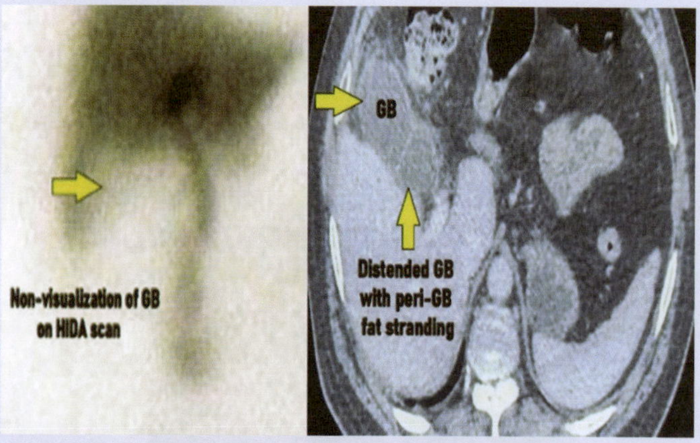

Acute Cholecystitis

Acute Cholecystitis:

IOC-USG[Q]:

- Over-distended GB with thickened/edematous walls and pericholecystic collection.
- Sonographic Murphy's sign[Q]—focal probe tenderness in right hypochondriac region

HIDA scan—Nonvisualization of GB on HIDA scan[Q].
Rim sign[Q]—increased uptake of the 99mTc-HIDA agent in the liver adjacent to the gallbladder fossa due to reactive hyperemia.

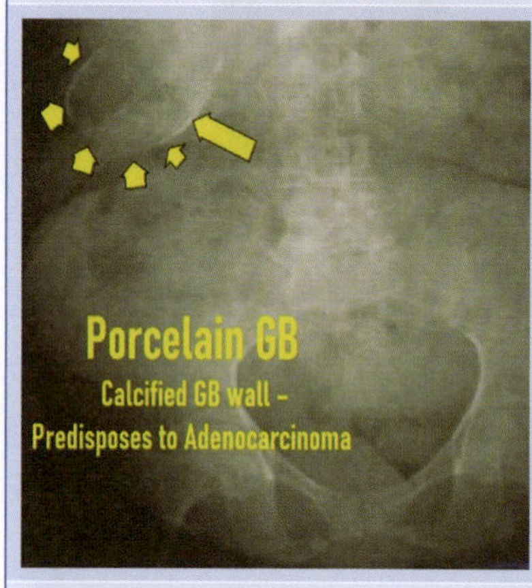

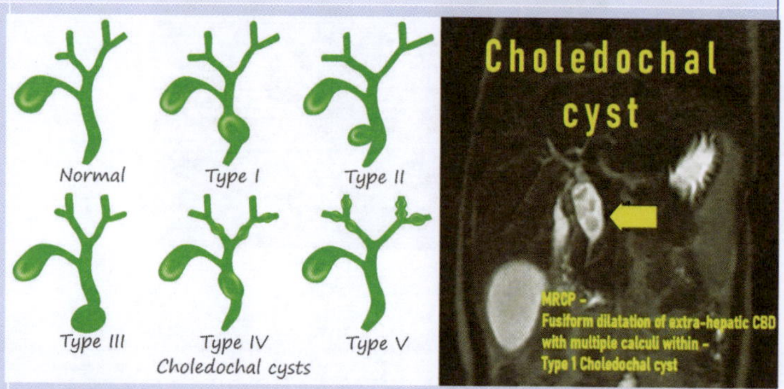

Choledochal cyst

Choledochal cyst:

Todani classification of choledochal cysts[Q]:

- Type I—Fusiform cystic dilatation of extrahepatic CBD
- Type II—Eccentric fluid-filled cyst/diverticulum
- Type III—Localized cystic dilatation of distal intramural segment of CBD—Choledochocele[Q]
- Type IVA—Multiple intrahepatic and extrahepatic bile duct cysts
- Type IVB—Multiple extrahepatic bile duct cysts
- Type V—Multifocal saccular dilatations of IHBR—Caroli's disease[Q]—shows Central dot sign[Q] on MRI.

IOC—MRCP/ERCP[Q]

PANCREAS SPOTTERS

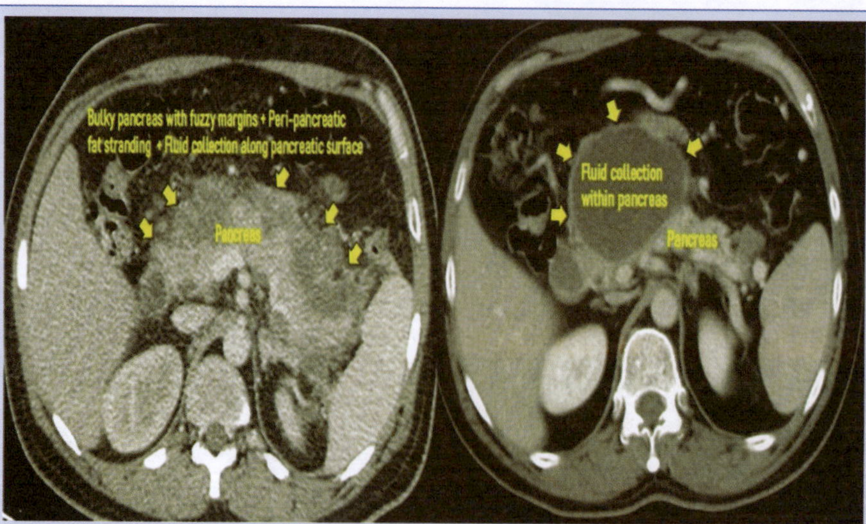

Acute pancreatitis   Pancreatic pseudocyst

Contd...

Acute pancreatitis

- Most common causes: Gallstones[Q] and alcoholism[Q]

Abdominal radiograph—Nonspecific

- Sentinel loop sign[Q]—dilated duodenal loop due to local ileus[Q]
- Colon cutoff sign[Q]—abrupt end of the gas column in transverse colon.[Q]

CE-CT[Q]—Investigation of choice[Q]

- Diffusely enlarged pancreas[Q] with fuzzy margins[Q] with peripancreatic fat stranding/fluid collections
- Uniform enhancement of pancreatic parenchyma seen in early/mild cases
- Pancreatic necrosis[Q] is suggested by – Nonenhancing areas in pancreas[Q]
- Pseudocyst formation[Q]—develop
  >4 weeks after an acute attack fluid collection (usually pancreatic secretions) lined by a wall of fibrous/granulation tissue — well-defined hypodense fluid collections in/around pancreas without any enhancement

Scoring of severity of pancreatitis:

- Balthazar Grading system[Q]—has prognostic implications
- CT Severity Index (CTSI)[Q]—Based on combination of Balthazar grading and Pancreatic necrosis. Correlates better with morbidity and mortality.

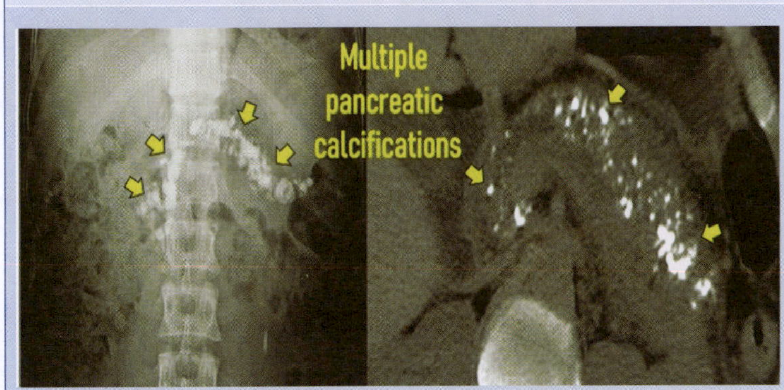

Chronic calcific pancreatitis

- MRCP/CRCP–Best for evaluation of pancreatic duct abnormalities. ERCP is better but is invasive.
- Chain of lakes appearance[Q]
- Duct penetrating sign[Q]–Non-obstructed main pancreatic duct seen penetrating an inflammatory pancreatic mass (it is compressed/obstructed in cases of neoplasm)

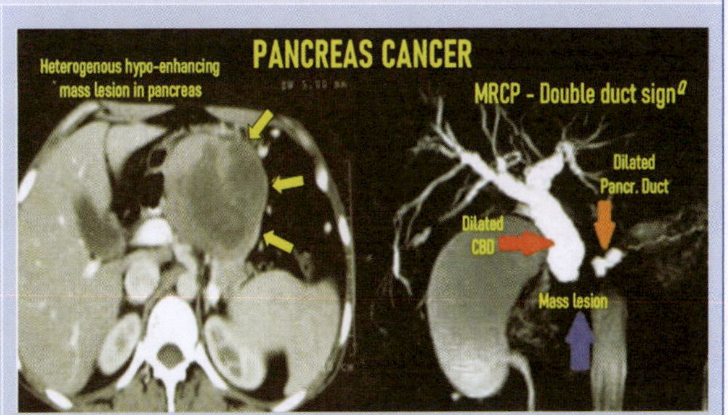

Pancreas cancer

MC type–Adenocarcinoma[Q]

Radiograph/Barium meal follow-through (BMFT).

- Widening of C loop of duodenum[Q]
- Reverse 3 sign of Frostberg/Frostberg inverted 3 sign[Q]

CE-CT[Q]–is IOC.

- Well defined lesion that enhances less[Q] than the normal pancreas parenchyma, most commonly in head of pancreas[Q]
- Teardrop sign[Q]–Alteration of the superior mesenteric from its normal round shape to a teardrop shape on axial images secondary to tumor in infiltration or peritumoral fibrosis

5. GENITOURINARY TRACT IMAGING

Urolithiasis Imaging

CLINICAL CLINCHER

- Acute pain in lumbar region – radiating from loin-to-groin
- Burning micturition +/- blood in urine
- Fever/Vomiting may be present

- 1st Investigation/Screening in acute renal colic patient—USG[Q]
- IOC for detection of Hydronephrosis—USG[Q]
- IOC for detection of renal ureteric calculi—NC-CT[Q]
- IOC for detection of Hydronephrosis—USG[Q]

Intravenous Urography/Pyelography (IVU/IVP) Patient with an obstructive right renal calculus

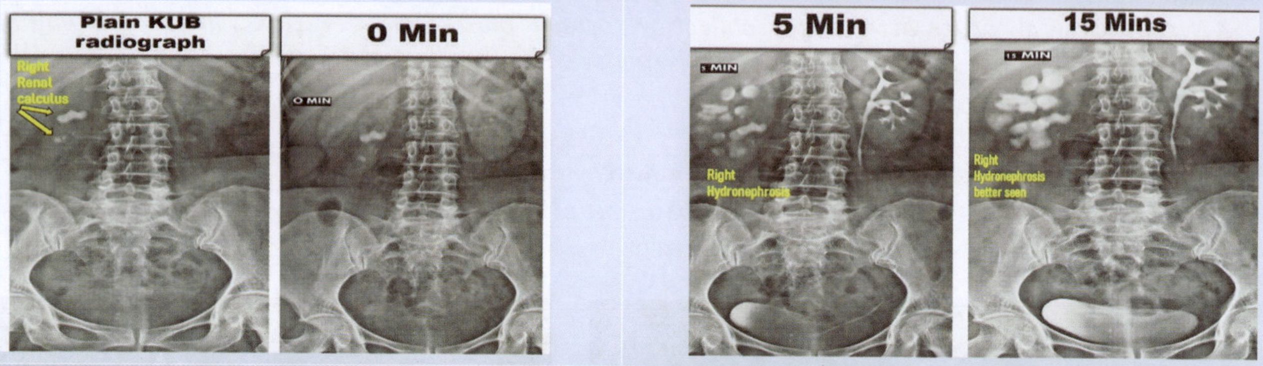

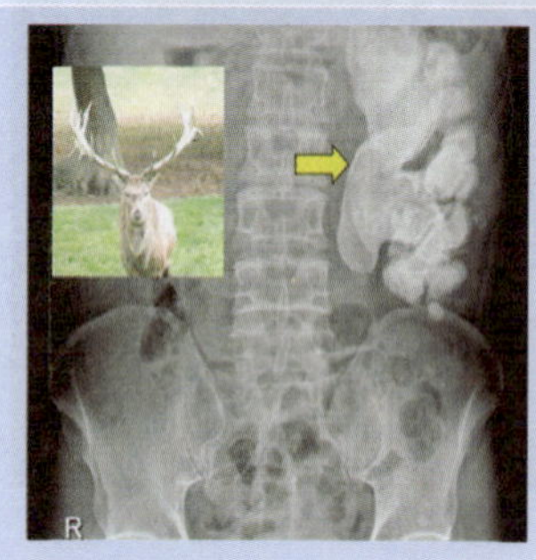

X-ray KUB–Staghorn Calculus

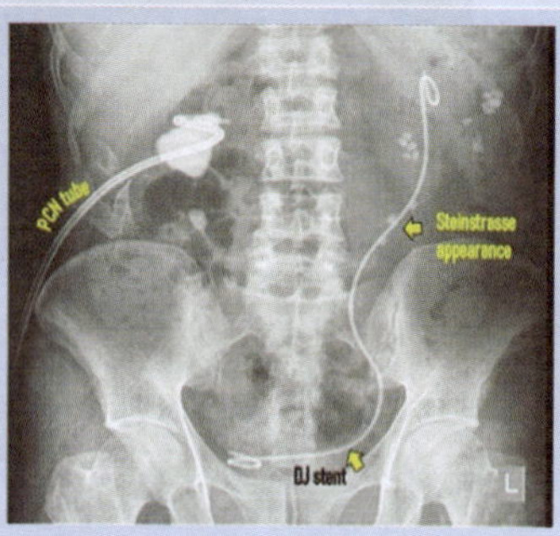

PCN tube + DJ stent + Steinstrasse appearance

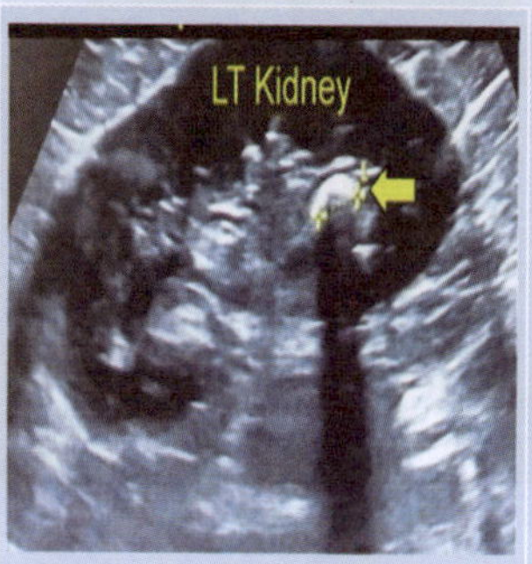

USG Calculus appears as a hyperechoic focus with posterior shadow

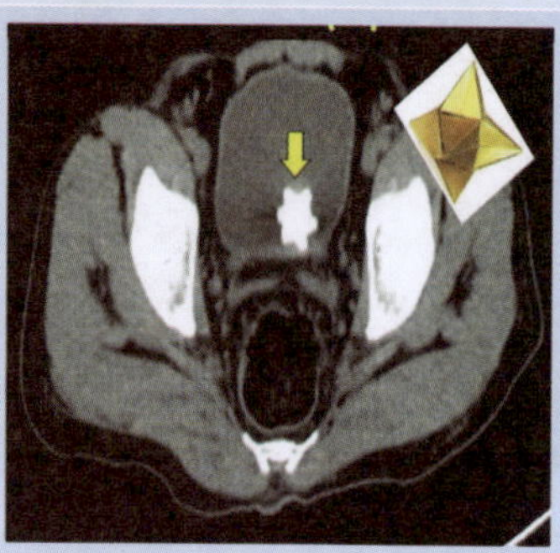

Jack-stone vesical (UB) calculus

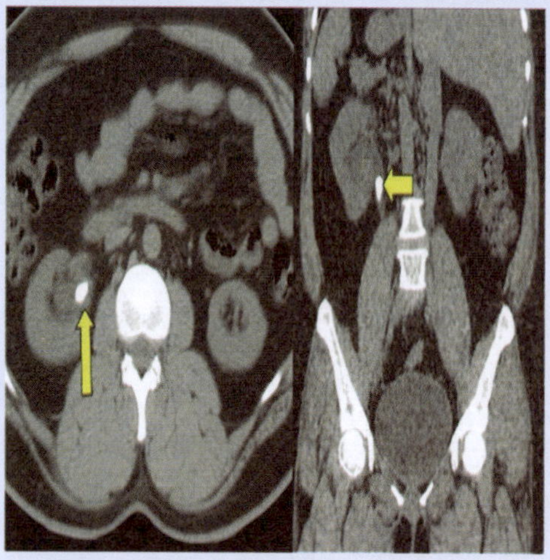

NC-CT-IOC for Renal/Ureteric calculi

PYQ ALERT "FMGE JAN 2023 PATTERN"

Urolithiasis Clinchers:

- MC renal calculus – **Ca oxalate**[Q]
- Staghorn calculus – is **Struvite/Triple-phosphate calculus**[Q] – a/w **Proteus infection**[Q]
- Hardest calculus – **Cystine calculus**[Q]
- MC primary bladder calculus – **Uric acid calculus**[Q] – also a/w **Gout**[Q]
- Radiolucent calculi (not seen on X-ray) – **Uric acid/Indinavir/ Pure matrix calculi**[Q]
- **Steinstrasse appearance**[Q] German-meaning street of stones.
  - Collection of multiple small stones/fragments of larger stone which collect around a DJ stent after Lithotripsy.
- **Soft tissue Rim sign**[Q]: A ureteric calculus appears as a hyperdensity surrounded by a soft tissue rim – the edematous ureteric wall. Used to distinguish a ureteric calculus from a phlebolith[Q].
- **Dual Energy CT (DE-CT)**: Can determine of calculus composition
- **Jack-stone calculus**[Q]**– Friable UB calculus**: Always **Calcium oxalate dihydrate**[Q] in composition

Congenital anomalies of urinary tract

Ureterocele

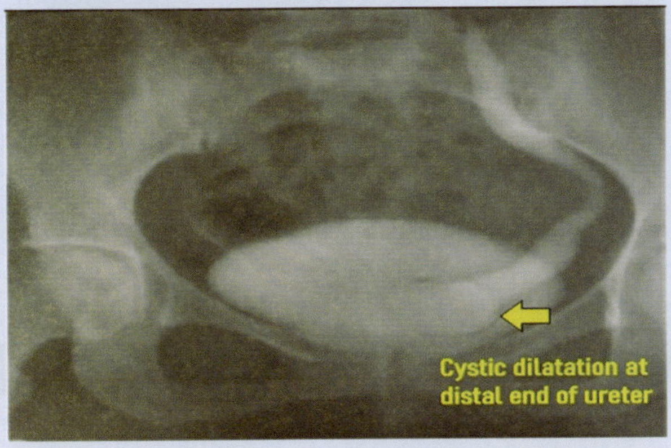

- Congenital dilatation of distal end of ureter.
- On IVU - **Cobra/Adder head/Spring onion appearance**[Q]

Duplex right pelvi-calyceal system

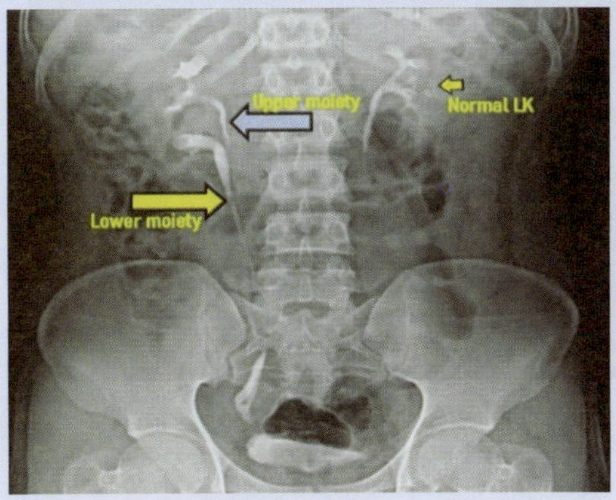

Duplex pelvicalyceal system:

- Two pelvises/ureters arising from one kidney
- **Weigert Meyer rule**[Q]:
  - **Upper renal moiety ureter (U-MI-U)** has ectopic insertion **Medial and Inferior**[Q] to the lower renal moiety ureter, and frequently ends in a **Ureterocele**[Q].
  - **Lower renal moiety ureter (Lower-Lax-Reflux)** has orthotopic insertion lateral and superior to the upper renal moiety ureter, and **vesicoureteral reflux**[Q] can occur
- IOC – CT Urography[Q] > IVU[Q].
- **Drooping Lily Sign**[Q]: Seen in Duplex pelvicalyceal system with obstructed upper pole moiety. The lower pelvis and ureter is displaced inferolaterally due to an obstructed (and unopacified) upper pole moiety.

Cross-fused ectopic kidney

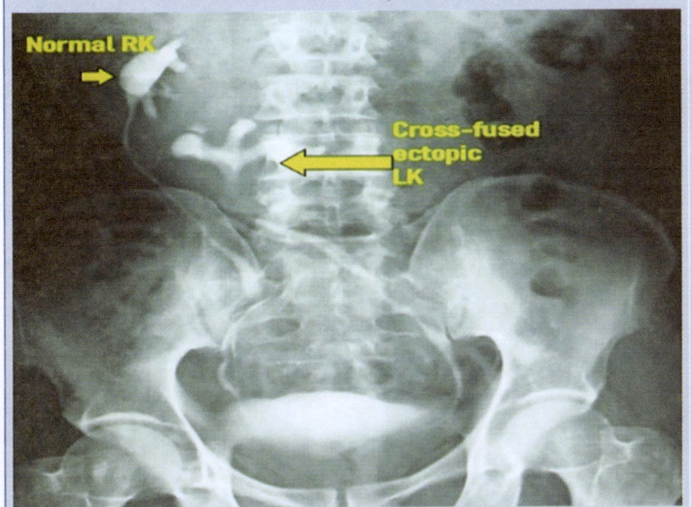

Horse-shoe kidney

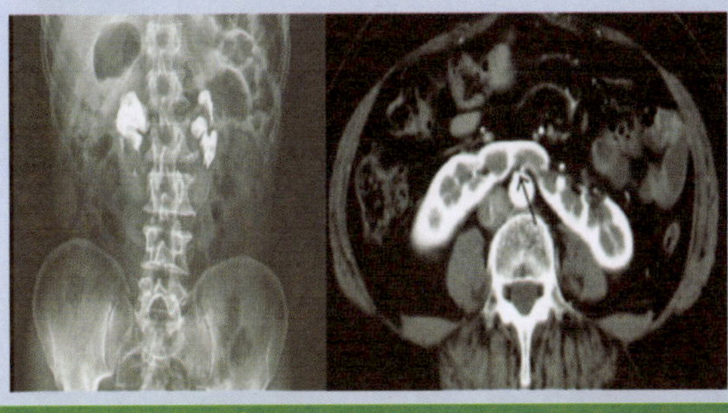

PYQ ALERT "FMGE JAN 2023 AND JULY 2023 PATTERN"

- **Most common type of renal fusion anomaly**[Q]: Results due to fusion of the lower poles of both kidneys in midline.
- **Sigmoid kidney**[Q]: Kidney fused at both the upper and lower poles
- **Pancake/Discoid kidney**[Q]: Fusion of both poles and pelvis

Contd...

MCU–Posterior urethral valve (PUV)

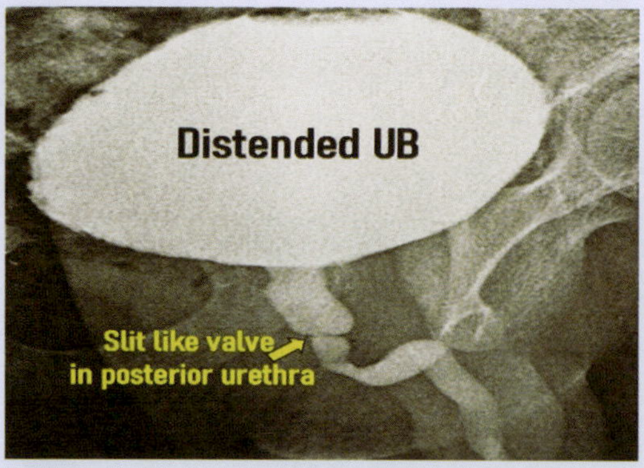

CLINICAL CLINCHER

Male neonate with narrow urinary stream[Q]

Key hole/Spinning top appearance[Q]: On antenatal USG

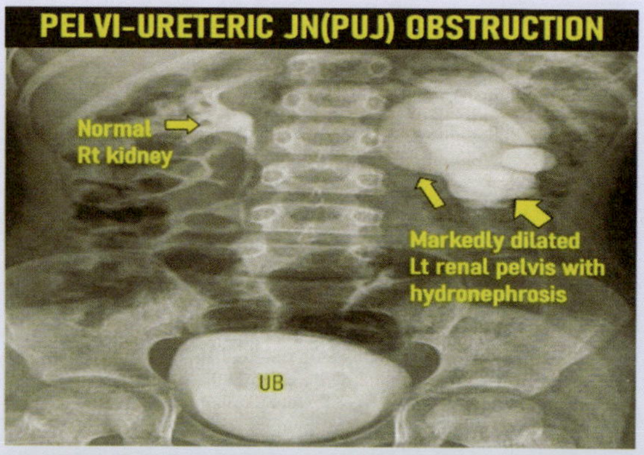

PYQ ALERT NEET-PG 2022 PATTERN

Pelvi-ureteric junction obstruction –

- MC cause of hydronephrosis in children
- **IVU:** Will show a dilated contrast filled renal pelvis with a normal ureter and a transition point at the PUJ.

MCU–Vesico-ureteric reflux (VUR)

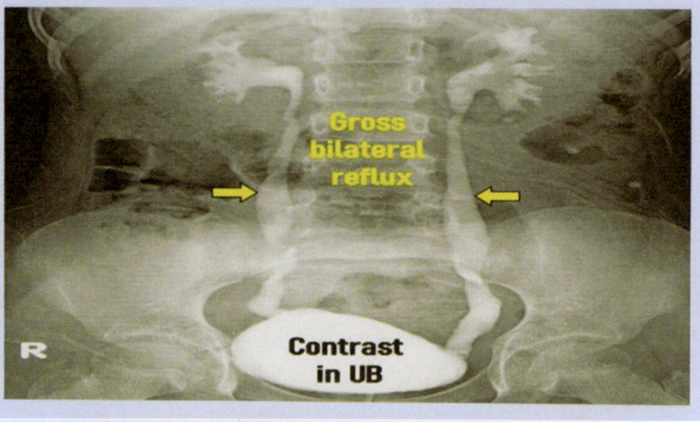

Vesico-ureteric Reflux:

- **Recurrent UTI in children**[Q]
- **USG is the 1st/screening modality**[Q]: May show some pelvicalyceal system or ureteric fullness/ dilatation.
- **Micturating cystourethrogram (MCU)**[Q] **is investigation of choice**[Q]: As it shows anatomical detail and helps in grading.
- **Radionuclide MCU**[Q] **is preferred for follow-up**[Q]: Due to less radiation exposure than MCU.
- **Best investigation for detection of Renal scars secondary to VUR:** DMSA scan[Q]

Urethral stricture

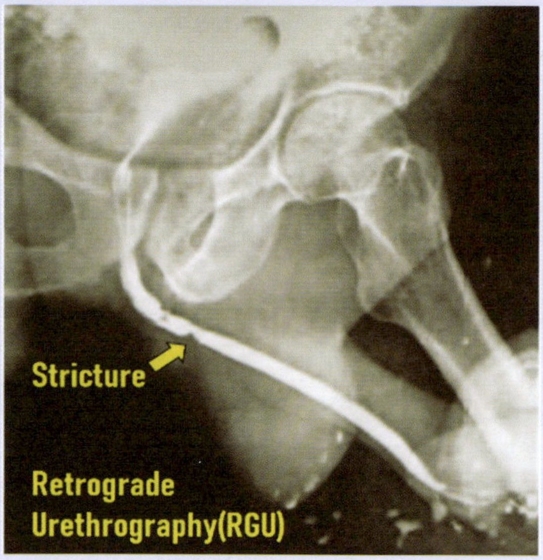

PYQ ALERT "NEET-PG 2020 PATTERN"

- Young sexually active male with recurrent urethritis
- Narrow urinary stream
- Incomplete evacuation of urine – recurrent micturition

Contd...

Pear shaped/Tear-drop UB

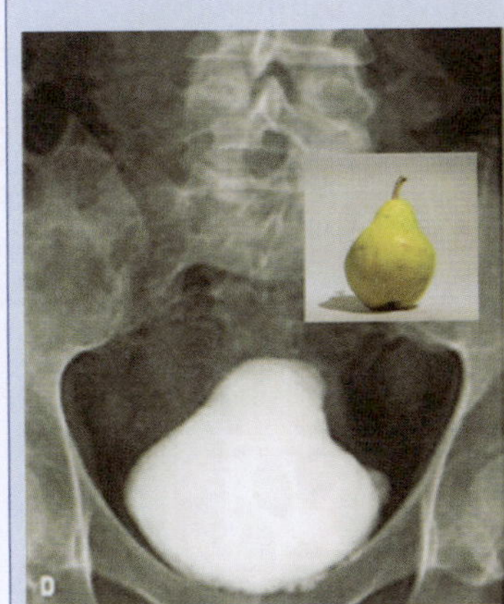

Extrinsic compression – Pelvic hematoma / lipomatosis / LN mass

Christmas tree/Pine cone UB

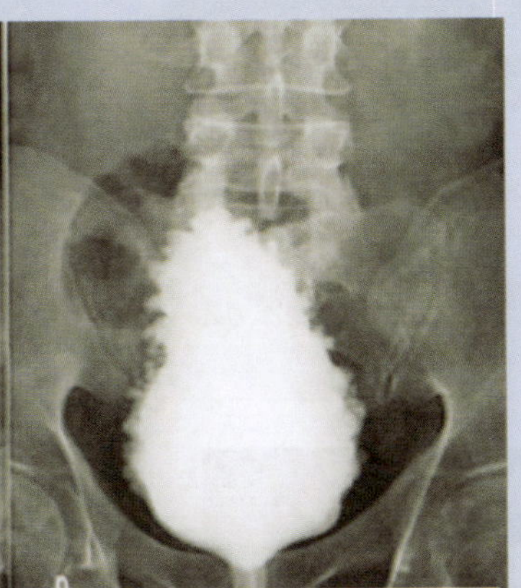

Neurogenic bladder with increased sphincter tone

CLINICAL CLINCHER

- H/o trauma with pelvic fractures
- Unable to pass urine
- Blood at external urethral meatus
- High-riding prostate on Digital rectal examination

Diagnosis – Urethral injury

IOC – Retrograde urethrogram to look for extravasation of contrast from urethra

Next step - Suprapubic catheterization to be done - Foley catheterization is contra-indicated

Intra-peritoneal UB rupture
Most common type

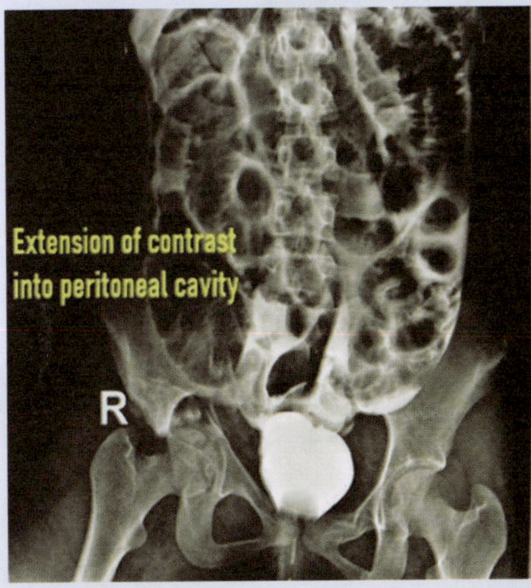

Extra-peritoneal UB rupture

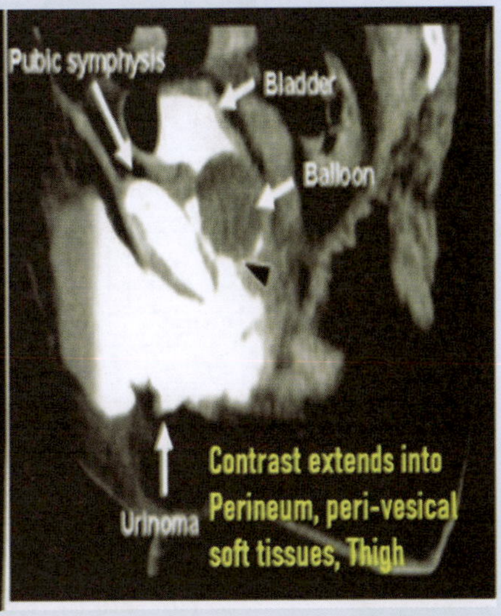

CLINICAL CLINCHER

Urinary bladder rupture: Intraperitoneal versus extraperitoneal rupture

Distinguishing features	Intraperitoneal bladder rupture	Extraperitoneal bladder rupture
Incidence	Uncommon—10–20%	Most common type[Q] — 80–90%
Etiology	Blunt trauma abdomen[Q] with distended, UB	Associated with penetrating injuries[Q]/ pelvic fractures[Q]
Site of rupture	Bladder dome[Q]—urine enters the peritoneal cavity	Bladder base anterolaterally[Q]—urine enters the prevesical soft tissues, scrotum, perineum, thigh and abdominal wall
Diagnosis	Conventional/CT cystography	
Imaging features	Contrast seen entering the peritoneal cavity[Q], filling the paracolic gutters and in between the bowel loops	Molar tooth sign[Q]: Ill-defined contrast extravasated in the prevesical space
Management	Immediate surgery[Q]	Usually conservative[Q]

Infections

Acute pyelonephritis

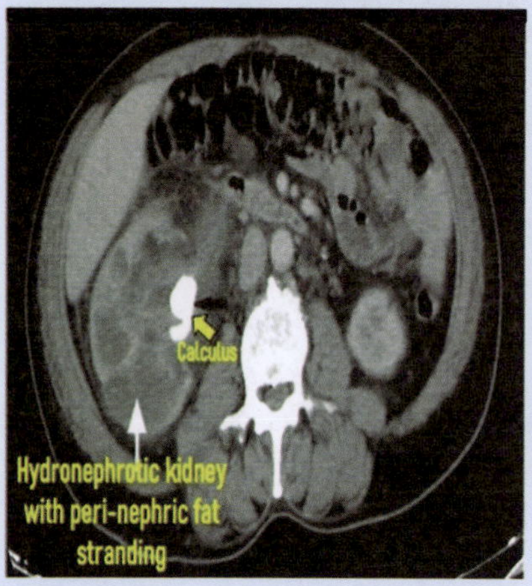

PYQ ALERT "FMGE JULY 2023 PATTERN"

- Known Diabetic
- High grade fever with flank pain
- UTI
- Gas shadows in the renal area on X-ray

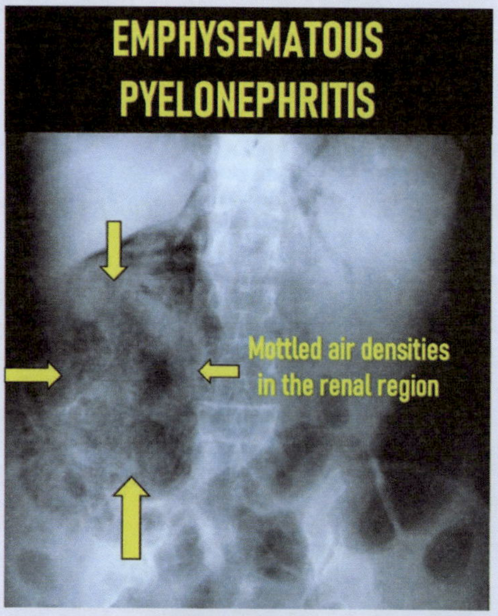

Xanthogranulomatous pyelonephritis

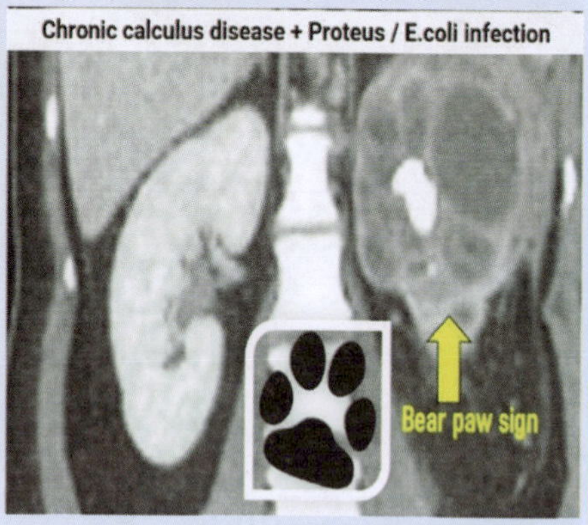

Putty kidney–Renal TB

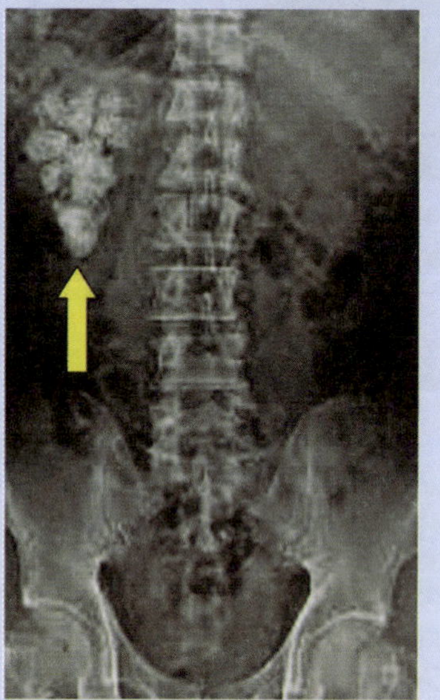

PYQ ALERT "NEET-PG 2021 PATTERN"

Renal TB:

Sterile pyuria[Q] is a characteristic feature.

IOC for early detection—Intravenous Urography/Pyelography (IVU/IVP)[Q]

Overall IOC — CE-CT Abdomen and pelvis[Q]

Most valuable radiologic feature - Multiplicity of findings[Q]

The most common CT finding - Renal calcification[Q]

Earliest finding on IVU - **"Moth-eaten"** calyx[Q] due to erosions

Hiked-up renal pelvis[Q]: Upward pulled pelvis

Kerr's kink[Q]: Deformity of pelvicalyceal system

Putty kidney[Q]: Homogeneous/uniform/ground glass-like calcification representing calcified caseous tissue.

Autonephrectomy[Q]: Small, shrunken, scarred, nonfunctioning kidney.

Pipe-stem ureter[Q]**/Beaded or Cork-screw appearance of ureter**[Q]

Thimble bladder[Q]: Scarred small bladder

Contd...

Renal masses

Renal cell carcinoma (RCC)/Hypernephroma/Grawitz tumor

Renal cell carcinoma

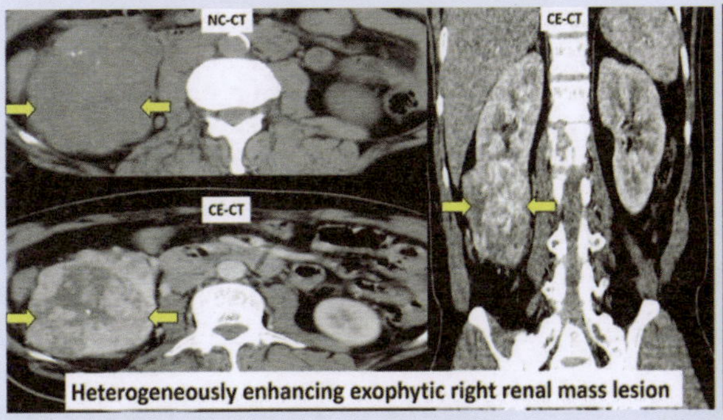

IVC extension–RCC

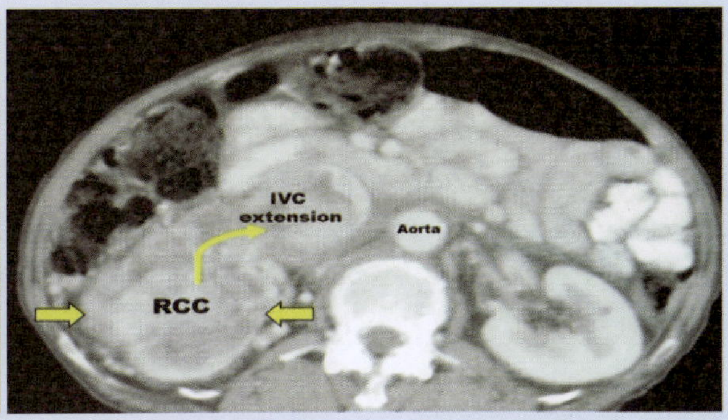

- Associated with Von Hippel-Lindau disease (VHL)[Q]
- Gross painless hematuria[Q] – is most common presentation
- **Ultrasound:** Variable echogenicity mass solid/cystic with internal vascularity on Doppler
- **IOC for renal masses:** CE-CT[Q] – Heterogenously enhancing lesion
- **IOC for renal vein/IVC involvement - MRI[Q]:** Best for distinguishing between a Bland thrombus versus Tumor thrombus[Q]

PYQ ALERT "INI-CET JULY 2021 PATTERN"

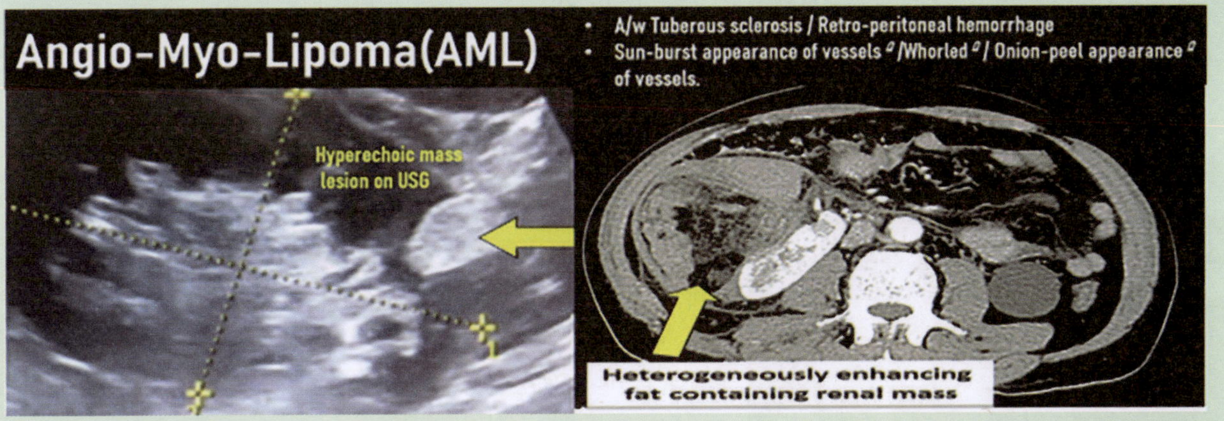

UB Cancer–Transitional Cell Cancer (TCC)

Bladder Cancer–Transitional Cell Cancer (TCC)

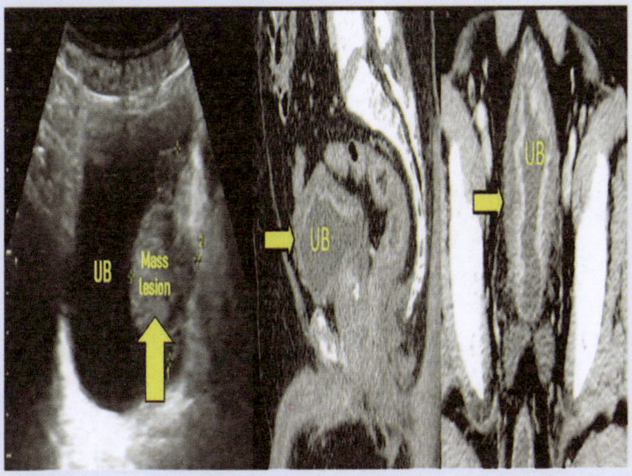

- Most common urothelial tumor is—Transitional cell carcinoma[Q].
- Bladder is most common site of TCC.
- **Stipple sign[Q] on IVU:** Seen in a papillary tumor as the contrast enters the lesion interstices.
- **Oncocalyx[Q]:** Dilated tumor filled renal calyx in renal TCC.
- **Phantom calyx[Q] on IVU:** A calyx that does not fill with contrast while rest of the pelvicalyceal system is well filled with contrast.
- **Goblet sign[Q]/Champagne glass sign of Ureter[Q]:** Ureteral dilatation below the site of an intraluminal ureteral filling defect, best seen at retrograde ureteropyelography.

CLINICAL CLINCHERS

Prostate Imaging	
MC site of BPH in prostate	Transitional zone[Q]
MC site of Ca prostate in the gland	Peripheral zone[Q]
Most common cancer in Men	Ca Prostate[Q]
MC site of prostate cancer	Peripheral zone[Q]
MC site of metastases from prostate cancer	Bone–vertebral column (Lumbar region)[Q]
MC primary tumor in sclerotic metastases in men	Ca Prostate[Q]
Earliest lymph node to be involved in prostate cancer	Obturator LN[Q]
Score used for grading of prostate Ca	Gleason score[Q]

Miscellaneous

Nephrocalcinosis

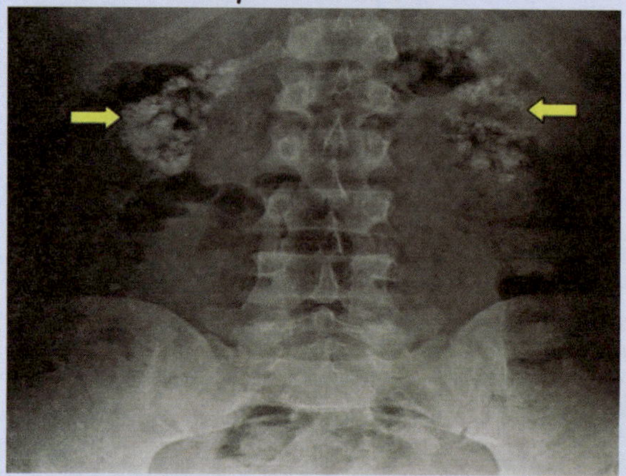

Nephrocalcinosis:

- Calcium deposition in the renal parenchyma, outside the pelvicalyceal system
- IOC – NC-CT[Q]
- **Medullary nephrocalcinosis:**
  - Most common type[Q]
  - Due to elevated serum calcium – Hyperparathyroidism, Medullary sponge kidney (Paint brush calcification[Q])
- **Cortical Nephrocalcinosis:**
  - Most common cause – acute cortical necrosis[Q] (due to any reason)
  - "Single pencil-line[Q]" or "Double tram-line[Q]" calcifications

Renal papillary necrosis

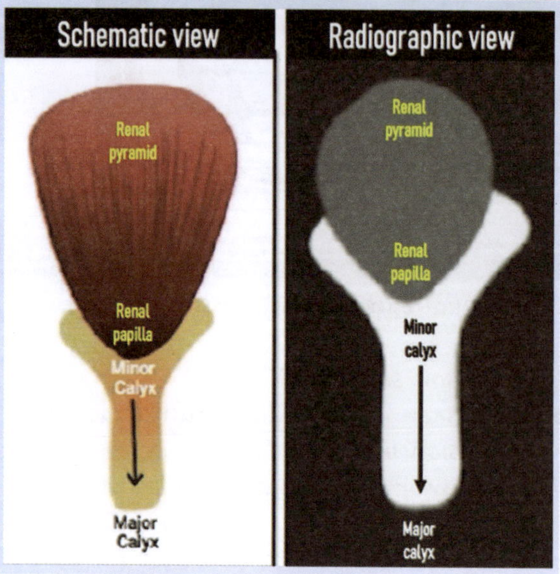

- Renal papilla is the tip of the renal pyramid. It is naturally prone to ischemic necrosis.
- Causes of papillary necrosis
  - P- Pyelonephritis
  - O- Obstruction
  - S- Sickle cell disease
  - T- TB
  - C- Cirrhosis
  - A- Analgesic abuse
  - R- Renal vein thrombosis
  - D- Diabetes mellitus
  - S- Systemic vasculitis

Contd...

Renal papillary necrosis

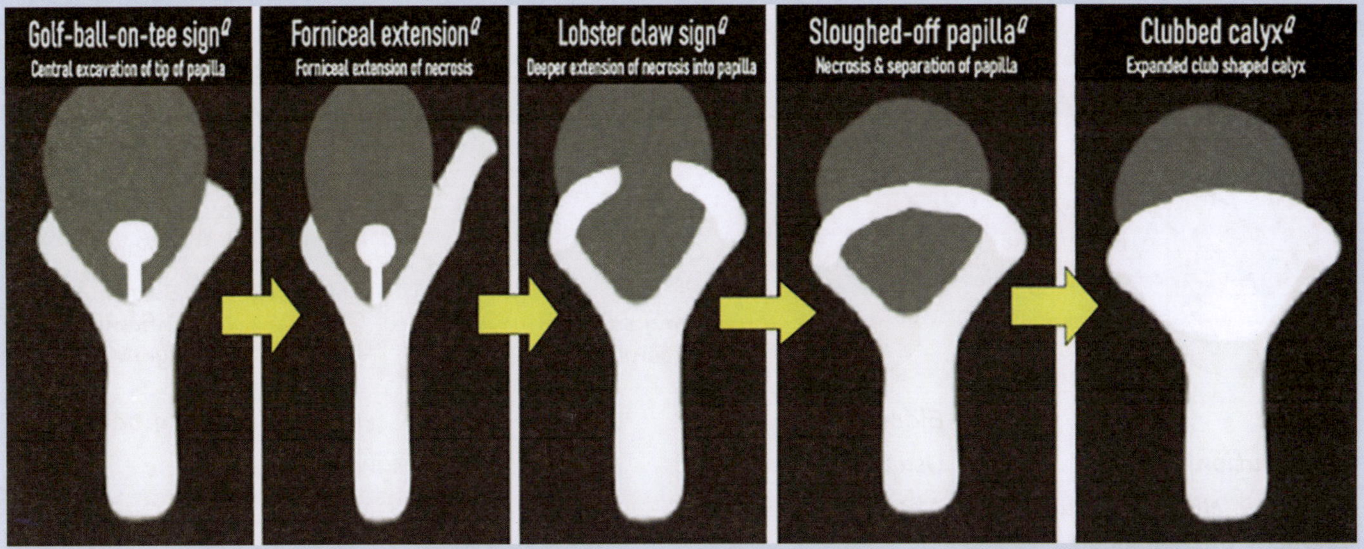

Renal artery stenosis

Renal artery stenosis—Angiography

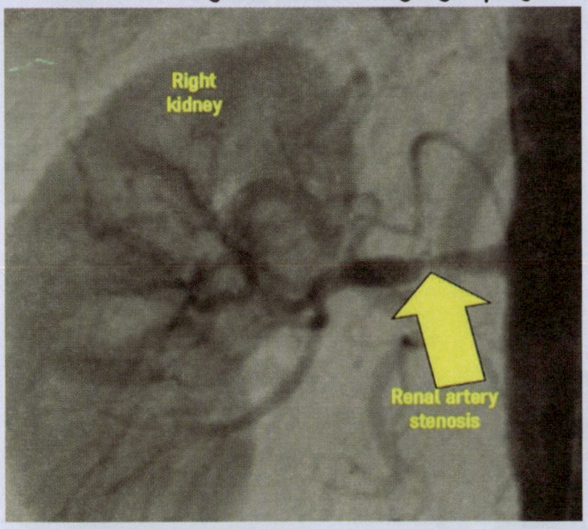

- Most common cause of secondary hypertension[Q]
- Most common cause of renal artery stenosis—Atherosclerotic narrowing[Q]
- Most commonly involved arterial segment—origin or proximal one-third of renal artery[Q]
- Most common non-atherosclerotic cause of renal artery stenosis - Fibromuscular dysplasia (FMD)[Q]—affects young females[Q] and shows "string-of-beads" appearance[Q]—on angiography as a result of multiple short stenosis.

CLINICAL CLINCHERS

Summary of Imaging Modalities for Renal Artery Stenosis/Renovascular Hypertension

1st investigation/screening investigation	USG with renal artery Doppler[Q]
Investigation of choice	CT angiography[Q]/MR angiography[Q]
Gold standard investigation	Invasive/Conventional angiography/Digital subtraction angiography[Q]
Functional significance of stenosis	Captopril ^{99}mTcDTPA scan[Q]

6. MUSCULOSKELETAL SYSTEM IMAGING

CLINICAL CLINCHER

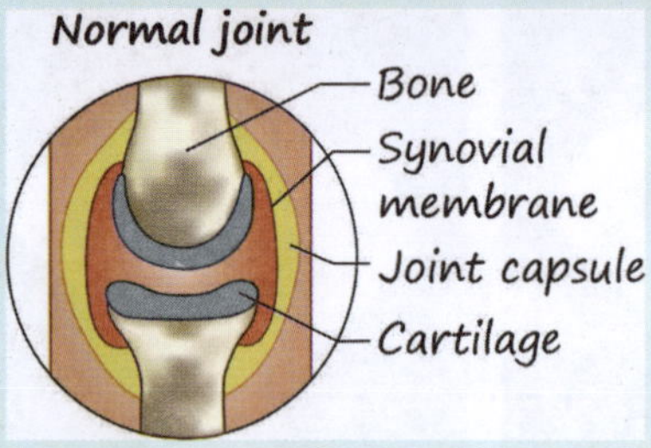

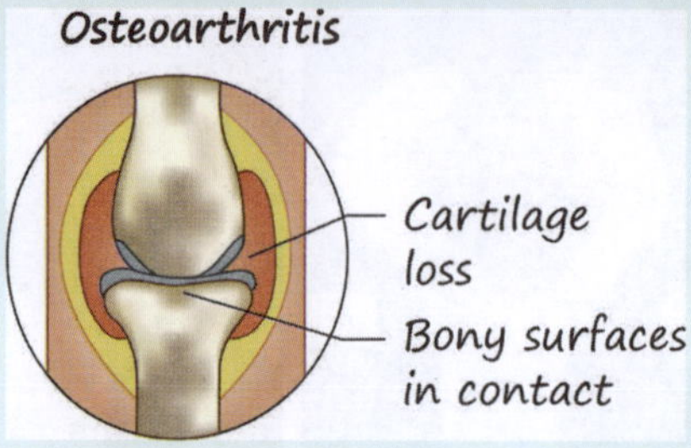

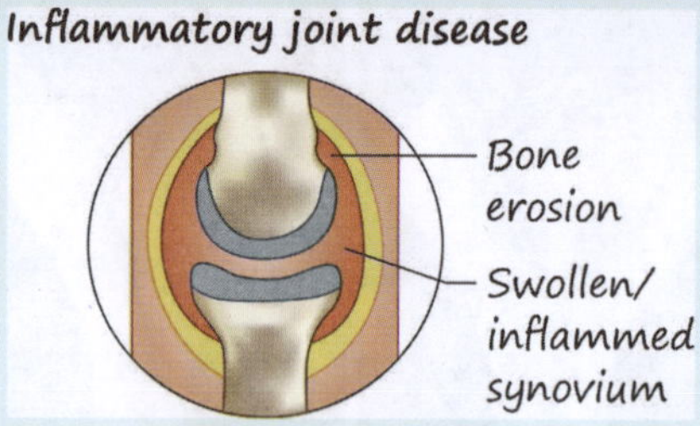

Features	Degenerative joint disease	Inflammatory joint disease
Age	Elderly	Varied–seen even in young patients
Distribution	Usually asymmetric	Usually symmetric
Systemic clinical features (clinic - pathological)	Absent	Present
Joint space loss	Nonuniform joint space loss	Uniform joint space loss
Sub/Periarticular changes	Subarticular sclerosis	Periarticular osteopenia
Intra-articular	Present	Absent
Subarticular cysts/Geodes	Present	Absent
Bone erosions	Absent	Present
Periosteal reaction/Periostitis	Absent	Present

Rheumatoid Arthritis- Seropostive arthritis - RA factor is positive in 70% cases

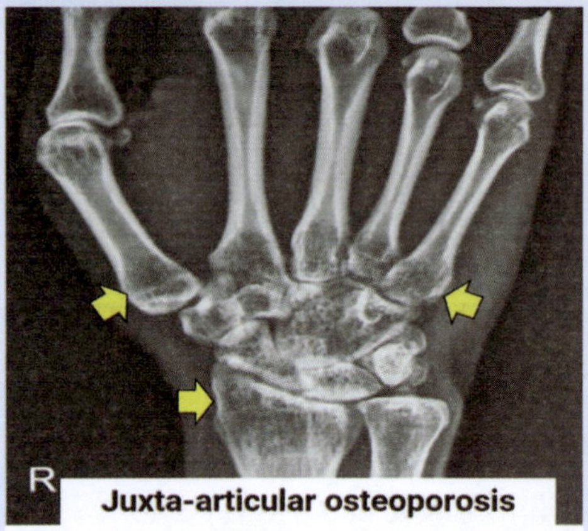

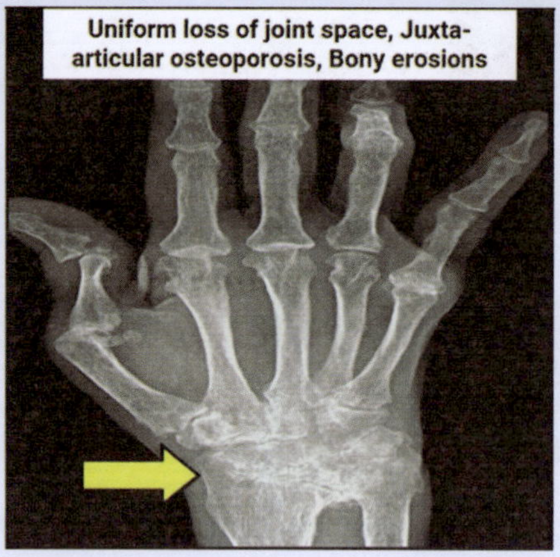

PYQ ALERT "NEET-PG 2019 PATTERN"

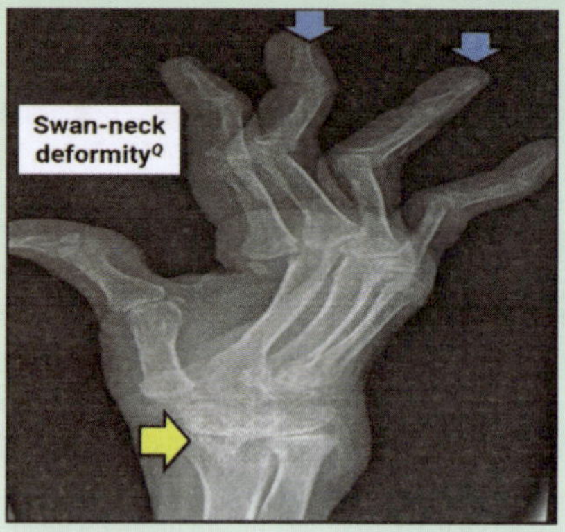

Hand and Wrist involvement in RA:

- **Earliest joints involved:** Metacarpophalangeal[Q] and Proximal interphalangeal joints[Q]
- **Earliest finding at wrist:** Erosion of ulnar styloid process
- **Boutonniere deformity[Q]:** Flexion of proximal interphalangeal joint, extension of distal IP joint, due to rupture of central slip of extensor digitorum communis at proximal IP joint
- **Swan neck deformity[Q]:** Flexion at DIP and extension at PIP joints
- **Hitchhiker thumb[Q]:** Boutonniere's deformity affecting thumb-hyperextension at IP and MCP joints
- **Dot:** Dash appearance[Q]—intermittent absence of articular cortex due to bone erosions and subarticular resorption
- **Ivory phalanx[Q]:** Homogenous sclerosis of distal phalanx

Contd...

Few more peculiar appearances are also seen—enlisted in the following table.

Arthritis mutilans[Q]	Severe polyarticular joint deformity with marked joint destruction
Lanois deformity[Q]	Fibular deviation of digits and dorsal subluxation of metatarsophalangeal joints
Mallet finger[Q]	Persistent flexion of distal phalanx due to rupture of Extensor digitorum communis
Spotty carpal sign	Characteristic appearance produced by multiple marginal erosions in the carpal bones
Summation effect[Q]	Decrease in neck length due to upward migration of odontoid, loss of C1-C2 disk height and osteolysis
Ulnar drift[Q]	Fingers of hand deviated toward the ulna at the MCP joint
Zigzag deformity[Q]	Combination of ulnar deviation of digits and radial rotation of carpal bones

CLINICAL CLINCHER

- Felty syndrome[Q]—RA, Leukopenia and Splenomegaly
- Caplan syndrome[Q]—Pneumoconiosis with RA[Q]

Ankylosing spondylitis/Bechterew's disease[Q]/Marie Strümpell disease[Q]

Prototype of Seronegative arthritis[Q]—RA factor negative[Q] and commonly associated with HLA B27[Q]

Ankylosing Spondylitis

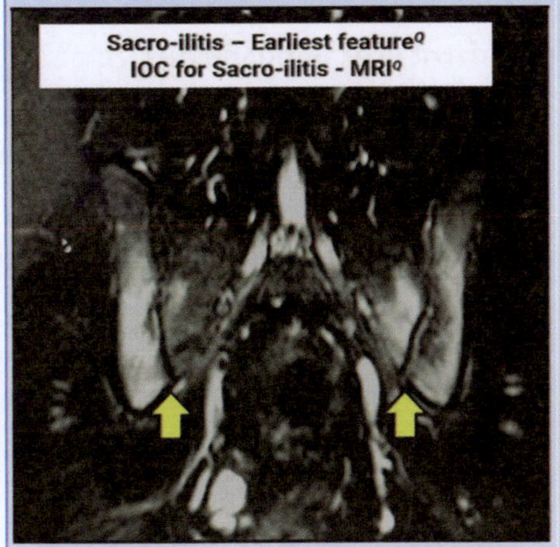

PYQ ALERT "FMGE JUNE 2022 PATTERN"

Ankylosing Spondylitis

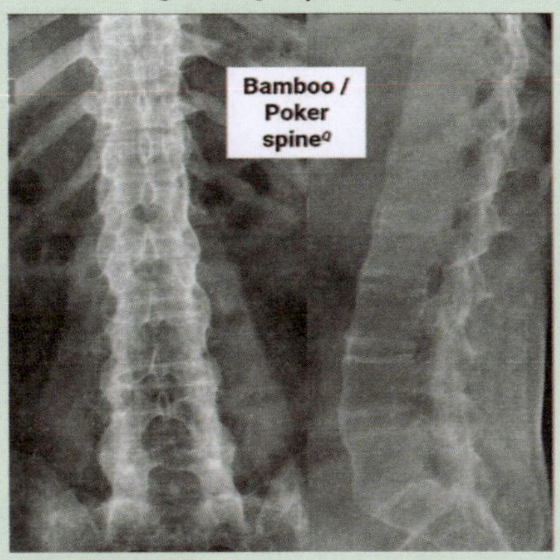

Ankylosing Spondylitis

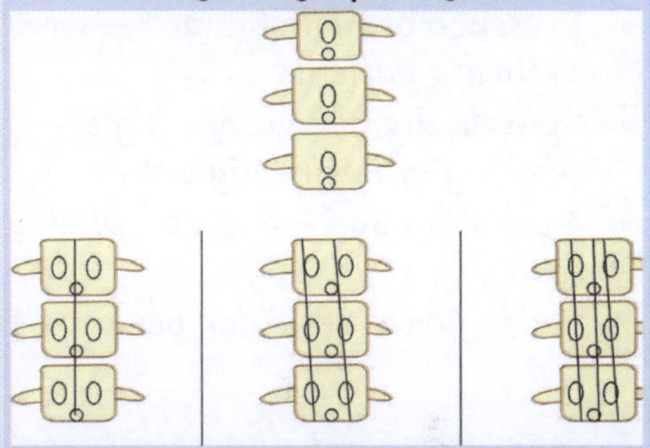

Dagger sign[Q]–Inter-spoinous ligament ossification[Q] | Rail road track sign[Q]–Para-spinous ligament ossification[Q] | Trolly track sign[Q]-Para-spinous ligament ossification[Q]

Enthesitis[Q]:

Inflammation of enthesis—the attachment of ligament/tendon to bone — is the imaging hallmark

Sacroilitis—Earliest clinical manifestation[Q]

- MRI—Imaging modality of choice for early sacroiliitis[Q]
- Early sacroilitis: Rosary bead appearance of SI joint[Q]
- Late sacroiliitis: Bony ankylosis[Q]

Spine Involvement:

- **Romanus lesions[Q]:** Vertebral body corner erosions
- **Shiny corner sign[Q]:** Vertebral body corner sclerosis
- Squaring of vertebral body[Q]/Barrel vertebra[Q]
- **Andersson's lesion[Q]:** Ankylosed previously fractured spinal segment resembling a noninfectious spondylodiscitis
- **Bamboo spine[Q]/Poker spine[Q]:** Diffuse marginal syndesmophytes ankylosis
- Carrot stick fractures of the spine[Q]
- **Enthesopathy:** The point of insertion of tendon on bone is known as enthesis.
- **Whiskering[Q]:** Seen at the enthesis as coarse spicules of bone extending away from bone–due to periostitis

Contd...

Gout Arthropathy-Tophi are seen	Calcium pyrophosphate deposition disease (CPPD)/ Pseudo-gout
Gout Arthropathy 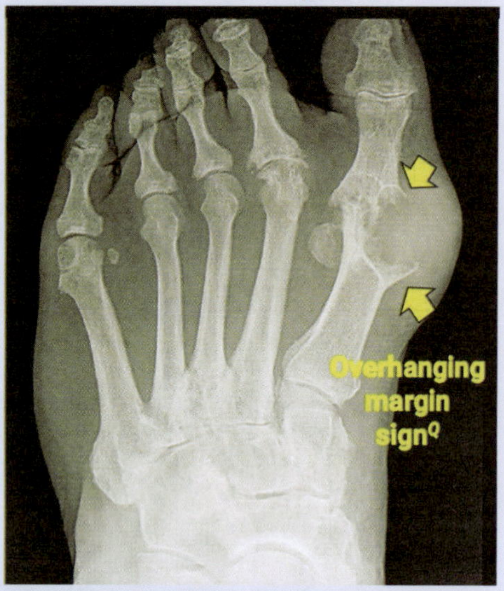	**Pseudo-gout (CPPD)** 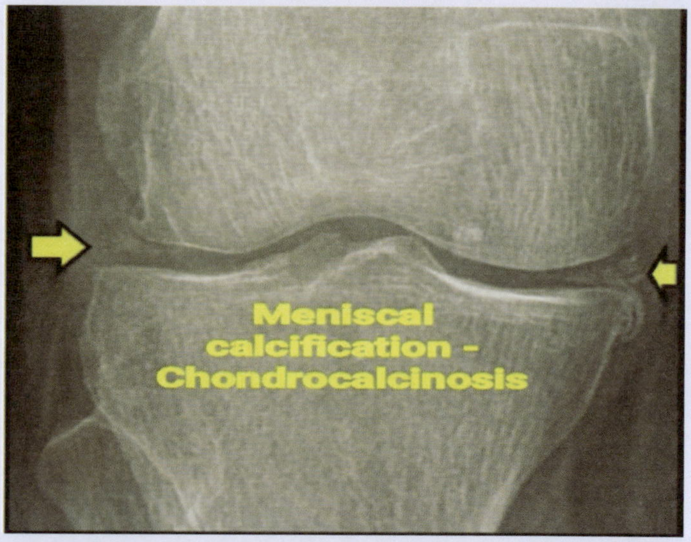

Other seronegative arthritis

Psoriatic arthritis:

- Presence of nail changes^Q—seen in 80% of arthritis patients
- Spindle digit^Q/Sausage digit^Q—soft tissue swelling of entire digit/toe
- Ivory phalanx^Q—sclerotic phalanx may be seen
- Fluffy juxta-articular periostitis^Q
- Mouse ears sign^Q—fluffy periosteal new bone formation adjacent to erosions
- Pencil-in-cup^Q/Pestle and mortar^Q/Mushroom and stem^Q/Cup and saucer^Q/Balancing pagoda deformity—Tapered end of a phalanx erodes into distal articular surface
- Opera glass hand^Q—Overall shortening of digit occurs

Degenerative joint disease/osteoarthritis:

- Most common type of arthritis overall^Q
- Knee and hip are the two most common joints affected

Early Osteoarthritis	Advanced Osteoarthritis
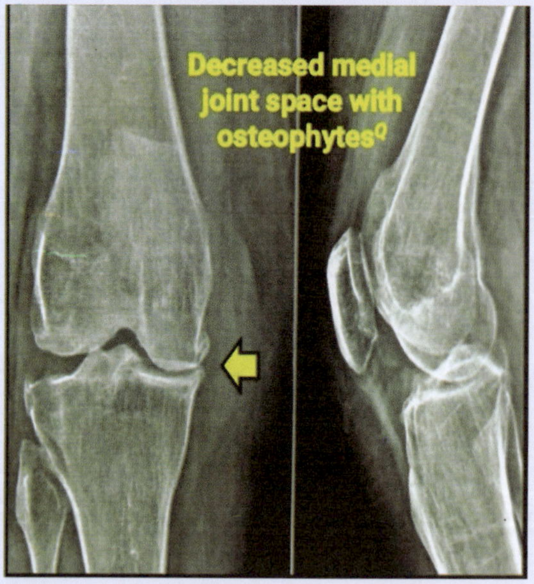	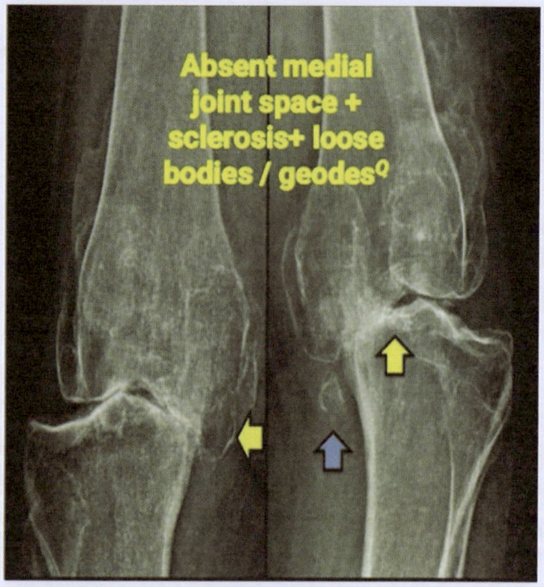

MISCELLANEOUS ARTHRITIS

Charcot's joint/Neuropathic joint

Licked candy stick appearance[Q]

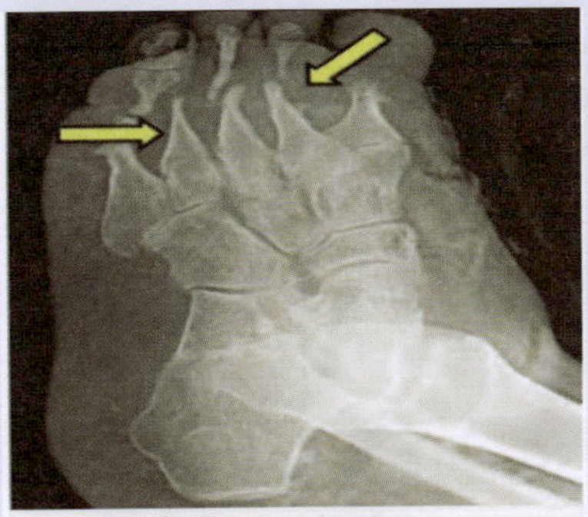

- 6D's[Q]: Disorganization, destruction, density (osteosclerosis), dislocation, debris and distension.
- Bag of bones[Q]
- Jigsaw vertebra[Q]
- Tumbling building block spine[Q]

Diffuse Idiopathic Skeletal Hyperostosis (DISH)

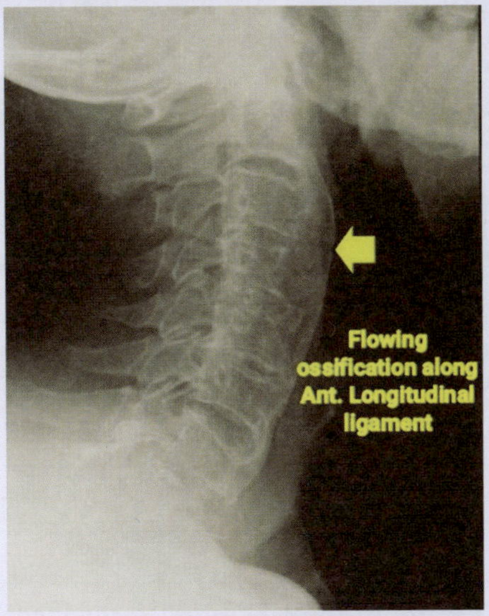

Ossified post-longitudinal ligament (OPLL)

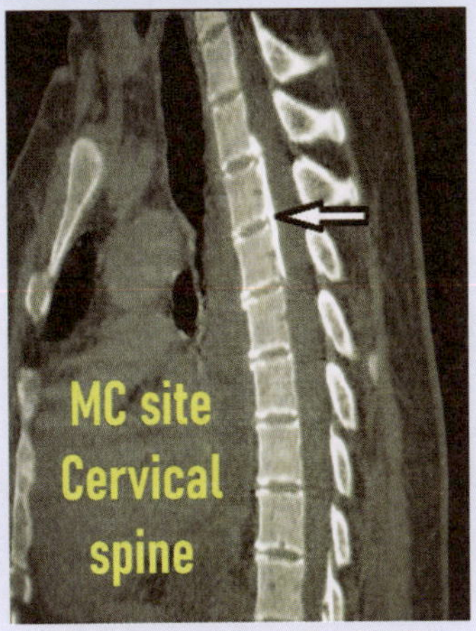

Ochronosis/Alkaptonuria

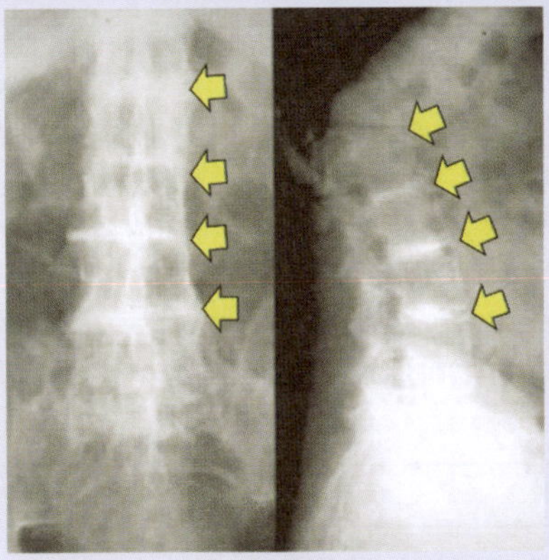

Intervertebral disk calcification

SYSTEMIC BONE DISORDERS

H-shaped vertebra-Sickle cell disease

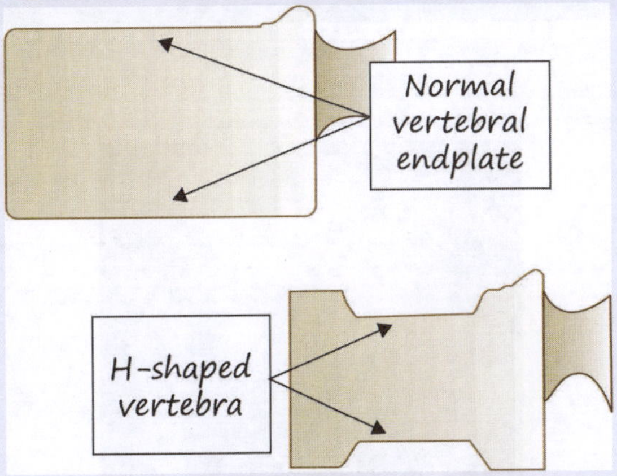

PYQ ALERT "FMGE AUG 2020 PATTERN"

Hair-on-end[Q]/Crew cut skull[Q]
Seen in hemolytic anemias

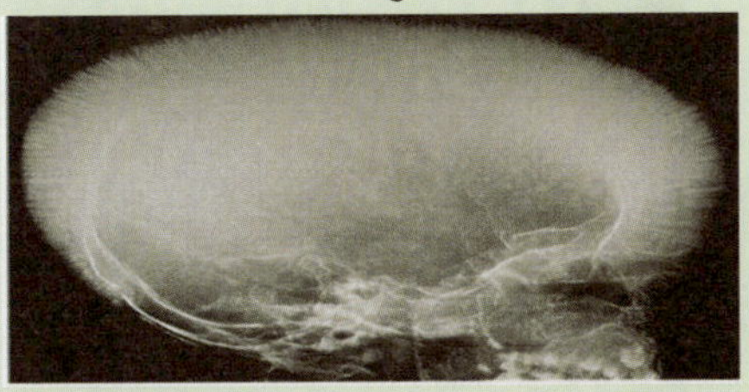

- Thalassemia major
- Hereditary spherocytosis
- Neuroblastoma
- Sickle cell disease
- G-6-PD deficiency
- Iron deficiency anemia

Contd...

Avascular necrosis femoral head

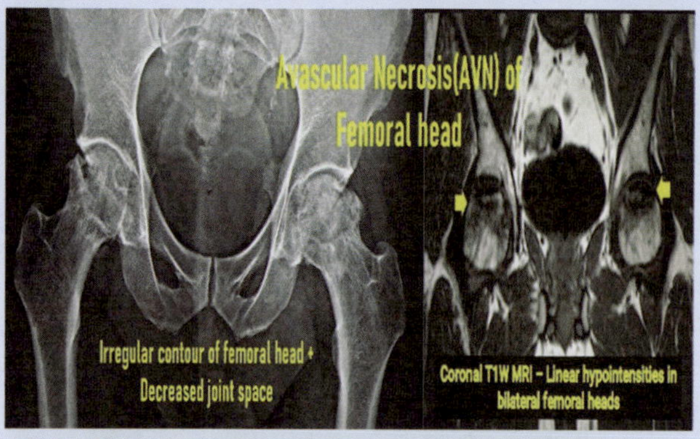

- Trauma (resulting in a fracture neck of femur) – Most common cause
- Ficat and Arlet classification[Q] is used.
- MRI[Q]—Best investigation
- Radiologic features:
  - Flattened/Irregular shaped femoral head
  - Snow cap sign[Q]/Bite sign[Q]/Crescent/Rim sign[Q]/Asterisk sign[Q]/Double line sign[Q]

Rickets

STEP 1: Chondroblast located at the physeal growth plate secrete chondroid matrix

↓

STEP 2: Vitamin D induces calcification of chondroid matrix towards the metaphyseal margin

↓

STEP 3: Calcification of chondroid matrix prevents diffusion of nutrients through the matrix. The nutritionally deprived chondroblasts are converted to chondrocytes and with furthur dense calcification eventually die through apoptosis

↓

STEP 4: Osteoblasts and osteoclasts appear at this site – ensure remodeling of calcified chondroid matrix and convert it into osteoid

RICKETS – VITAMIN D DEFICIENCY

- No provisional zone of calcification at metaphyseal margin-
  - Indistinct metaphyseal margin-fraying[Q] /paint-brush metaphysis[Q]
  - Weak metaphysis – widening[Q] and cupping[Q]
  - Excess physeal cartilage – Widened physeal plate[Q] & Rickety rosary[Q]
- Generalized poor bone calcification and softening of bones – bowing of weight bearing bones[Q]
- Generlized poor bone calcification-radiolucent bones with coarsened trabecular patters[Q]
- Healing rickets – re-appearence of provisional zone of calcification at the metaphyseal margin

PYQ ALERT "FMGE DEC 2020 PATTERN"

Rickets—Widening + Cupping + Fraying of metaphysis	Osteomalacia-Adult rickets–Lack of osteoid mineralization leading to generalized bone softening
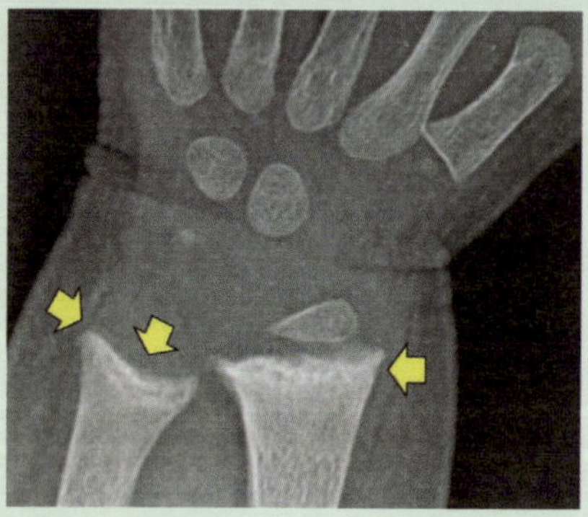	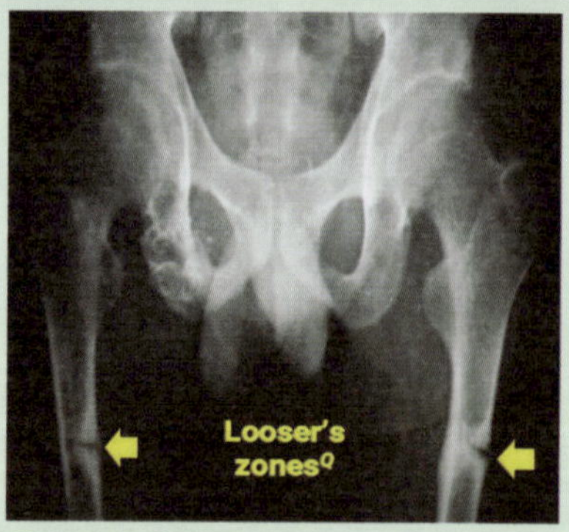

Scurvy—Vitamin C Deficiency—Weak collagen due to lack of Cross-linking/lack of hydroxylation of Lysine and proline residues of collagen

PYQ ALERT "NEET-PG 2021 PATTERN"

Scurvy

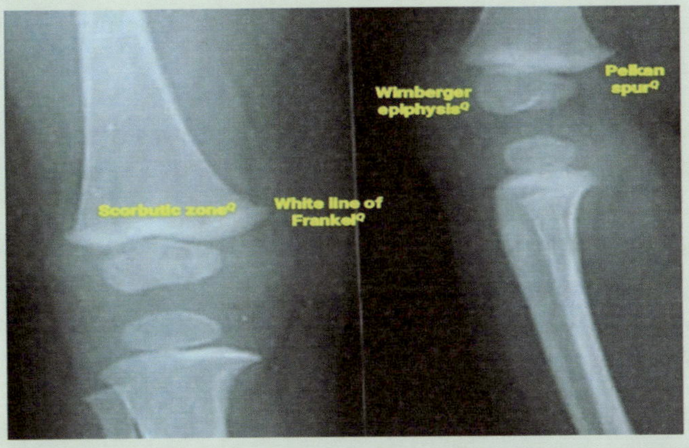

Radiologic findings:

- Generalized osteopenia
- Wimberger sign[Q]/Ring epiphysis[Q]: Radiolucent central area surrounded by a dense margin
- White line of Frankel[Q]—dense zone of provisional calcification at metaphyseal margin
- Trummerfeld zone of rarefaction[Q]/scorbutic zone[Q]—lucent band just below the metaphyseal zone of provisional calcification
- Pelkan spurs[Q]: Lateral metaphyseal spurs
- Corner sign[Q]/Angle sign[Q]
- Subperiosteal hemorrhages[Q]

Osteopenia/Osteoporosis—Reduction in bone quantity[Q], with the bone quality remaining normal[Q].

PYQ ALERT "NEET-PG 2021 PETTERN"

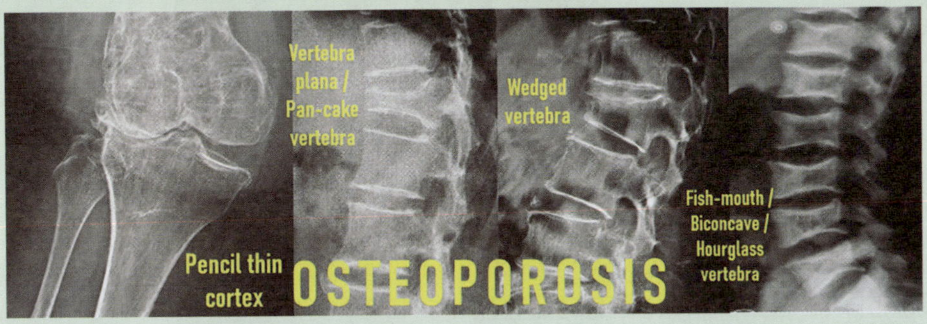

Dual energy X-ray Absorptiometry[Q]—most common and Most reliable modality used. Quantitative CT (Q-CT may also be used)

Dual energy X-ray absorptiometry (DEXA)

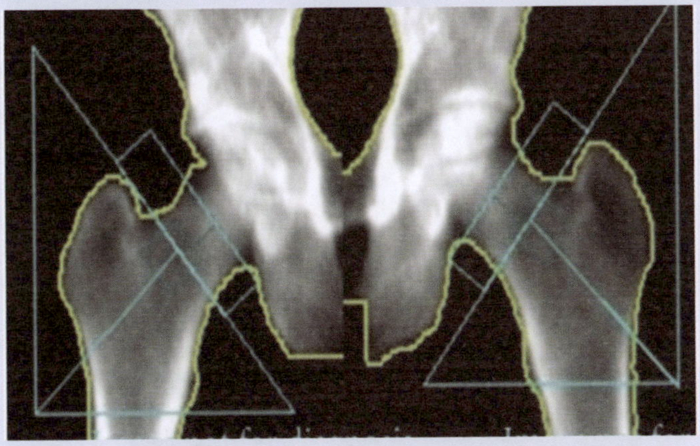

- Values calculated for the lumbar vertebrae and femur
- Bone mineral density (BMD) is calculated in g/cm^2
- **T-score**:
  - **Used for** postmenopausal women and men >50 years
  - **Comparison** by standard deviation (SD) to a young adult population, matched for sex and ethnicity
- ≥-1.0: Normal
- <-1.0 to >-2.5: Osteopenia
- ≤-2.5: Osteoporosis
- ≤-2.5 + fragility fracture: Severe osteoporosis
- **Z-score**:
  - Used for premenopausal women, men <50 years, and children
  - Compared by SD to an age, sex, and ethnicity population
  - <-2.0: Below expected range/low bone density for age

Contd...

Hyperparathyroidism—Excess of parathormone results in excess of osteoclastic activity– leading to peculiar skeletal findings

Hyperparathyroidism subperiosteal resorption

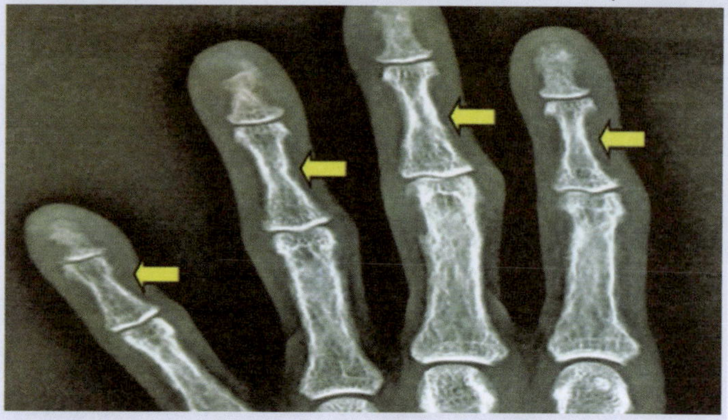

Imaging features:

- Subperiosteal bone resorption[Q]—hallmark/Single most definitive diagnostic sign of HPT[Q]. Most common sites–radial margins of middle and proximal phalanges of 2nd digit.[Q]
- Salt and pepper skull[Q]/Pepper pot skull[Q]–granular appearance of skull due to resorption
- Brown tumors[Q]
- Rugger-Jersey spine[Q]:
- Floating teeth[Q]: Resorption of Lamina dura (cortical bone) around the tooth socket
- Acro-osteolysis[Q] – distal phalanx resorption
- Rib notching–usually superior margin

Osteomyelitis

Investigations for osteomyelitis:

X-rays:

- Poor sensitivity
- Normal in early cases
- Latent period[Q]–No finding seen on radiographs in spite of osteomyelitis. This latent period of around 10 days[Q] for extremities and around 3 weeks[Q] for the spine

99mTc—MDP Bone scan is earliest to detect[Q], but is nonspecific

MRI – IOC/Overall best investigation[Q]

Penumbra sign-sub-acute osteomyelitis

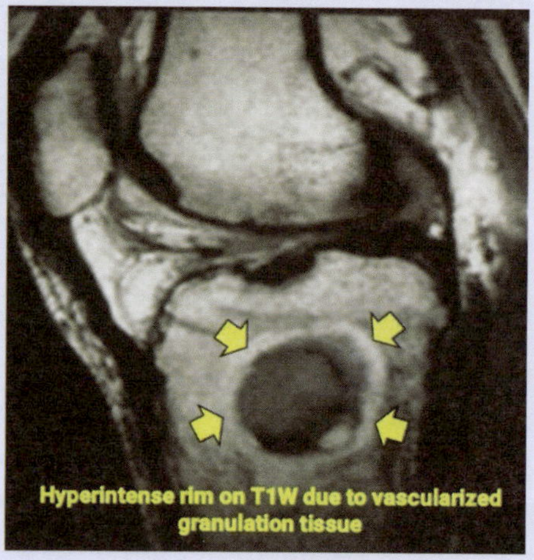

Acute osteomyelitis peripherally enhancing lesion in metaphysis on CE-MRI

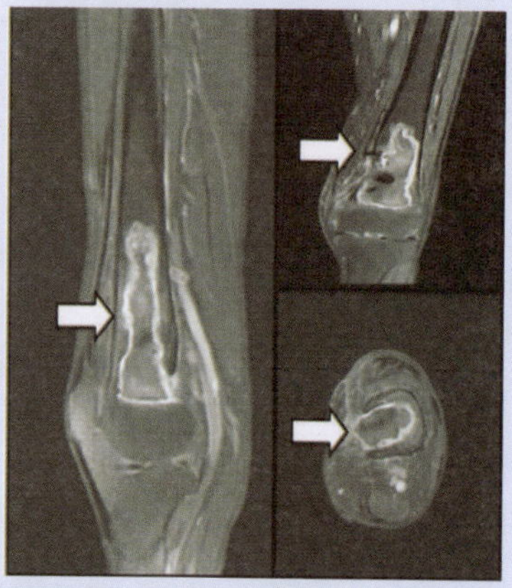

Chronic osteomyelitis

- Mixed pattern of bone destruction, followed by healing and periosteal reaction
- Sinus tracts[Q] may open into the skin draining the infected/necrotic material
- **Sequestrum[Q]**: Dead bone as a result of cortical and medullary infarcts. Needs excision for definitive treatment of infection
    - Button sequestrum[Q]: Small sequestrum surrounded by a lucent rim. Seen in osteomyelitis and eosinophilic granuloma[Q]
- **Involucrum[Q]**: Thick layer of periosteal new bone formation around the sequestrum
- **Cloaca[Q]**: Defect developing in an involucrum
- Also known as empyema necessitans[Q]

Chronic osteomyelitis sequestrum–involucrum–cloaca

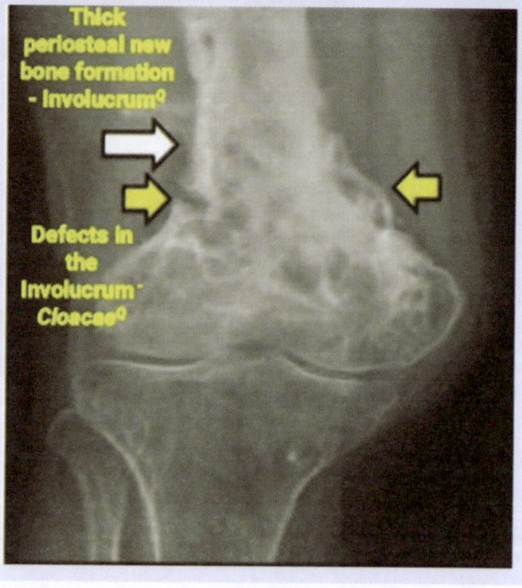

Contd...

Osteomyelitis specifics

Brodie's abscess

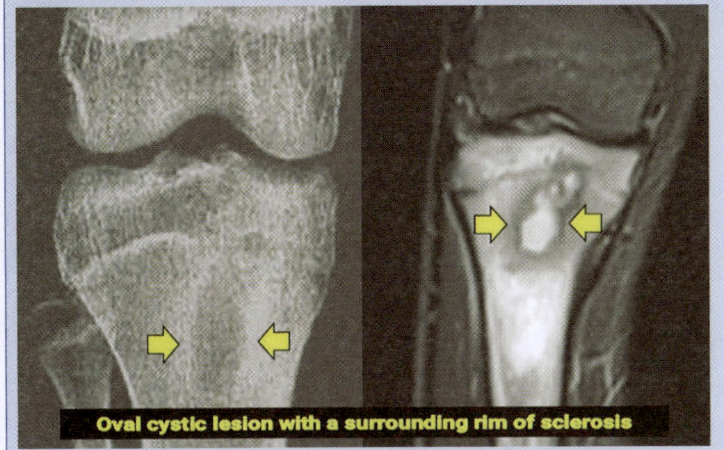

- Localized, aborted form of subacute osteomyelitis
- Abscess surrounded by sclerosis[Q]
- Tibia[Q]—most common site
- X-ray findings—oval, elliptical radiolucency >10 mm[Q]—abscess cavity
- Halo/Doughnut rim of surrounding reactive sclerosis[Q]

TB Spondylitis/Pott's spine

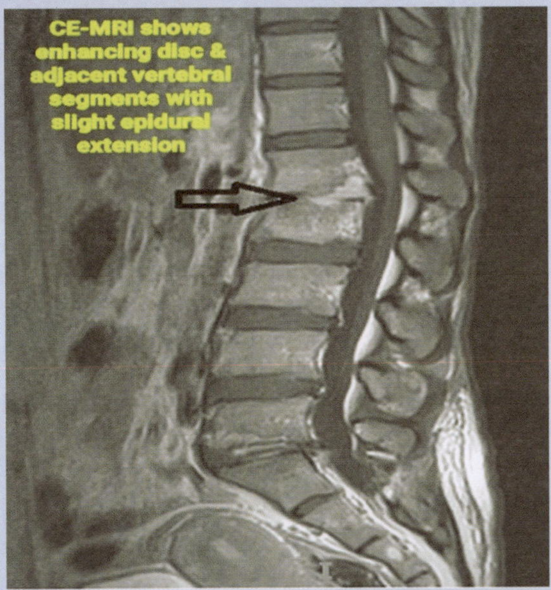

- Spine involvement is most common site involved in MSK TB[Q]
- Lower thoracic and upper lumbar are the most commonly involved regions[Q].
- MRI with gadolinium enhancement is best imaging technique[Q]
- Classic pattern of involvement is of more than one vertebral body together with the intervening disks[Q].
- Pott's abscess[Q]—paravertebral TB abscess.

TB dactylitis/spina ventosa

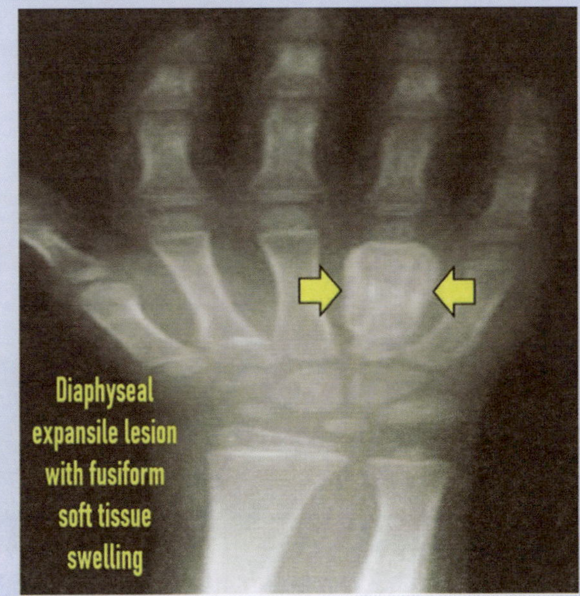

SKELETAL DYSPLASIAS – TREASURE OF NAMED SIGNS AND APPEARANCES!

Achondroplasia

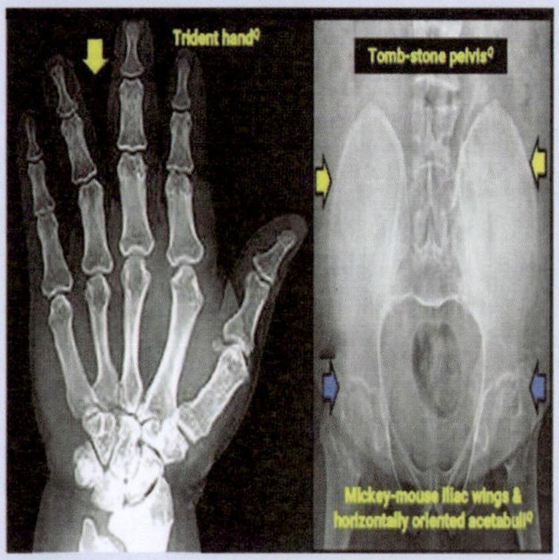

Most common congenital dwarfism[Q]

Imaging features:

- (Remember Tyrion Lannister in Game of thrones!!) Foramen magnum stenosis
- Brachycephaly[Q]—large cranium with a short AP dimension
- Rhizomelic dwarfism[Q]—symmetric shortening of all long bones resulting in short stature
- Trident hands[Q]
- Tombstone pelvis[Q]/Champagne glass pelvis[Q]
- Mickey mouse ear iliac wings[Q]
- Bullet-nosed vertebral bodies[Q] with gibbus formation

Cleido-Cranial Dysplasia (CCD)

Absent clavicles[Q]

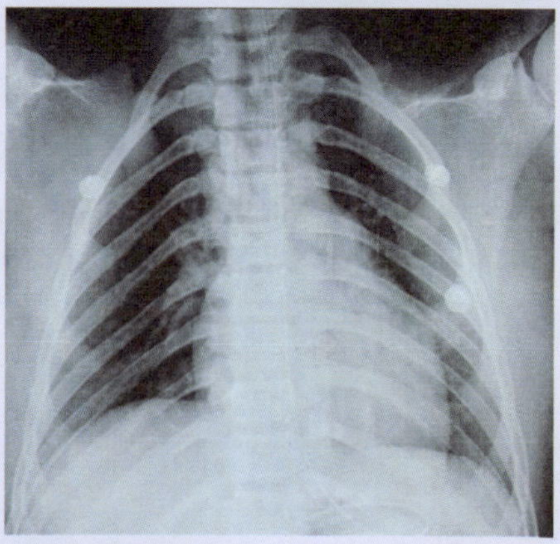

Characterized by:

- Skull abnormalities
- Clavicle abnormalities
- Midline defects

Imaging findings:

- **Hot-cross-bun skull**[Q]–due to widening of sagittal and coronal sutures
- Persistent metopic suture
- Multiple Wormian bones[Q]
- Absent/Hypoplastic clavicles[Q]
- Midline defect at pubic symphysis
- Chef's hat femoral head[Q]

Osteogenesis Imperfecta (OGI)

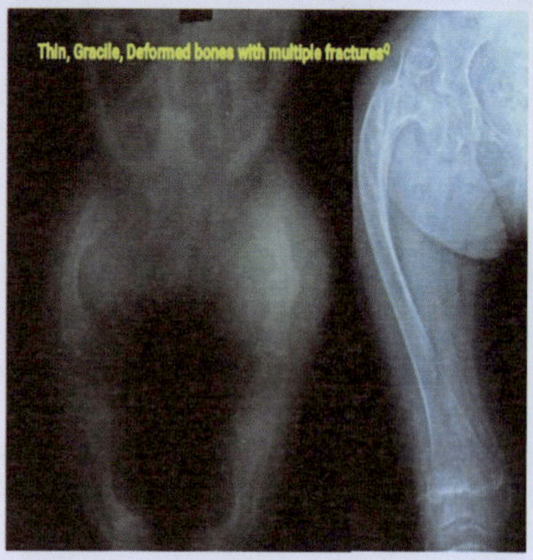

Quantitative and qualitative defects in synthesis of collagen type 1[Q]

Imaging findings:

- Thin and Gracile bones[Q]—diffuse osteopenia with pencil thin cortices.
- Multiple fractures[Q]—transverse fractures especially involving lower limb bones–is characteristic
- Antenatal detection of fractures–is pathognomonic
- Persistent Wormian bones
- Shepherd's crook deformity of proximal femur[Q]
- Zebra stripe sign[Q]–Cyclical treatment with bisphosphonates produces band like sclerotic growth arrest lines in long bones

Melorheostosis

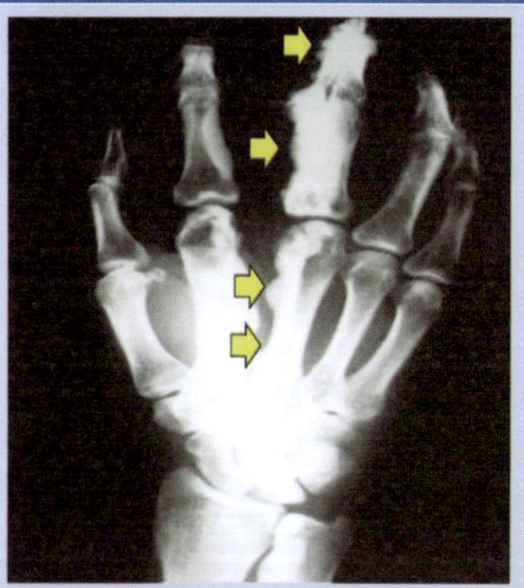

Flowing/Molten/Dripping candle wax appearance[Q]

Osteopetrosis/Marble/Chalk bone disease

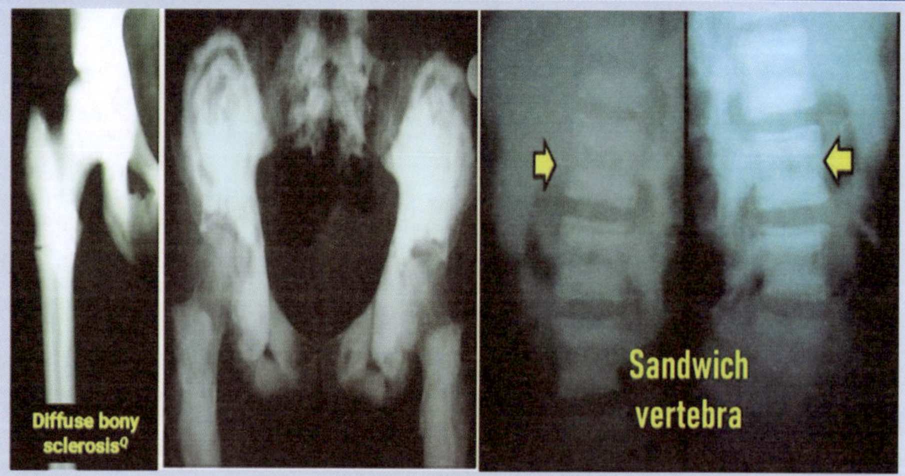

Bone-within-bone appearance[Q]/Endo-bones[Q]

BONE TUMORS

Age-based bone tumor occurence		
<20 years	20–40 years	>40 years
• **Benign tumors:** Eosinophilic granuloma, simple bone cyst, aneurysmal bone cyst, fibrous dysplasia, osteoid osteoma, osteoblastoma, chondroblastoma • **Malignant tumors:** Ewing's sarcoma, osteosarcoma	• **Benign tumors:** Enchondroma, osteoma, Osteoblastoma • **Malignant tumors:** Giant cell tumor, parosteal osteosarcoma	• Chondrosarcoma • Metastases • Multiple myeloma

Location: Distribution of neoplasms based on site of bone involved		
Epiphyseal lesions	Metaphyseal lesions	Diaphyseal lesions
• Chondroblastoma • Infection • Giant cell tumor (in adults) • Geode/Subchondral cyst	• NOF—Nonossifying fibroma • SBC • CMF—Chondromyxoid fibroma • Osteosarcoma • Chondrosarcoma • Enchondroma • Infections	• Ewing's sarcoma • Enchondroma • Fibrous dysplasia • SBC • ABC • Osteoblastoma

Transition Zone/Margins	
Narrow zone of transition — Well-defined margins	Wide zone of transition — Ill defined margins
Narrow zone of transition 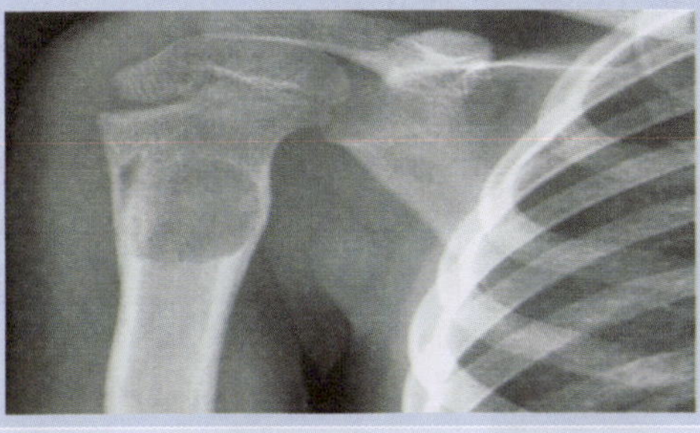	**Wide zone of transition** 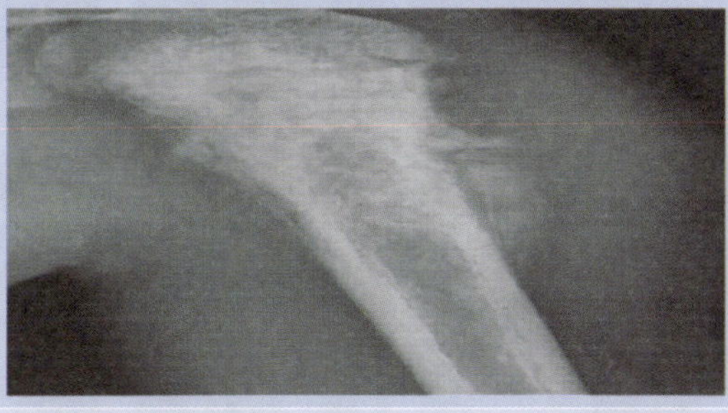
• Usually indicates a benign lesion—simple bone cyst. • **Exceptions:** In patients aged >40 years—metastases and multiple myeloma lesions are malignancies that show a narrow zone of transition.	• Usually indicates a Malignant lesion – Osteosarcoma • **Exceptions:** Infection and Eosinophilic granuloma – are benign lesions that may show wide zone of transition

Appearance—Periosteal reaction

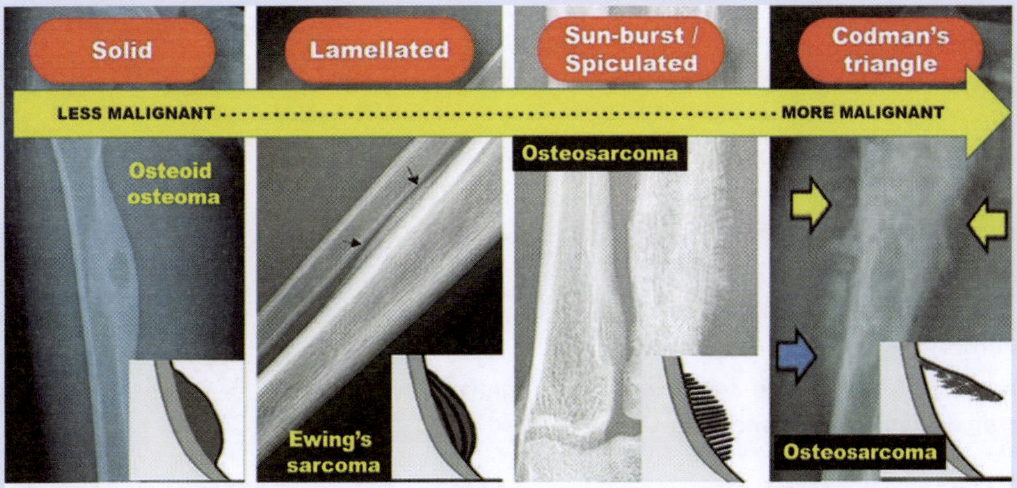

BENIGN BONE TUMORS

Osteoid Osteoma

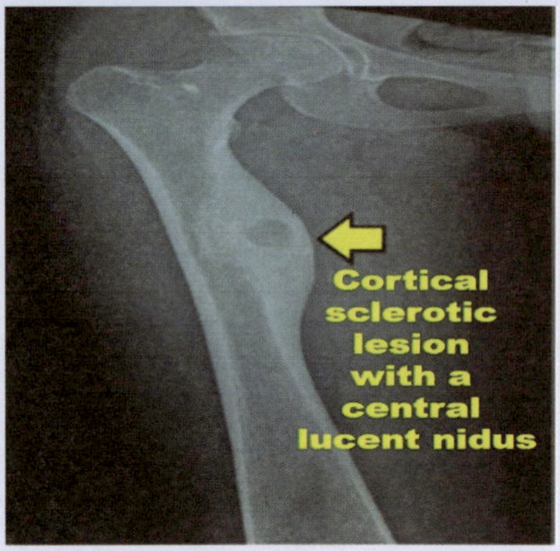

Osteochondroma/Exostosis

PYQ ALERT "FMGE JULY 2023 PATTERN

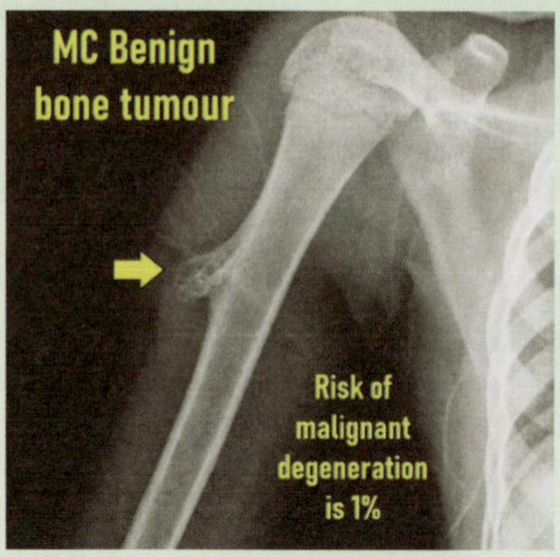

Vertebral Hemangioma

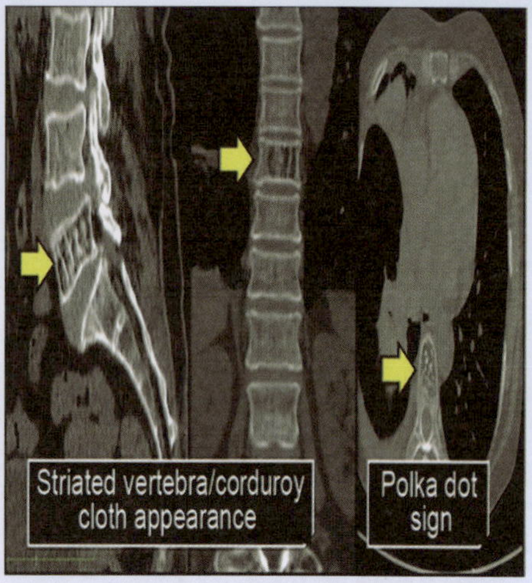

Aneurysmal Bone Cyst (ABC)

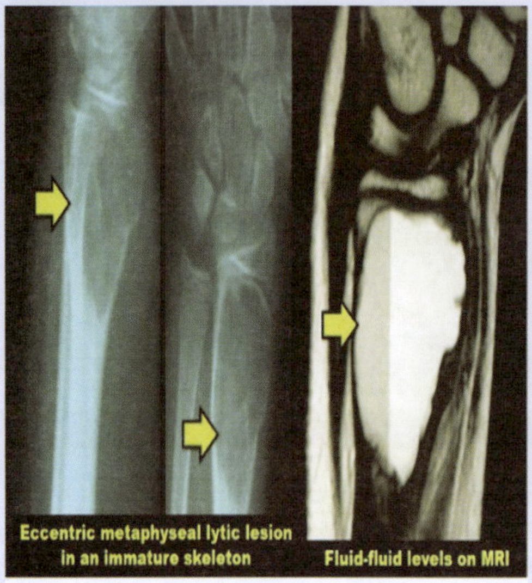

Enchondroma

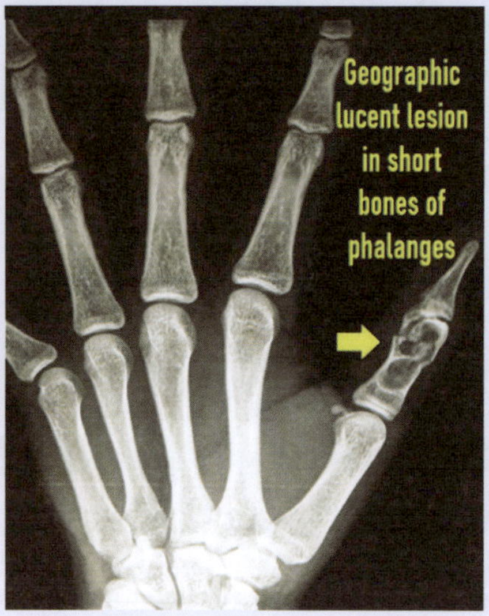

Simple bone cyst

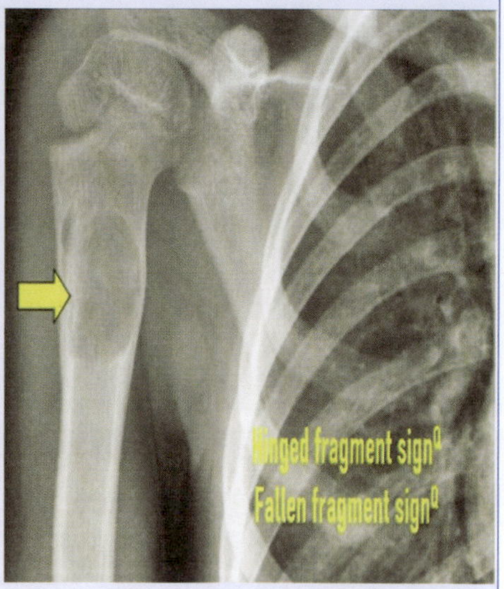

Simple bone cyst

MC Proximal Humeral Lesion in a Child

Bone tumor syndromes:

Gardner syndrome:

- GI polyposis
- Multiple osteomas, epidermal cysts, desmoid tumor and fibromatosis
- Extra-intestinal manifestations precede the colonic polyps

Olier's disease:

- Multiple enchondromas
- Higher rate of malignant degeneration – 10%

Maffucci syndrome:

- Enchondromatosis + Soft tissue cavernous hemangiomas
- Higher rate of malignant degeneration –15%

MALIGNANT BONE TUMORS

Bone Metastasis

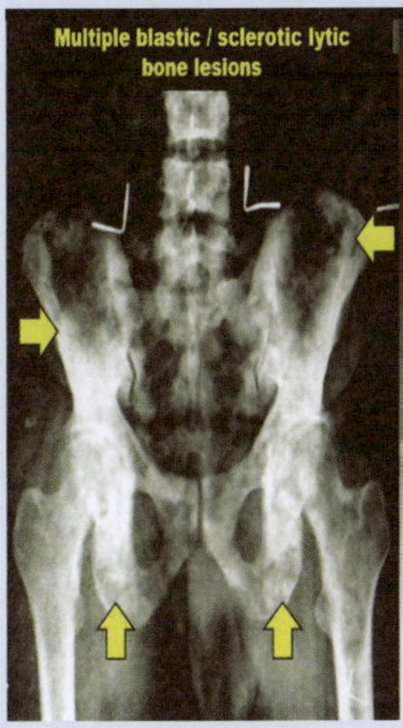

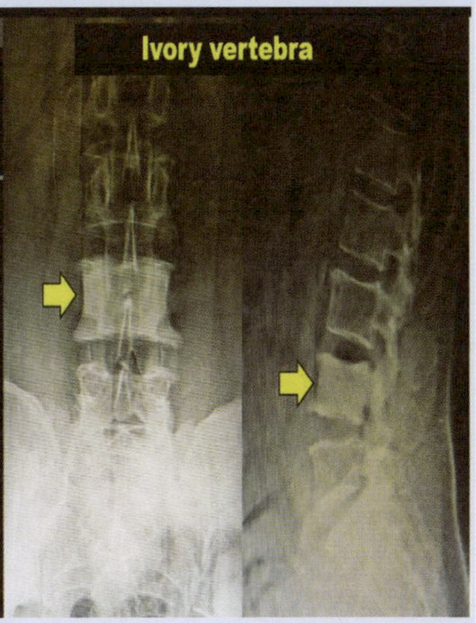

CLINICAL CLINCHER

Bone metastases specifics:

- Most common malignant bone tumor[Q]
- Breast cancer[Q]–most common primary in females
- Prostate cancer[Q]—most common primary in males overall. Also most common cause of Blastic metastases[Q]
- Lung cancer[Q]–most common cause of lytic bone metastasis
- 99mTc–MDP Bone scan[Q]—most sensitive/Best technique for detection–appear as Hot spots
- Central/Axial skeleton[Q]—most commonly involved

Bone metastases appearances:

- Blow out lesions[Q]—highly expansile bone lesions. Seen in primaries form RCC/Thyroid/Lung malignancy
- Cookie bite lesion[Q]—cortical metastatic deposit with scalloping of cortex. Seen in Lung–Breast–Kidney cancer
- Lytic lesions[Q]—permeative/Moth-eaten destructive lesion
- Snowball appearance[Q]—multiple blastic/radiodense lesions
- One-eyed pedicle[Q]/Winking owl sign[Q]—destruction of single pedicle, pedicle not seen on AP radiograph
- Blind vertebra[Q]—bilateral pedicle destruction
- Ivory vertebra[Q]—densely sclerotic vertebra
- Extrapleural sign[Q]—obtuse angled opacity due to deposit in chest wall/ribs
- Sunburst lesion[Q]/Spiculated lesion of skull vault[Q]—seen in Neuroblastoma metastasis

Multiple myeloma

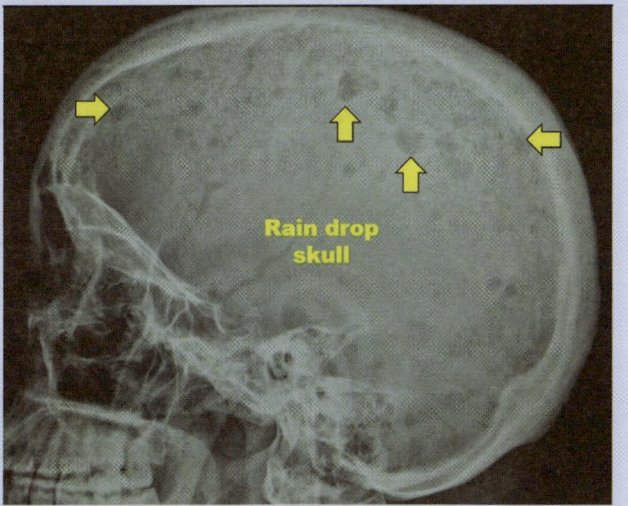

Multiple Myeloma

Multiple punched-out lytic lesions in skull in an elderly patient

Multiple myeloma:

- Most common primary malignant bone tumor[Q]
- Spine[Q]—most common site
- 99mTc–MDP Bone scan[Q]—appear as cold spots[Q]
- Raindrop skull[Q]multiple uniformly sized punched-out lytic lesions in skull
- Vertebra plana/Wrinkled vertebra[Q]—vertebral body collapse
- Pedicle sign of myeloma[Q]—as pedicles are poor in red marrow, hence are spared
- Solitary plasmacytoma[Q]—localized plasma cell proliferation. Geographic lucent expansile lesion—soap bubble internal architecture[Q]

Contd...

Osteosarcoma

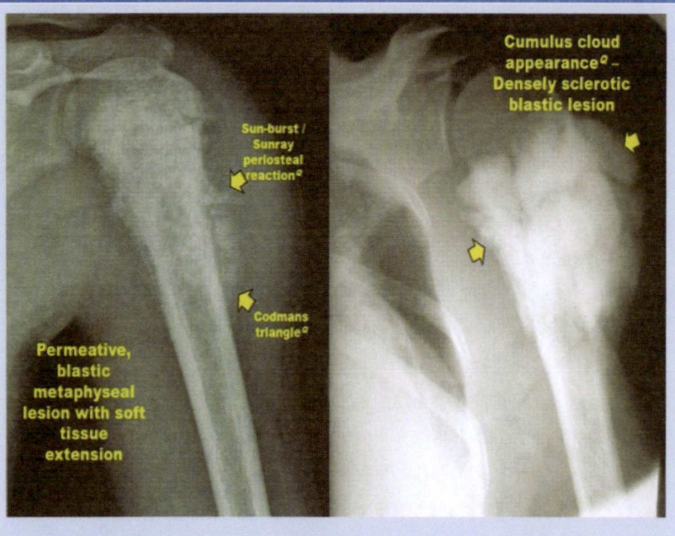

Osteosarcoma:

- 2nd most common primary malignant bone tumor[Q]
- 10–25 years age group—Metaphyseal location[Q]
- Femur[Q]—most common site
- Permeative/Ivory medullary lesion in metaphysis[Q] with cortical disruption[Q] and soft tissue extension[Q]
- Sunray/Sun-burst periosteal reaction[Q] seen
- Codman triangle[Q]—elevated periosteum–not specific for osteosarcoma
- Cumulus cloud appearance[Q]—eccentric lobulated soft tissue mass adjacent to bone
- Cannonball ossifying lung metastasis[Q]—may be seen
- Parosteal/Juxtacortical osteosarcoma—cleavage plane sign/String sign[Q]—seen as a radiolucent cleft between the mass and underlying cortex

Ewings sarcoma

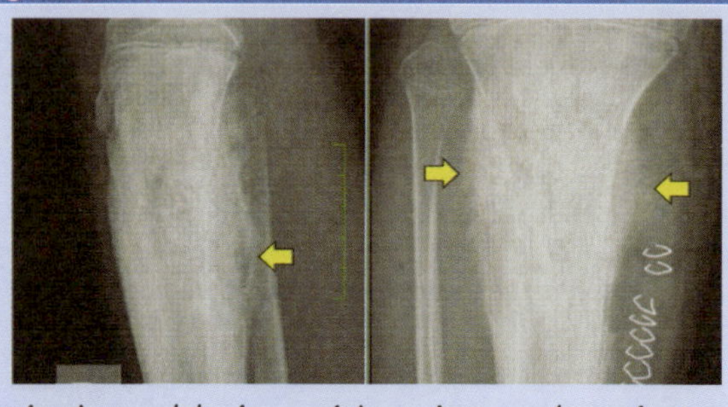

Diaphyseal lesion with onion peel periosteal reaction

Ewings sarcoma:

- Diaphyseal lesion presenting at 10–25 years
- Femur[Q]–most common site
- Permeative lesion in diaphysis[Q] with Laminated/Onion peel periosteal reaction[Q]
- Cortical saucerization[Q] seen
- Groomed/Trimmed whiskers effect[Q]—spiculated periosteal reaction

Skip lesions[Q] may be seen

Chondrosarcoma

MC site – Pelvis and Proximal femur

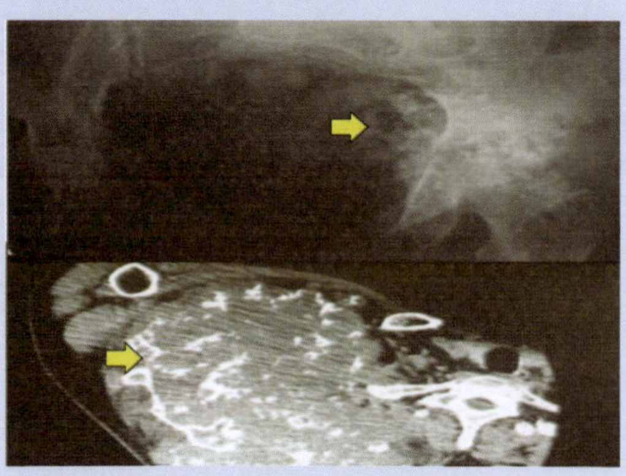

Popcorn/Fluffly/Stippled/Cotton-wool/ Rings and broken arcs calcification

PYQ ALERT "NEET-PG 2021 PATTERN"

Giant Cell Tumor

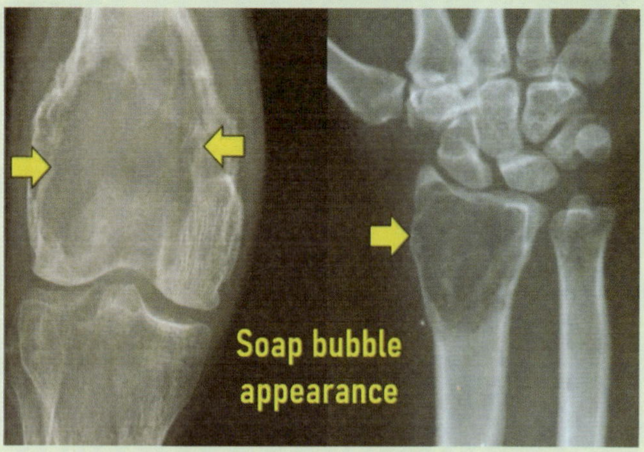

Eccentric epimetaphyseal lytic lesion in adults

Quasi-malignant tumor–most are benign, some are malignant

HEAD AND NECK TRAUMA

Nasal bone fracture

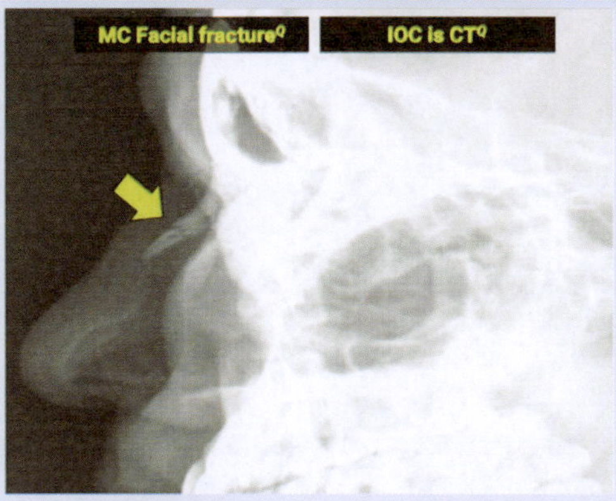

Tripod/trimalar fracture of zygoma

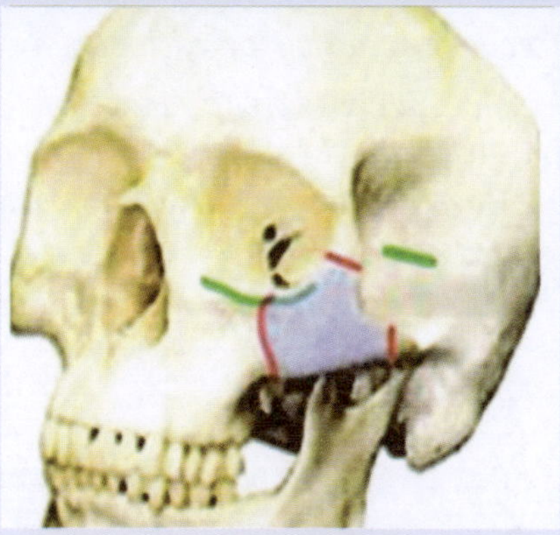

CT Reconstructed Image

Involves – Zygomatic arch[Q] + Orbital process[Q] + Maxillary process[Q]

Orbital Floor Fracture/ Blow-out Fracture

PYQ ALERT "FMGE JAN 2023 PATTERN"

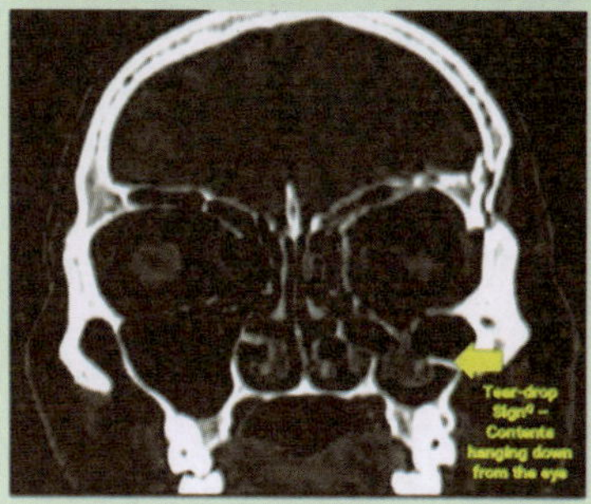

Fracture of Infraorbital plate of Maxilla[Q] – Fist blow on the eye

SPINAL INJURIES/FRACTURES

Jefferson's fracture/burst fracture of atlas C1

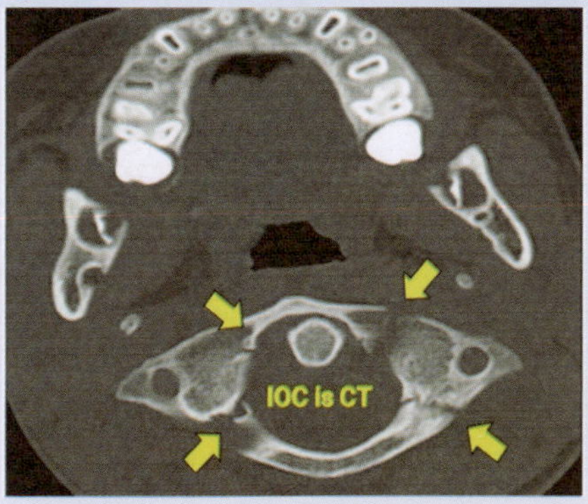

Hangman's/hangee's fracture/pars interarticularis fracture of C2

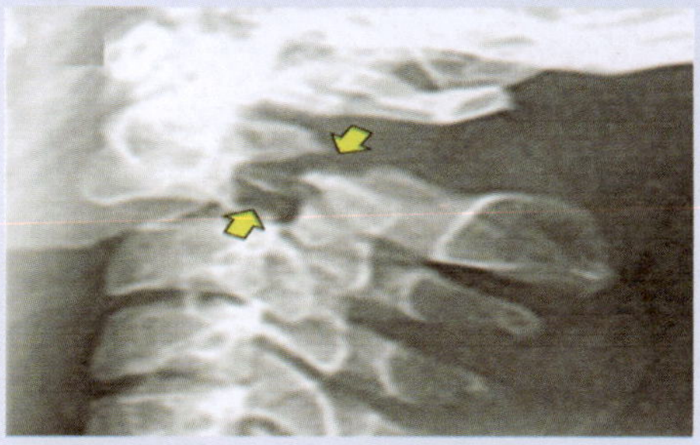

- Seen in Judicial hanging[Q]
- MC cause is – Motor vehicle accident[Q]
- Not associated with any neurological deficits[Q]

Clay shoveler fracture

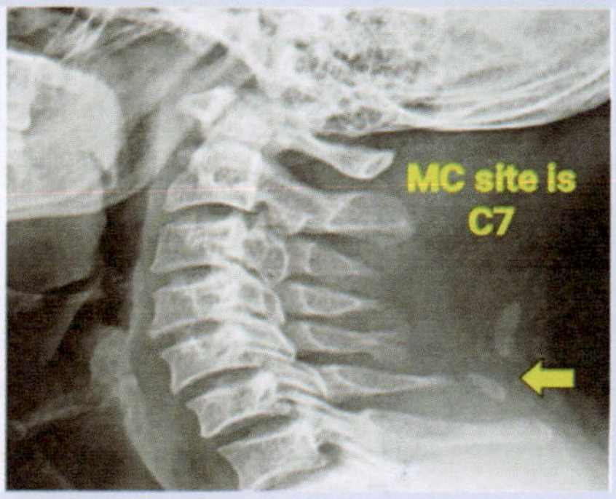

Avulsion fracture of lower cervical spinous processes

SHOULDER AND UPPER LIMB INJURIES

Clavicle fracture

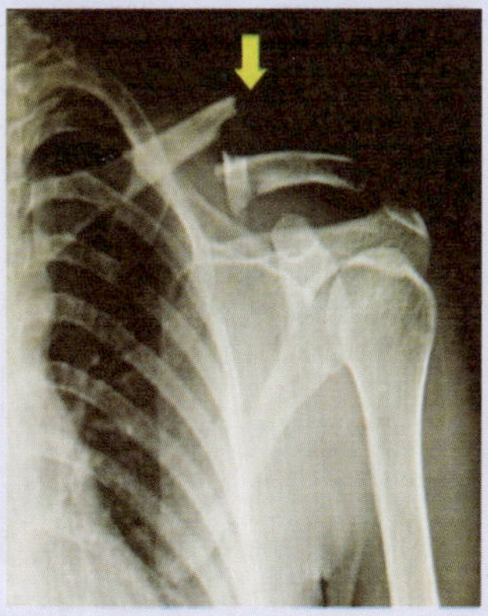

Altman classification used

Acromioclavicular joint dislocation

PYQ ALERT "INI-CET MAY 2023 PATTERN"

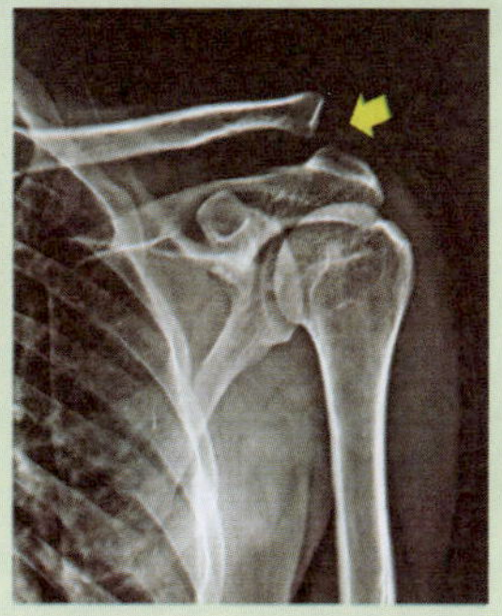

Anterior/subcoracoid shoulder dislocation

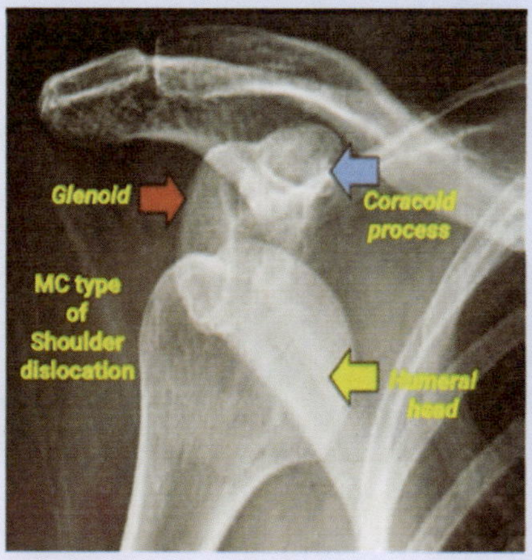

Contd...

Posterior shoulder dislocation (fluoroscopic spot film)

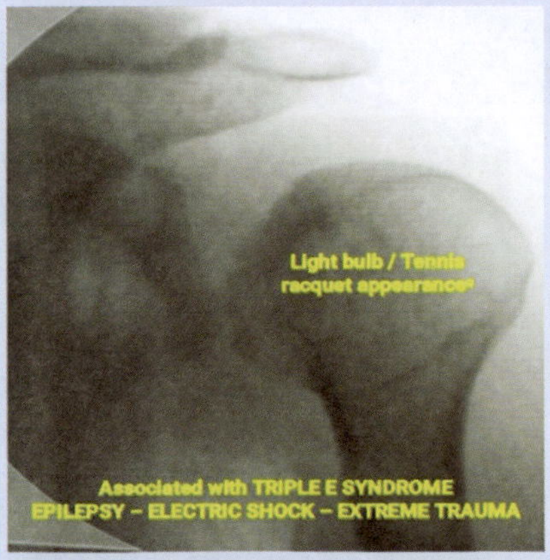

CLINICAL CLINCHER

Recurrent anterior shoulder dislocation—associated injuries

Recurrent anterior dislocation is associated with:

- Hill-Sachs defect[Q]/Hatchet defect[Q]–Impaction injury on posterolateral aspect of humeral head
- Bankart lesion[Q]–Avulsion injury of anteroinferior glenoid rim
- Greater tuberosity fracture
- HAGL lesion[Q]–Humeral avulsion of glenohumeral ligament

Humeral fractures Neer classification[Q]

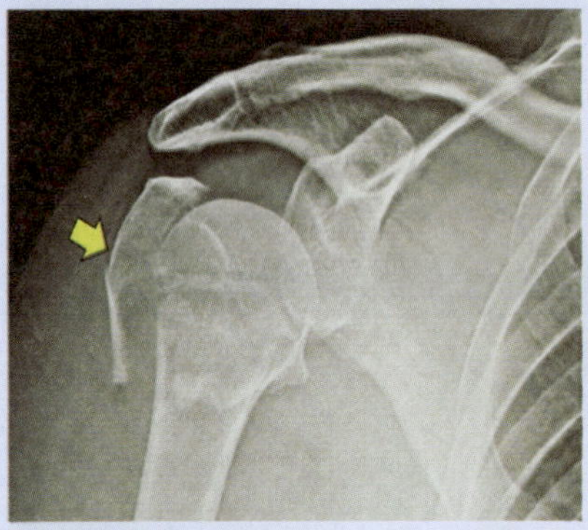

Neer Classification

Based on - Number of fracture parts and fragment displacement

Supracondylar fracture of humerus MC fracture around elbow in children

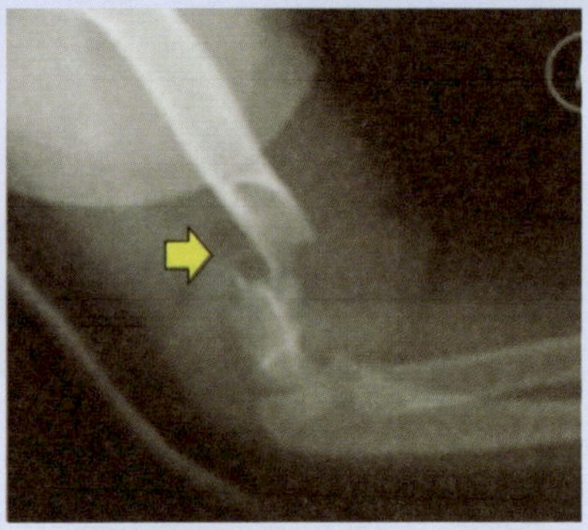

- MC type – Extension type[Q]
- MC nerve injured – AIN[Q]
- MC artery injured – Brachial artery[Q]
- MC long-term complication – Malunion[Q] (Gunstock deformity[Q])

Scaphoid fracture MC carpal fracture[Q]

PYQ ALERT "NEET-PG 2019 PATTERN"

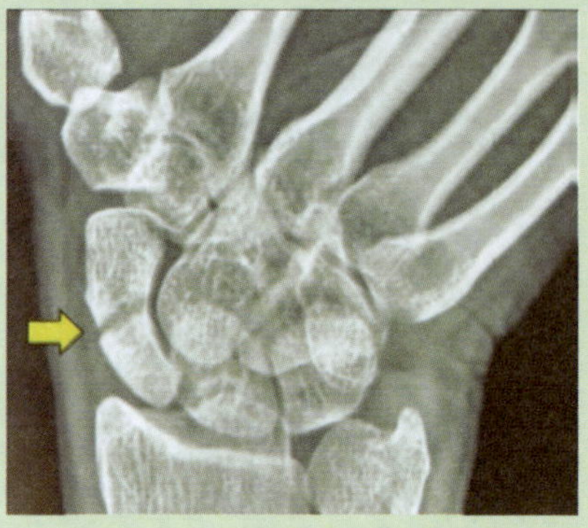

MC Carpal Fracture[Q]

- Tenderness at anatomical snuff box[Q]
- MC site – Waist of scaphoid[Q]
- Avascular necrosis[Q] – More proximal the #- greater the risk of AVN[Q]
- Herbert screw technique used for Rx[Q]

Colles' fractures

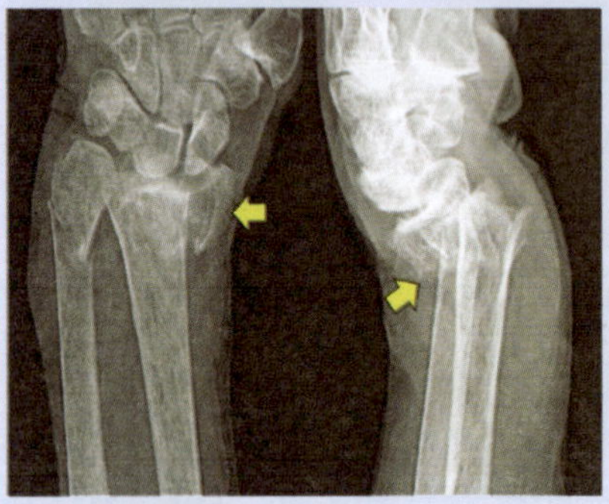

Distal Radius Fracture with Dorsal Tilt and Impaction

Monteggia fracture dislocation

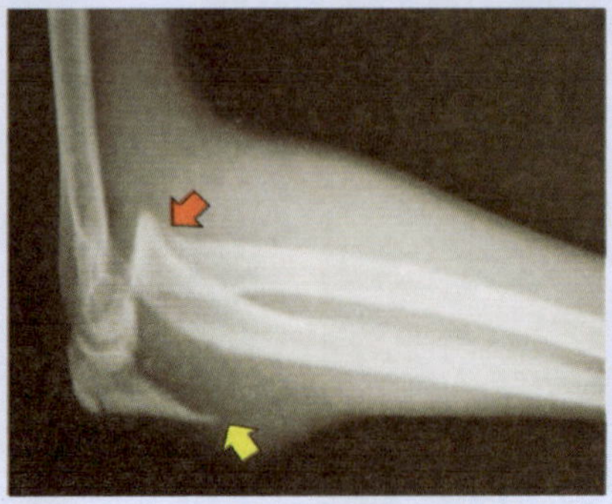

Fracture Ulna + Dislocation of Radius

Galeazzi fracture dislocation

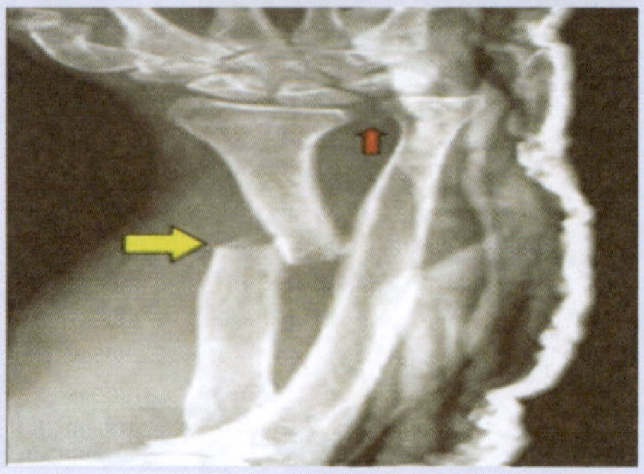

Fracture Radius + Dislocation of Ulna

Contd...

Barton fracture

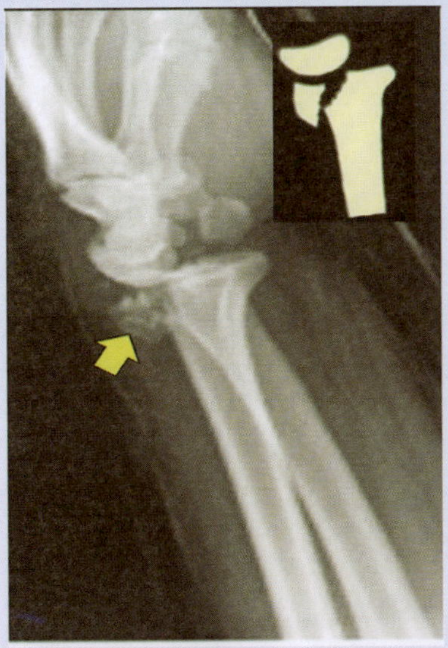

Volar barton fracture

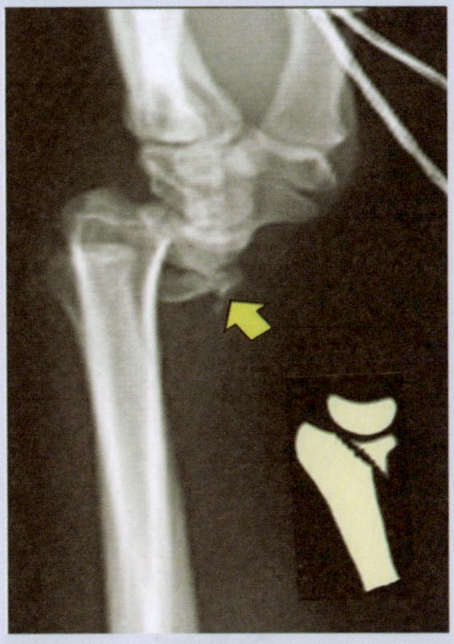

Bennett's fracture

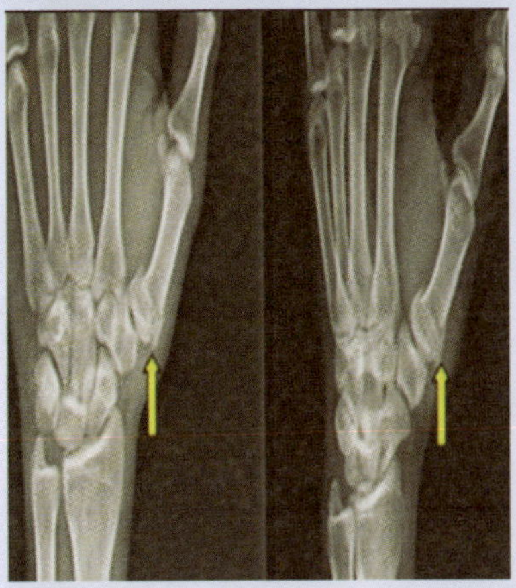

Intra-articular fracture of proximal 1st metacarpal[Q]

Gamekeeper's fracture

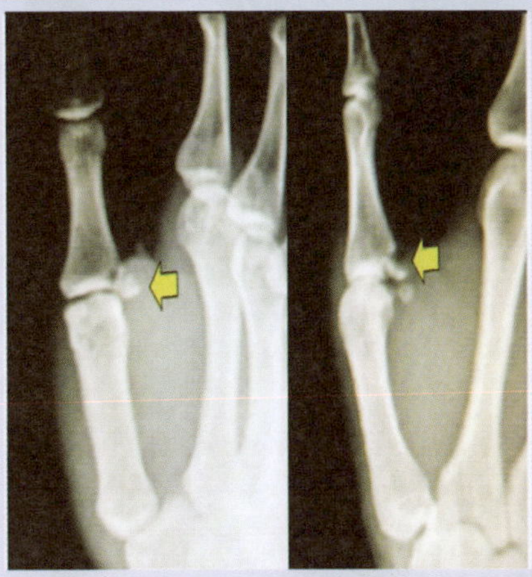

Avulsion fracture of Ulnar collateral ligament at proximal phalanx of thumb[Q]

Normal

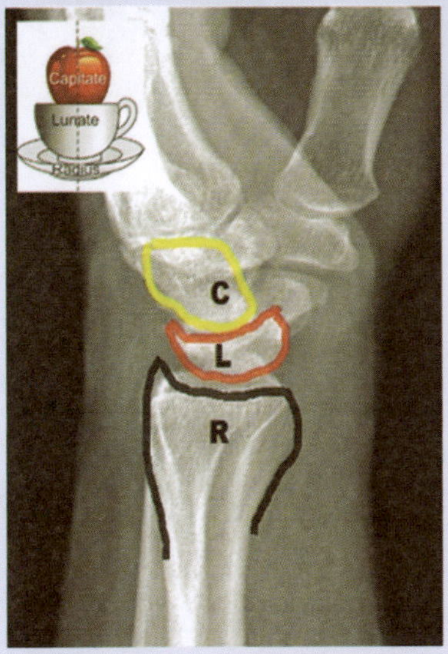

Radius-Lunate-Capitate in a straight line

Lunate dislocation

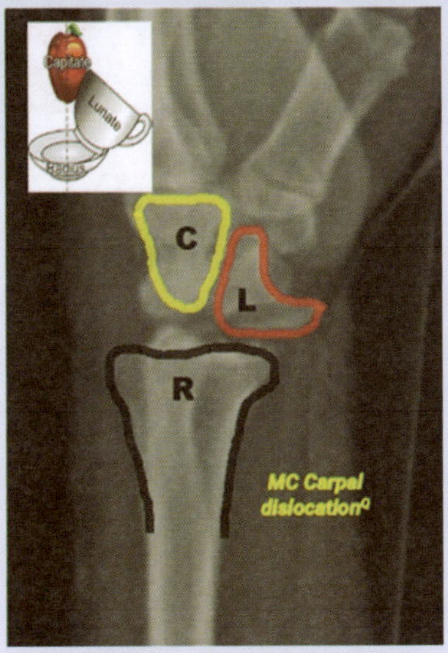

Lunate tilts forward – "The cup spills"

Perilunate dislocation

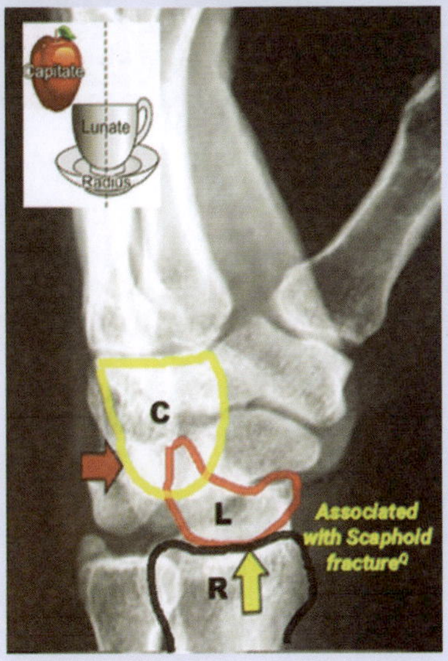

Capitate displaced dorsally

PELVIC AND LOWER LIMB FRACTURES

Neck of femur fracture

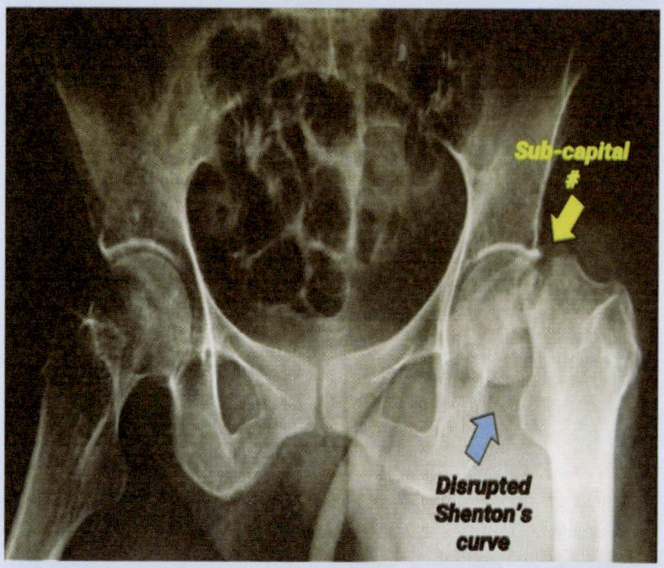

Intertrochanteric femur fracture

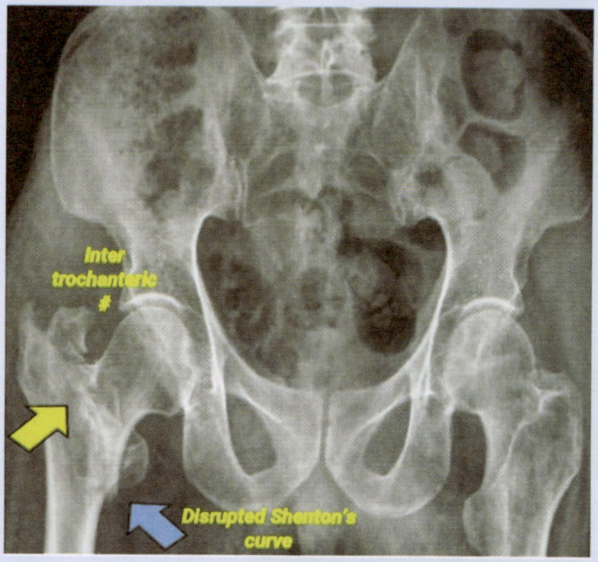

Patellar fracture

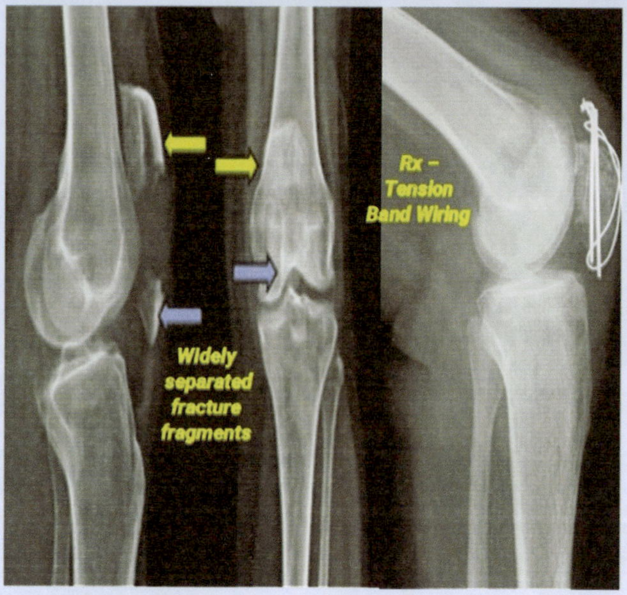

Hip Joint Dislocation

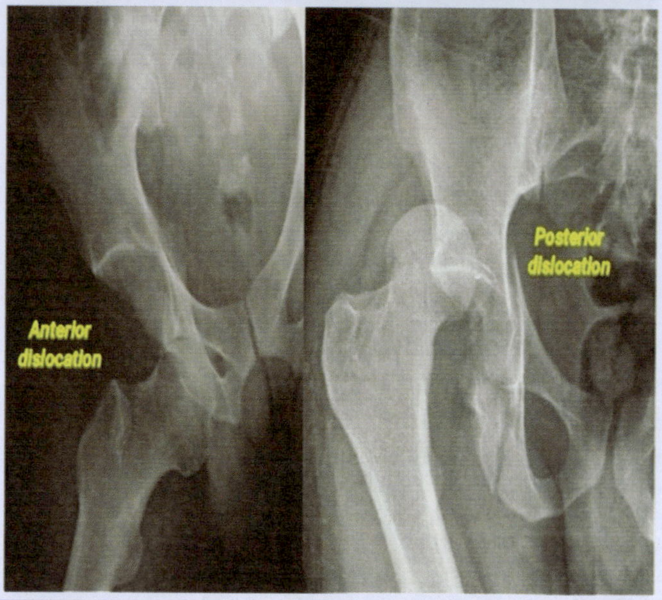

MISCELLANEOUS

Stress fracture—Bone injury due to repetitive stress of lower intensity than that required for an acute traumatic fracture	Sciwora–spinal cord injury without obvious radiographic abnormality
Stress fracture 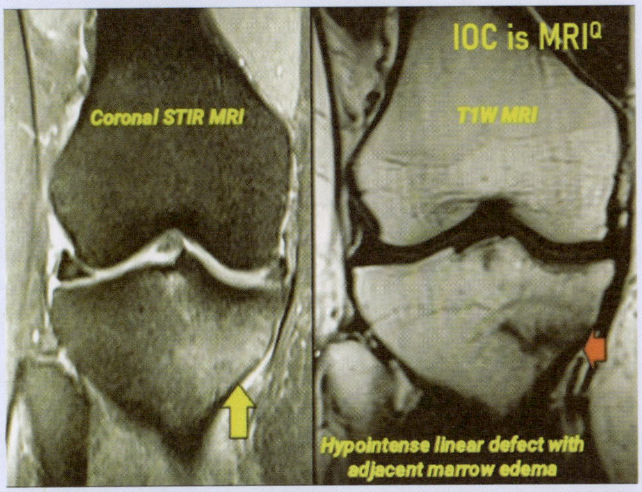	• Seen in pediatric age group[Q] • Most commonly seen in Cervical spine[Q] • **Concept:** ▪ Spine is comprised of two components—Musculoskeletal (muscles/ligaments/disks) and neurological (spinal cord and nerve roots). ▪ The MSK component is highly elastic in children—hence, as a result of spinal trauma, fracture dislocations do not occur. Hence, X-rays are normal. ▪ But spinal cord/nerve roots are not elastic – so though there is no fracture externally—there is neurological injury in the form of cord contusion/hematoma/laceration. ▪ Thus the child develops neurological deficits (paraplegia) but X-rays are normal. **Hence, IOC is MRI[Q]**

Pediatric trauma specifics

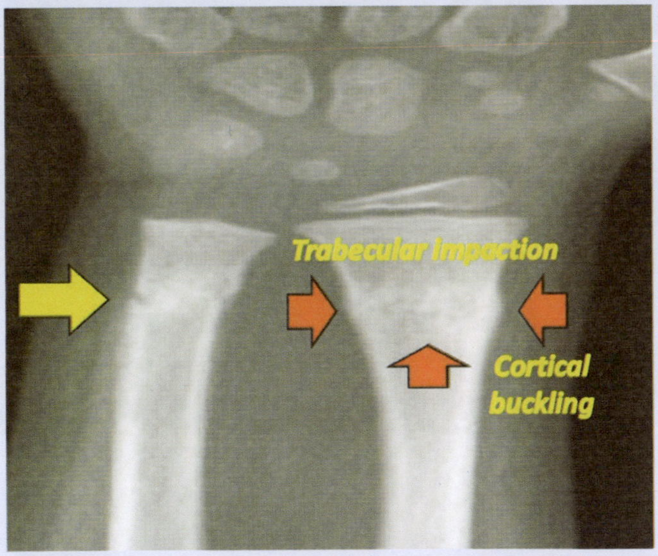

Torus/Buckling Fracture[Q]—cortical buckling[Q] and trabecular impaction[Q]—without cortical break[Q]

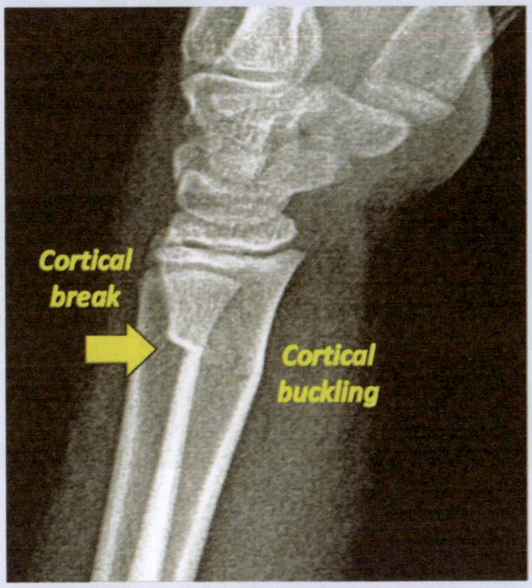

Greenstick/hickory stick fracture[Q]—one cortex broken–one cortex buckled/normal

7. CENTRAL NERVOUS SYSTEM IMAGING

Acute stroke imaging

CONCEPT

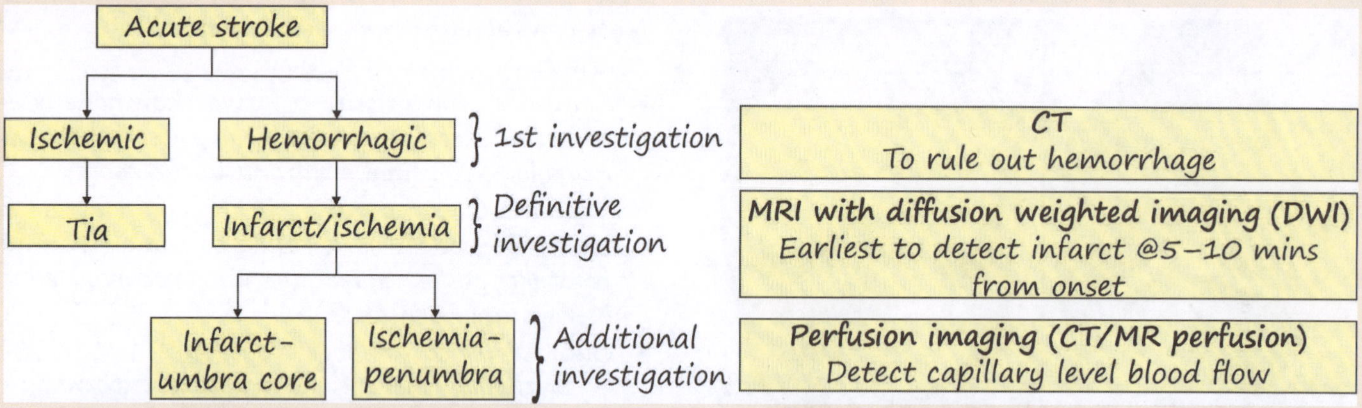

Ischemic stroke—hyper-acute infarct

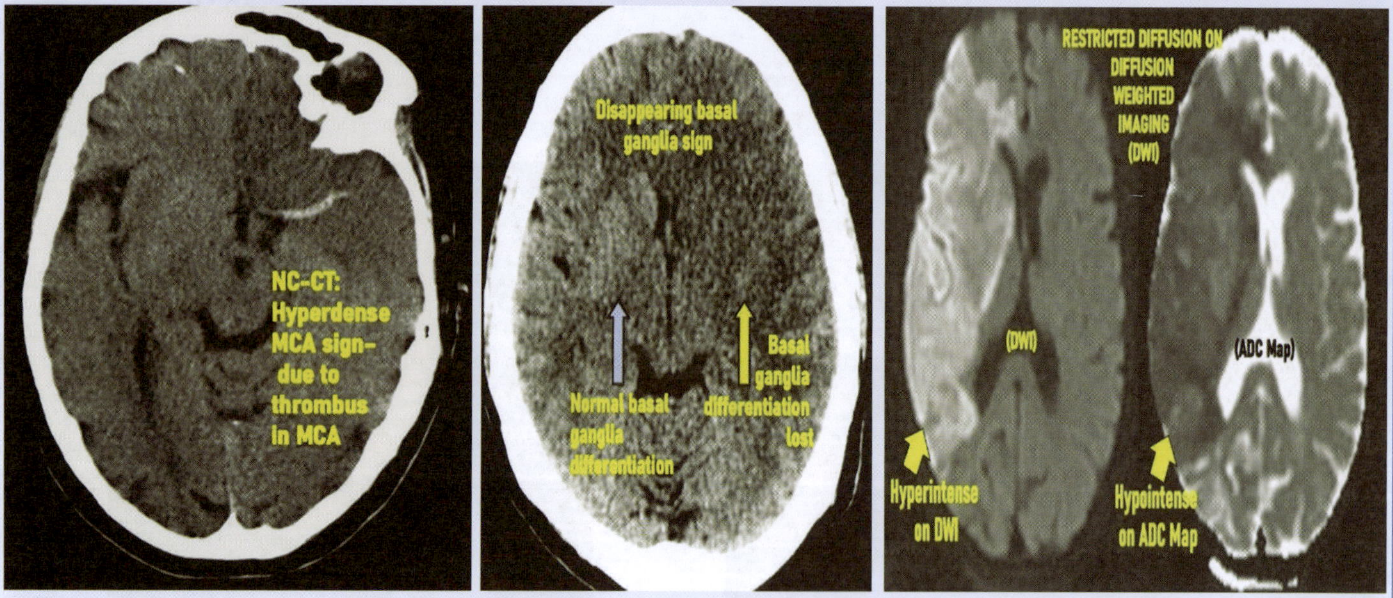

- **Hyperacute infarct—CT**
  - Dense artery sign[Q]: Earliest imaging sign
  - Hyperdense MCA[Q]/Sylvian dot sign[Q]: Hyperdense thrombus within the middle cerebral artery—correlates with large infarcts distally.
  - Early parenchymal signs: Decrease in gray matter density[Q]– with obscuration of lentiform nucleus[Q]/ disappearing basal ganglia sign[Q]—loss of insular ribbon sign[Q]
- **Hyperacute Infarct – MRI**
  - Restricted diffusion on DWI[Q]: Hyperintense appearance on diffusion weighted imaging (DWI) and corresponding area appearing hypointense on apparent diffusion coefficient (ADC) map.

Contd...

Ischemic stroke—acute infarct

PYQ ALERT "FMGE DEC 2020 PATTTERN"

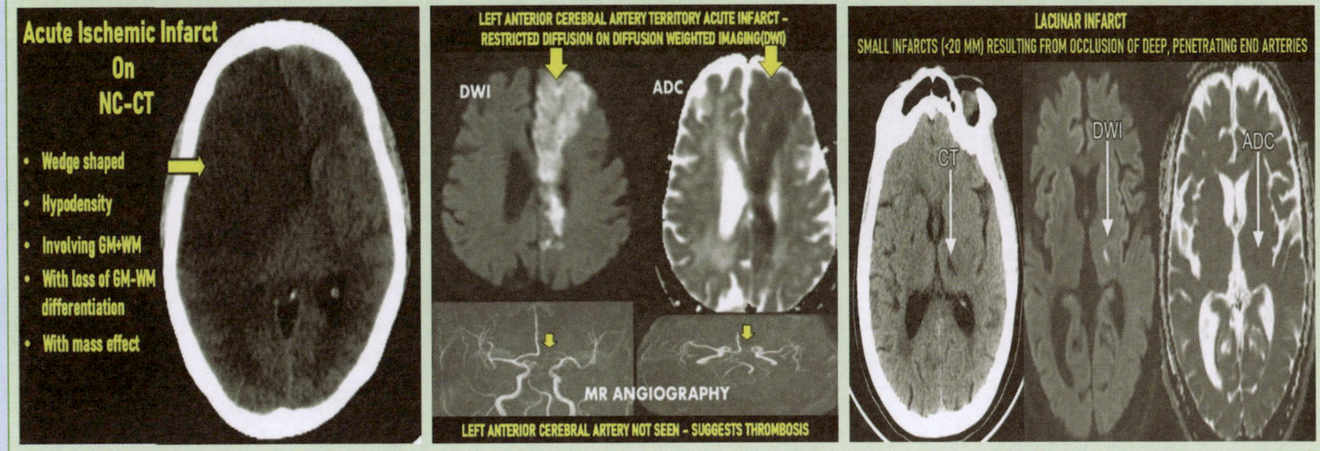

- Acute infarct on CT:
  - **Wedge-shaped area**[Q]: Corresponds to the arterial territory.
  - **Diffuse hypodensity**[Q]: Due to edematous affected brain parenchyma.
  - **Involving gray and white matter**[Q]: As both are supplied by the same artery.
  - **With loss of gray-white differentiation**[Q]: As both GM and WM are involved.
  - **With evidence of mass effect**[Q]: Due to edematous brain parenchyma.
- Subacute infarct on CT–**CT Fogging phenomenon**[Q] **– due to subcortical hemorrhages**
- Chronic Infarct on CT–**Gliosis**[Q] **and ex vacuo dilatation of ventricles/sulci**[Q]
- **Lacunar infarcts**[Q]:
  - Small infarcts (<20 mm) resulting from occlusion of deep, penetrating end arteries(lenticulostriate arteries, thalamo-perforating, and pontine perforating arteries, recurrent artery of Heubner).
  - **Most common locations:** Basal ganglia, internal capsule, thalamus, and the corona radiata.
- Time-of-Flight (TOF) MR-Angiography is preferred over CE-CT Angiography for vascular imaging
- Alberta Stroke Program Early CT (ASPECTS) Score
  - Affected middle cerebral artery territory is divided into ten segments, 1 point is deducted for each area that shows early ischemic changes of swelling or reduced attenuation/hypodensity.
  - A lower total score carries a worse prognosis.
  - Can be used to predict outcome and risk of post-thrombolysis hemorrhage[Q].

Venous sinus thrombosis/venous infarcts

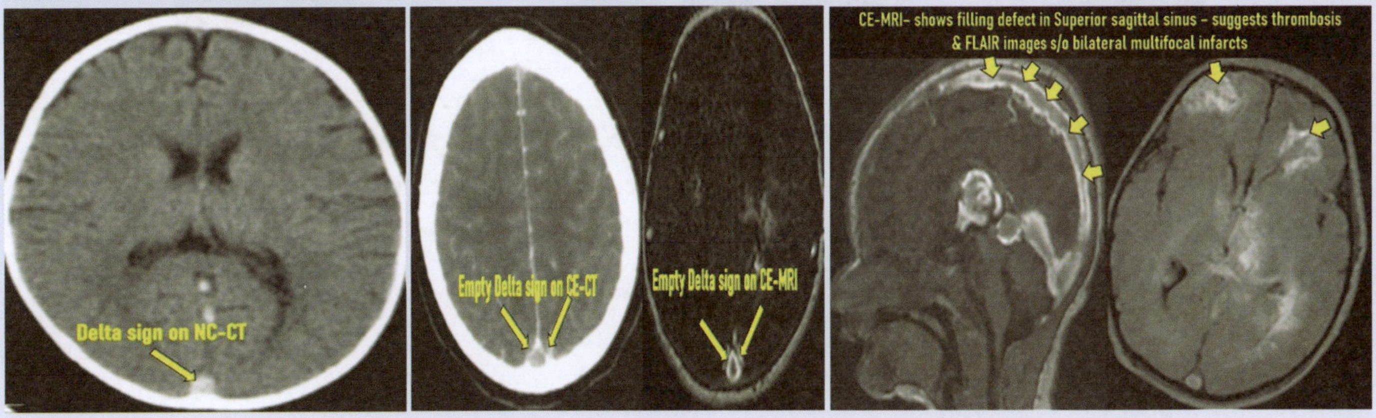

Contd...

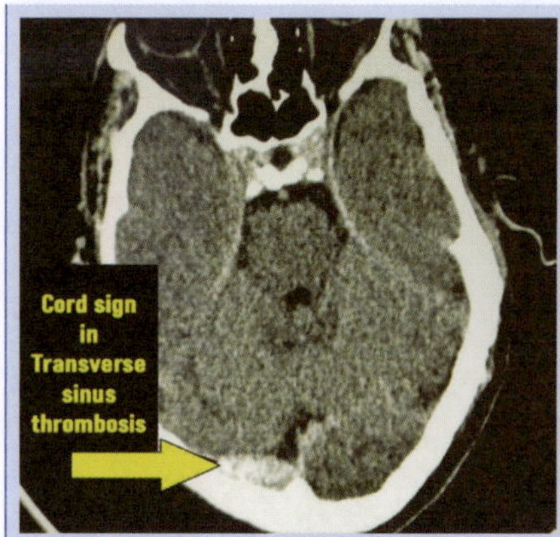

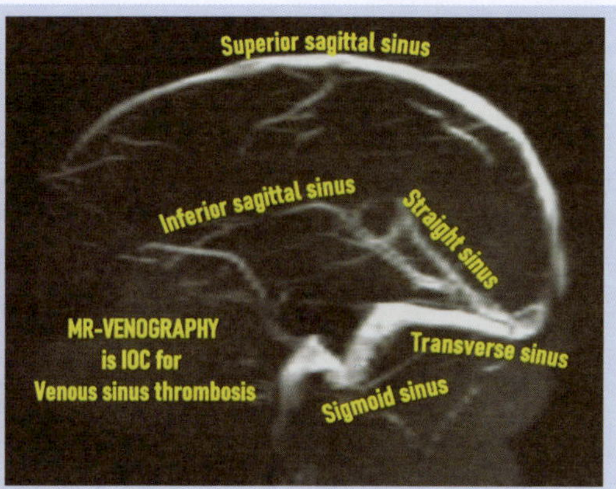

Venous sinus thrombosis/venous infarcts:

- Venous infarcts are hemorrhagic and multifocal.
- IOC - MRI and MR Venography[Q].
- MC sinus involved superior sagittal sinus[Q] – results in bilateral para-sagittal infarcts
- Delta sign[Q] on NC-CT – sinus appears hyperdense due to thrombus
- Empty delta sign[Q] on CE-CT/ CE-MRI - The sinus walls enhance but the contents (thrombus) do not.
- Cord sign[Q]: Cord-like hyperattenuation within a dural venous sinus on NC-CT. Most commonly seen in the transverse sinus.

Hemorrhagic stroke - Acute hemorrhage appears hyperdense on CT

PYQ ALERT "FMGE AUG 2020 PATTERN"

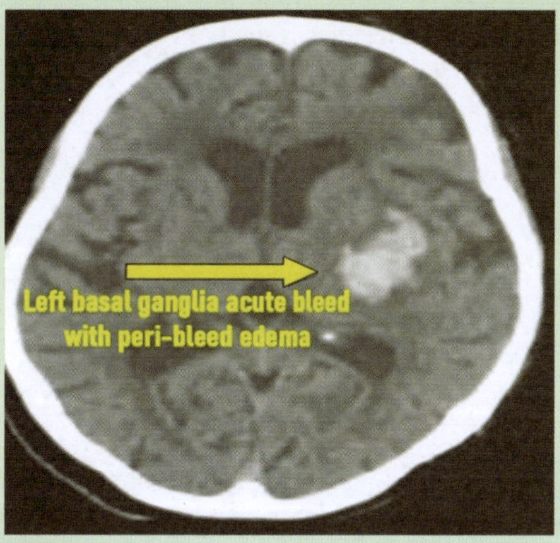

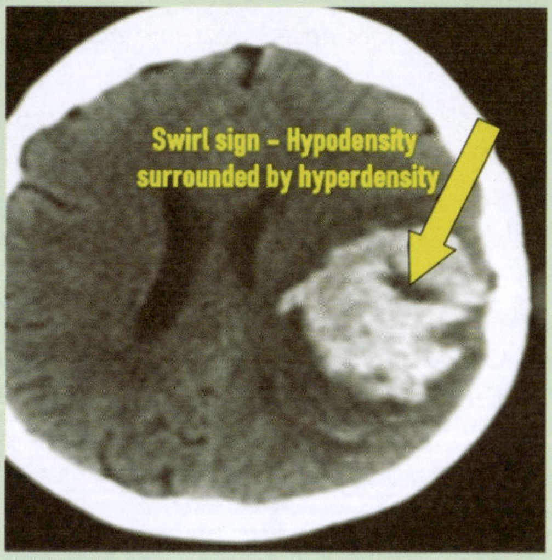

CONCEPT

CLINICAL CLINCHER

Acute hemorrhage in the basal ganglia-is hypertensive bleed unless it proven otherwise

- The most common sites of Hypertensive bleeds in a decreasing order are:
  - Putamen
  - Thalamus
  - Pons
- Thus, 1st two the most common sites, putamen and thalamus are actually components of the Basal ganglia.
- This is a very important diagnostic clue the next 40-50 years of your clinical practice ahead.

Contd...

Sub-Arachnoid Hemorrhage (SAH)

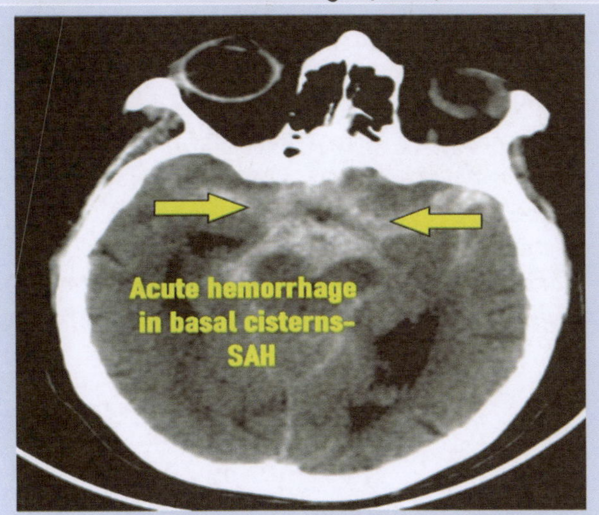

PYQ ALERT "FMGE DEC 2021 PATTERN"

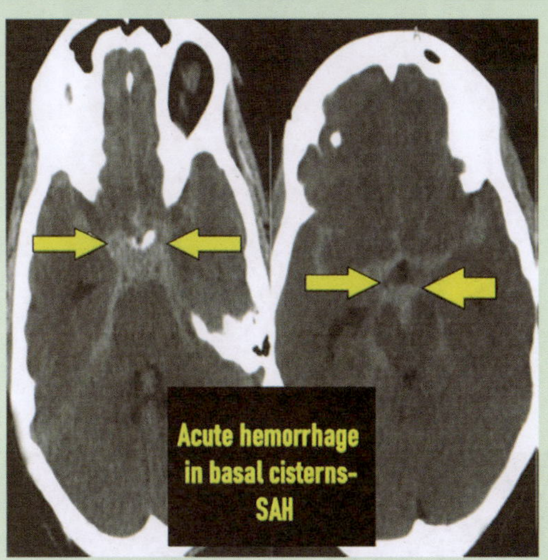

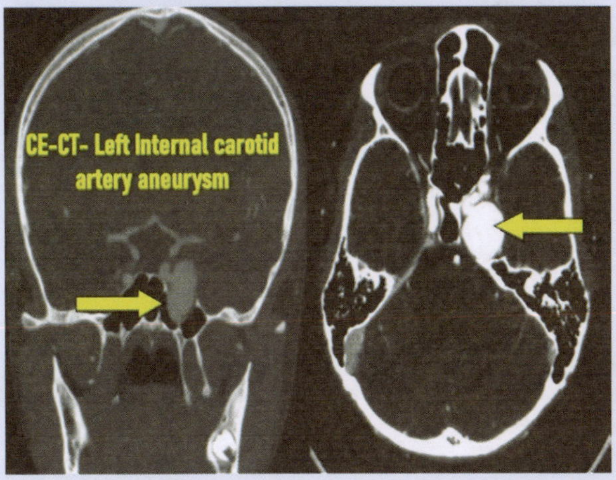

MC cause of SAH–Trauma[Q]

- MC cause of non-traumatic SAH—rupture of berry aneurysm[Q]
- MC site of berry aneurysm-anterior communicating artery (ACom)[Q]

CLINICAL CLINCHER

History:

- Middle-aged patient
- Thunder-clap headache[Q]/worst headache of my life[Q]
- Altered sensorium
  - Hunt and Hess grading system[Q] is used—predicts outcome
  - IOC for acute SAH — CT
  - IOC for subacute SAH — MRI
  - Best MRI sequences — Gradient Echo (GRE) and Susuceptibility Weighted Imaging (SWI)

Stroke specifics

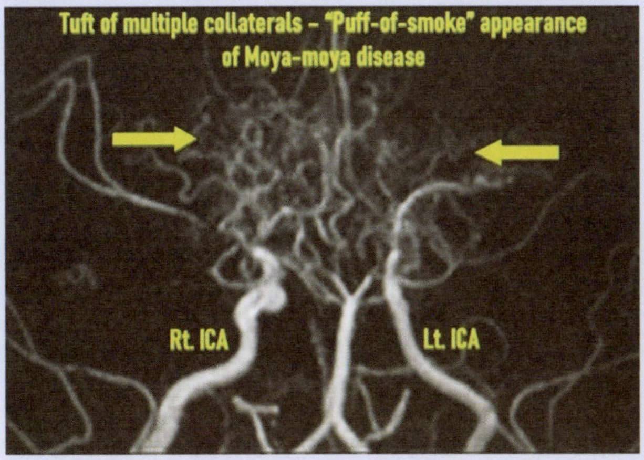

Moyamoya disease:

- Idiopathic arteriopathy, common in Japan - characterized by progressive narrowing of supraclinoid internal carotid artery.
- Gradual ICA narrowing leads to multiple small abnormal net-like collaterals seen on Digital Subtraction Angiography (DSA)—as if a **"Puff-of-smoke"**[Q] is rising up—hence, the name.

Contd...

Stroke specifics

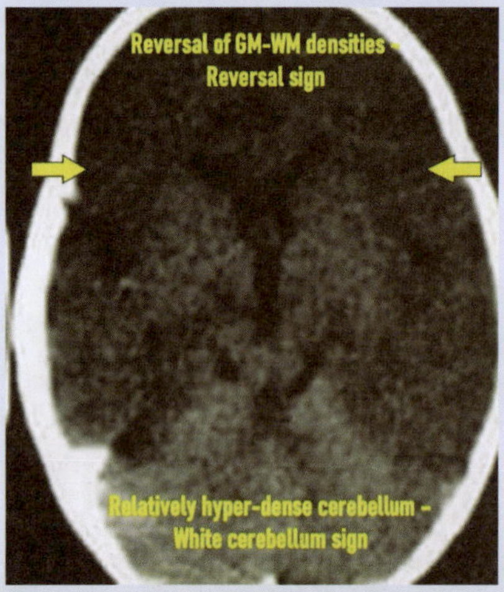

Global cerebral hypoperfusion/Anoxia

- Due to severe hypotension/cardiac arrest/ hypoxia/anoxia/CO poisoning.
- **Reversal sign**[Q]: Diffuse reversal of gray and white matter densities on.
- **White cerebellum sign**[Q]: Relative high density of the Cerebellum (and also the central gray matter nuclei) is maintained and appear brighter relative to the hypodense cerebrum on CT.

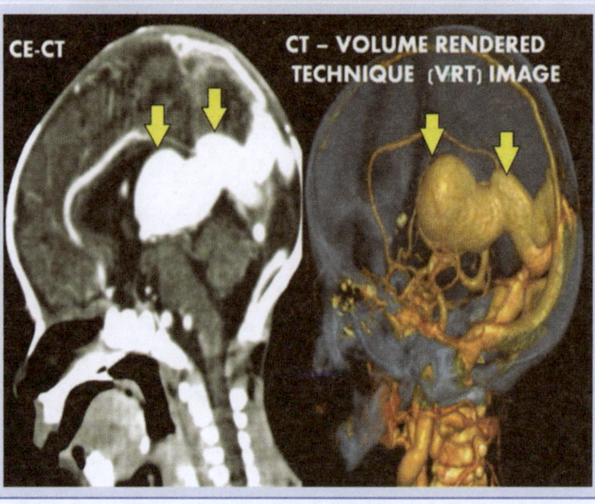

Vein of galen malformation

- A misnomer — actually involves the median prosencephalic vein (MPV) of Markowsky.[Q]
- Clinically — neonate/infant with hydrocephalus and high cardiac output failure — most common extracardiac cause of CHF in neonates[Q].

Head trauma imaging

CT brain – Diagnostic Protocol in Head Trauma Imaging

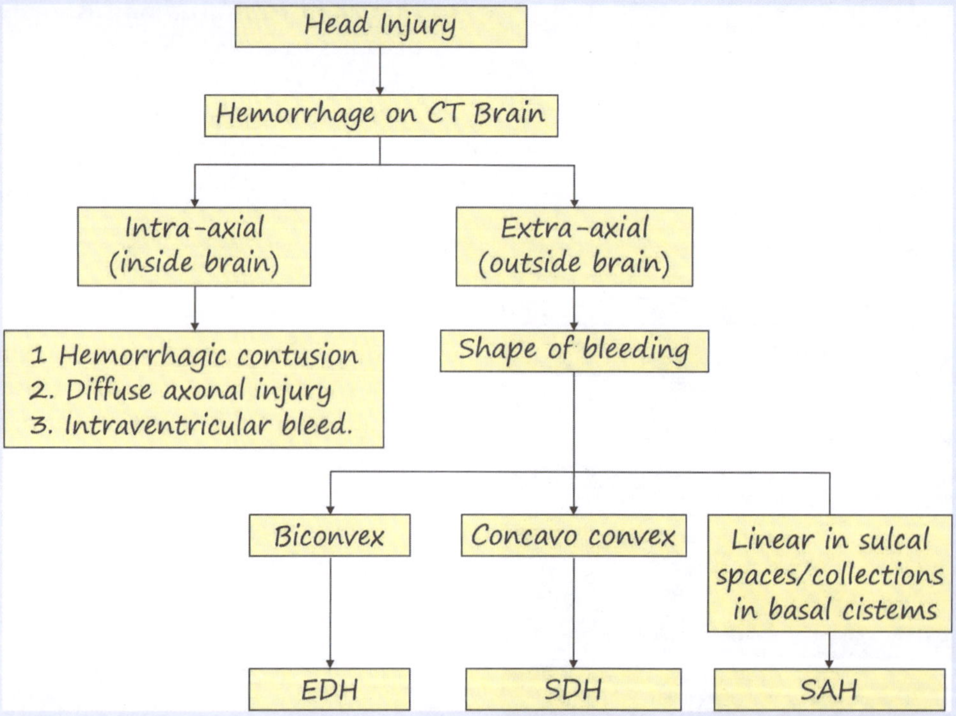

Extradural versus intradural bleed

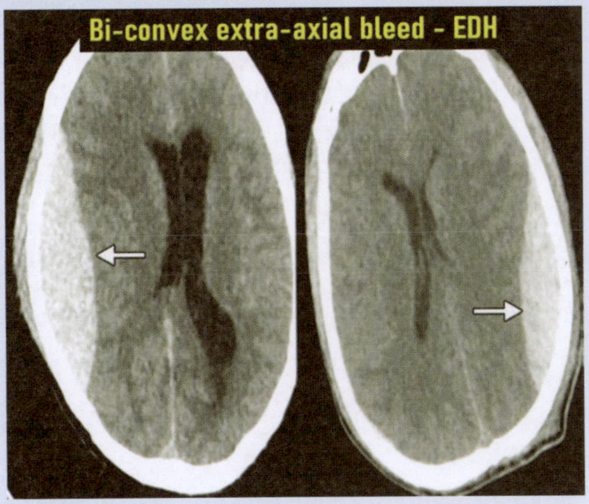

- Origin– Middle meningeal artery (MMA)[Q].
- Usually, associated with a skull fracture[Q] –the bone fragments cause damage to an MMA branch – results in EDH
- Clinically associated with lucid interval[Q] and talk-and-Die syndrome[Q]
- **Shape:** Typically Bi-convex[Q]/Lentiform[Q] in shape.
- Does not cross the cranial sutures.
- Not limited by venous sinuses – they can cross and elevate/displace venous sinuses.
- MRI is preferred in case of suspected spinal EDH[Q].

PYQ ALERT "FMGE JAN 2023 PATTERN"

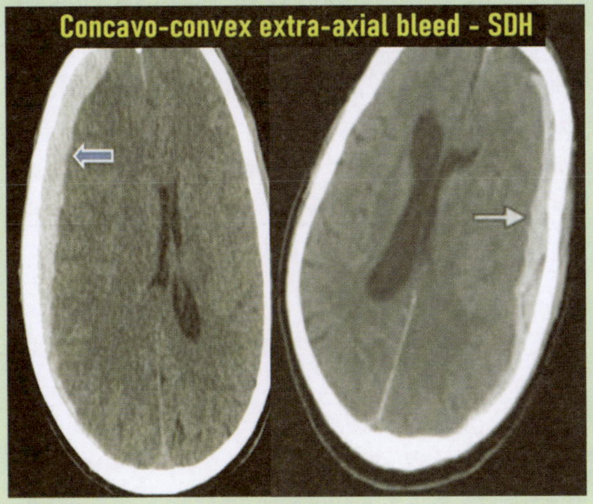

- Origin—Bridging cortical veins[Q]
- **Spontaneous SDH in the Elderly:** May be asymptomatic or present with mild headache or transient but repetitive neurological deficits—termed pseudodementia[Q].
- **Concavo-Convex shape**[Q]: Inner margin is concave, outer margin is convex.
- Not limited by cranial sutures but limited by dural folds like falx cerebri, falx cerebella, tentorium cerebelli
- SDH in neonates and infants should raise suspicion of Non-accidental injury/Battered baby syndrome[Q].

CT appearance of bleed overtime

Acute bleed	Sub-acute bleed	Chronic bleed
0 to 3 days from onset	**3 to 21 days from onset**	**>3 weeks from onset**
Acute hematoma – high density	Partially disintegrated clot – intermediate density	Completely disintegrated clot – low density
Acute bleed is hyperdense	**Sub-acute bleed is isodense**	**Chronic bleed is hypodense**
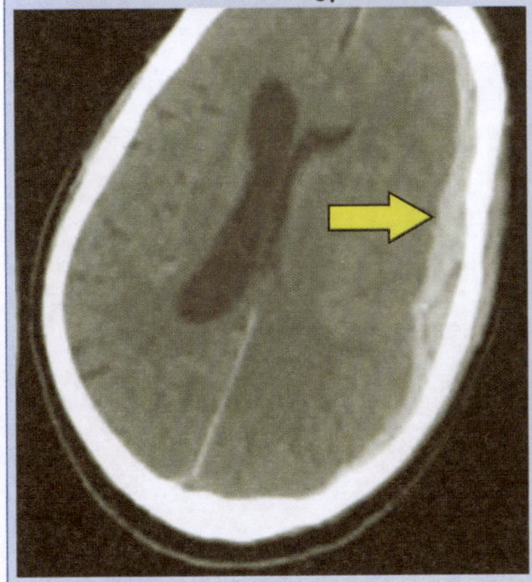	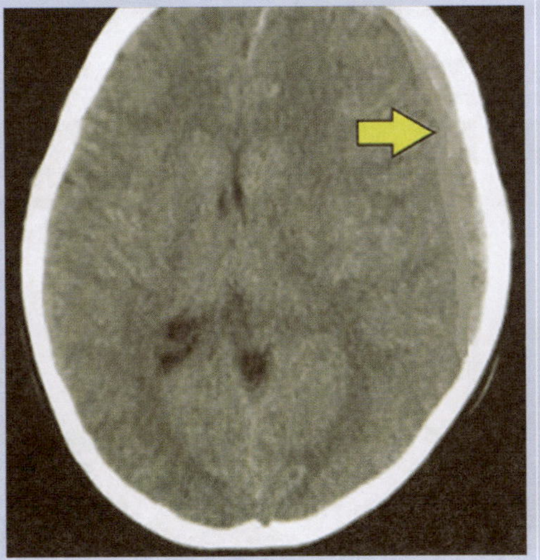	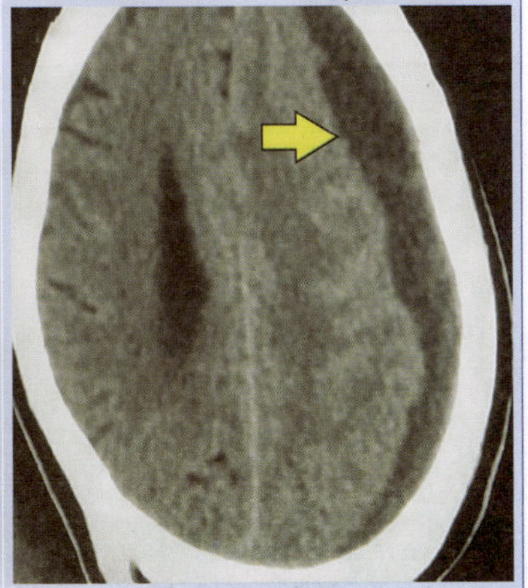

Diffuse Axonal Injury (DAI)

PYQ ALERT "INI-CET JULY 2021 PATTERN"

CLINICAL CLINCHER

History Clincher of DAI –

Head injury - with immediate loss of consciousness

↓

Early CT brain — normal/mild generalized cerebral edema

↓

Treated conservatively steroid/mannitol does not improve or many deteriorate

↓

Delayed MRI done for furthur investigation

↓

Diagnosis — diffuse axonal injury

- **What is DAI:**
  - Shearing stress/force exerted on the brain, caused due to rotational acceleration and deceleration forces—cause a neuron to break permanently at the junction of cell body and neurofilament.
  - So this, Axonal level injury[Q] occurring in a Diffuse manner[Q] is called as Diffuse Axonal injury!
- **IOC for DAI – MRI (GRE - Gradient Echo and SWI – Susceptibility Weighted Imaging)**
  - Small petechial bleeds seen mainly at three sites:
    1. Gray-White matter junction[Q]—Most common site[Q]—corresponds to the site of neuronal break/ discontinuity – Stage 1[Q]
    2. Corpus callosum[Q] – Stage 2[Q]
    3. Dorsolateral brainstem[Q] – Stage 3[Q]

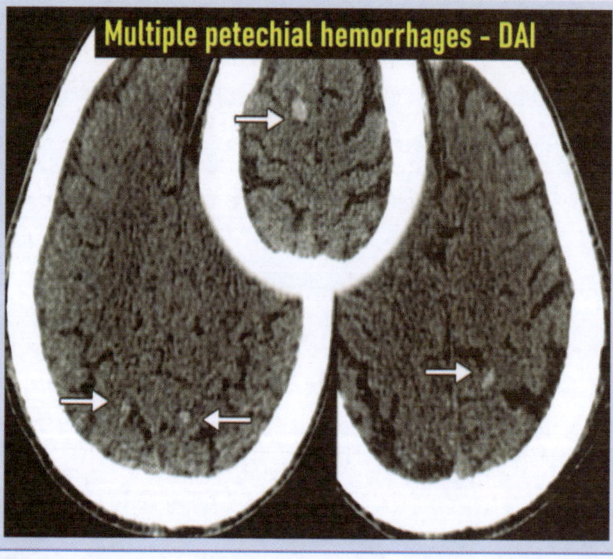

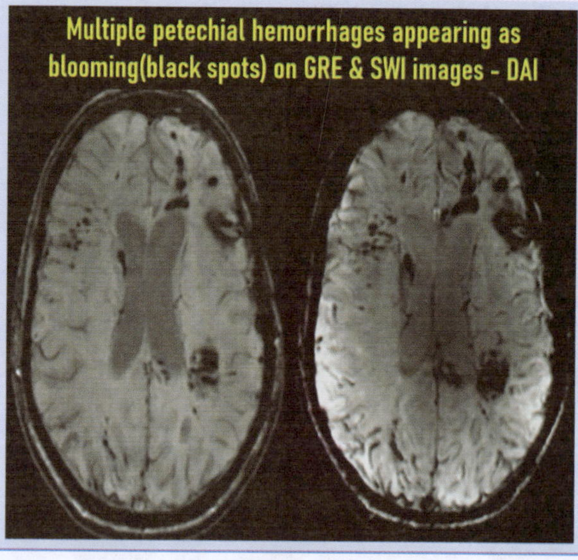

Head Trauma Miscellaneous

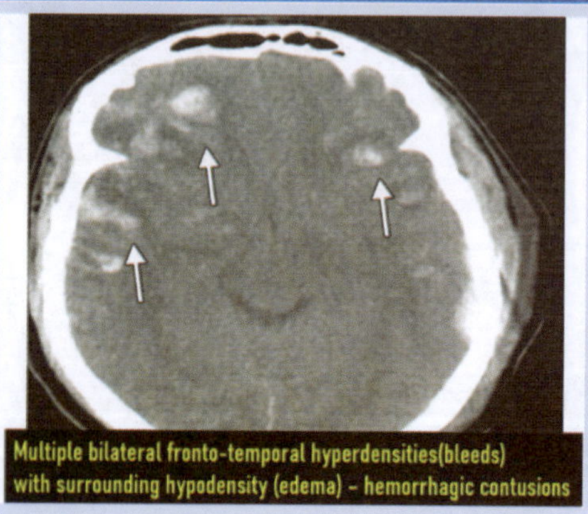

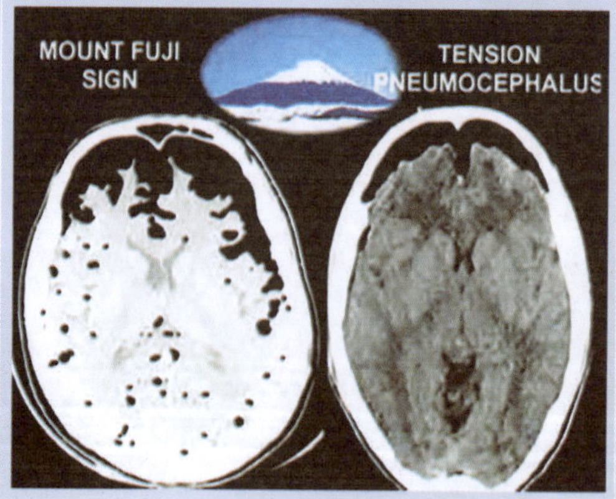

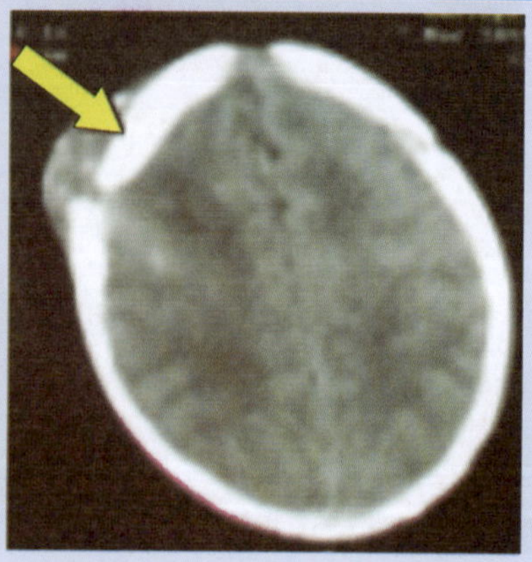

Contd...

Head Trauma Miscellaneous

Parenchymal contusions:

- May be hemorrhagic/ nonhemorrhagic.
- Seen in areas of brain close to rough bony surfaces, hence commonly seen in Orbitofrontal[Q] and temporal regions of brain[Q].

CT-ill-defined hyperdensities (blood) with surrounding hypodensities (peribleed edema)

Pneumocephalus- IOC is CT

- Suggests basal skull fracture with air coming from the paranasal sinuses.
- Tension pneumocephalus[Q] — Subdural air causes a mass-effect over the underlying brain parenchyma. **Mount Fuji sign**[Q]
- May separate and compress the frontal lobes, creating a widened interhemispheric space that mimics a picture of a volcano just like Mount Fuji in Japan.
- Treatment is emergent surgical decompression.

Growing skull fractures[Q]/ Craniocerebral erosion[Q] (leptomeningeal cysts[Q])

- Seen in children <3 years age[Q]
- Secondary to skull fractures causing dural tears allowing the leptomeninges and/or cerebral parenchyma to herniate into it.
- Pulsations from CSF erode the fracture margin, resulting in eventual expansion and nonunion.
- IOC-CT scan[Q]

Basic Approach to Brain Tumors

Intra-Axial tumors

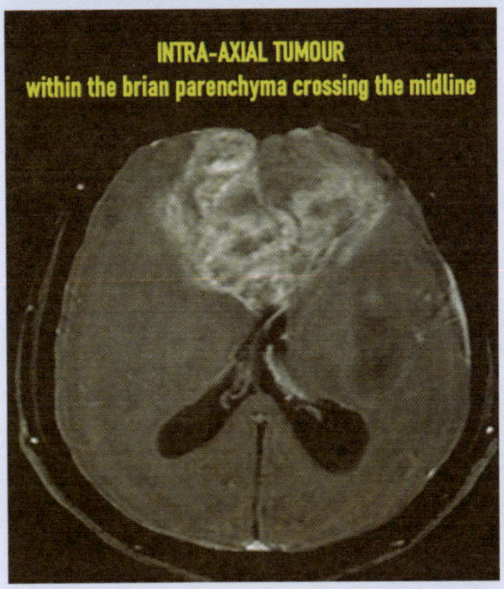

Extra-axial tumors

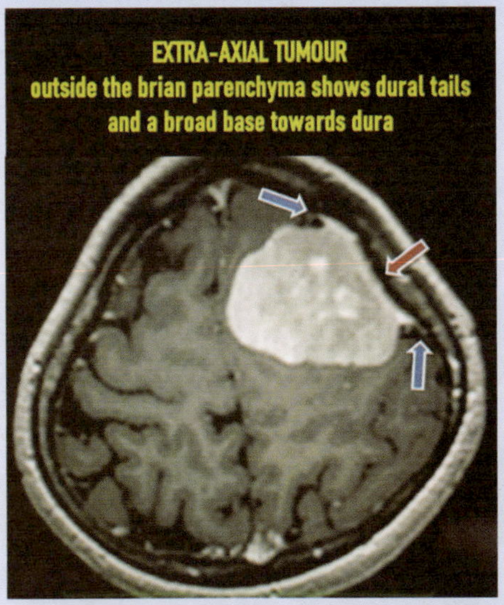

Location	Inside the brain parenchyma	Outside the brain parenchyma
Broad base toward dura	Absent	Present
Dural tail	Absent	Present
CSF cleft between tumor and brain parenchyma	Absent	Present
Cortical buckling	Absent	Present
Displacement of blood vessels	Absent	Present
Sclerosi/Scalloping of adjacent bones	Absent	Present

Location Clinchers

For your exam, when you see a tumor at a specific site—there is a specific and only 1 specific diagnosis!! This hold true for almost all the questions asked on this topic till date. So, why not use it as a **SMART-WORK** strategy and use to your advantage!!

Contd...

Cerebellopontine (CP) angle

- Most common tumor at CP angle is an Acoustic schwannoma[Q]/Vestibular schwannoma[Q].
- 2nd most common tumor is a Meningioma[Q].

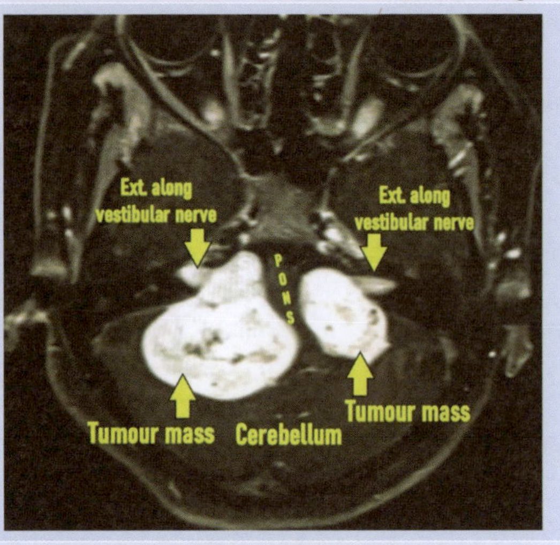

Acoustic shwannoma/Vestibular schwannoma-

- **Icecream-cone appearance[Q]:** Icecream is the mass in the CP angle cistern, cone is its extension into the internal auditory meatus.
- Bilateral Ac.schwannoma—is a clincher for Neurofibromatosis type 2[Q]/Multiple Inherited Schwannoma Meningioma and Ependymoma (MISME) syndrome[Q]

Sellar and Para-sellar region

- Most common tumor in children—Craniopharyngioma[Q].
- Most common tumor in adults—Pituitary macroadenoma[Q].

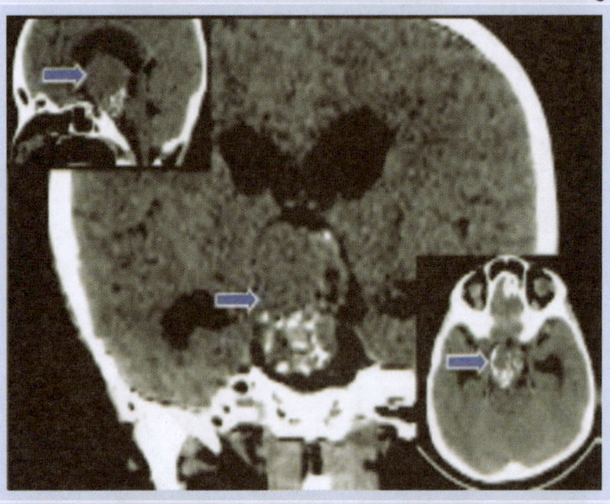

Craniopharyngioma

- Benign tumor derived from Rathke's pouch epithelium[Q]
- Solid-cystic, calcified suprasellar lesion in child[Q]—is diagnostic
- Compresses on the optic chiasma—results in typical bitemporal hemianopia[Q]

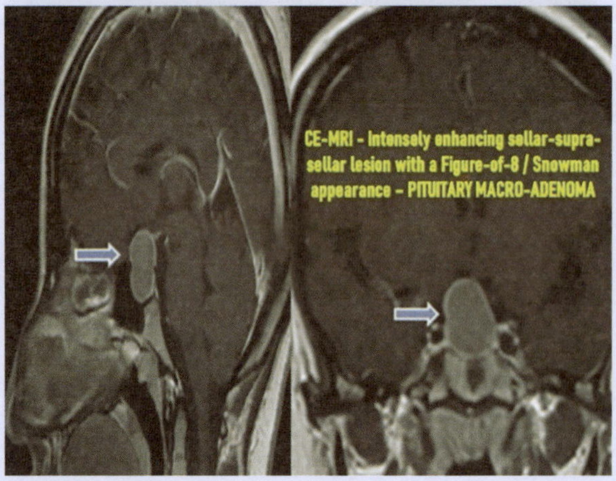

Pituitary macroadenoma

- >10 mm diameter[Q]
- Sellar mass without separate identifiable pituitary gland
- Snowman[Q] or figure-of-eight[Q] appearance
- Intense enhancement

Pituitary microadenoma

- <10 mm diameter[Q]
- Intrapituitary lesion that enhances less rapidly than normal pituitary[Q]
- Dynamic contrast enhanced MRI[Q] is used for diagnosis

Intra-ventricular tumors:

- Tumors seen in the lateral ventricles — Central neurocytoma, Choroid plexus papilloma, Ependymoma
- Tumors seen in the 4th ventricle — Ependymoma, Medulloblastoma

Contd...

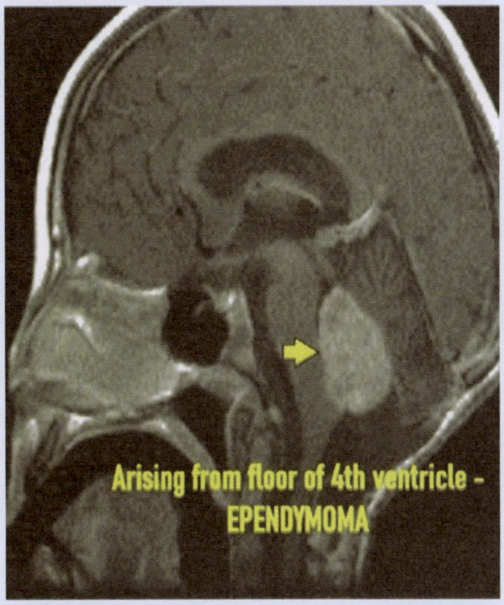

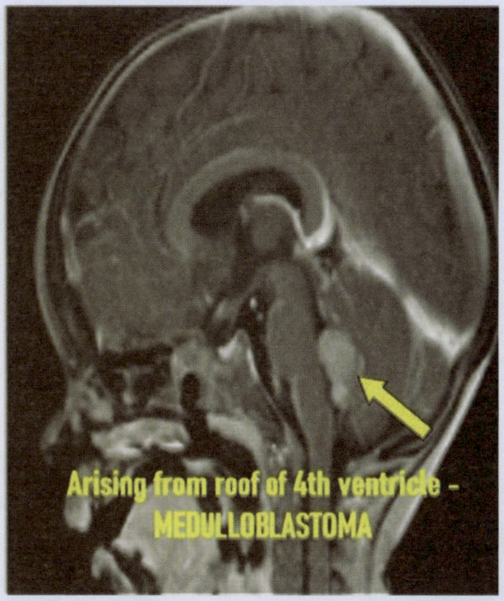

Ependymoma

- Most common site – 4th ventricle[Q] plastic tumor[Q] – squeezes out through 4th ventricle into CSFcisterns
- Arises from floor of 4th ventricle[Q]

Medulloblastoma/Primary Neuroectodermal Tumor-MB (PNET – MB)[Q]

- WHO Grade IV tumor
- Most common tumor of posterior fossa in children[Q]
- **Site of origin:** Roof of 4th ventricle[Q] from superior medullary velum – appears as a solid 4th ventricle mass causing hydrocephalus
- **High cellularity:** Hyperdense on NC-CT[Q]
- **Zuckerguss[Q]:** Cake icing like deposits on brain surface due to CSF metastasis

Glial tumors

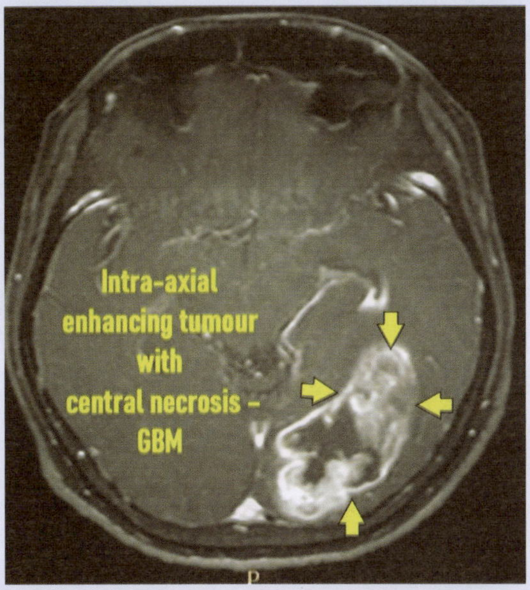

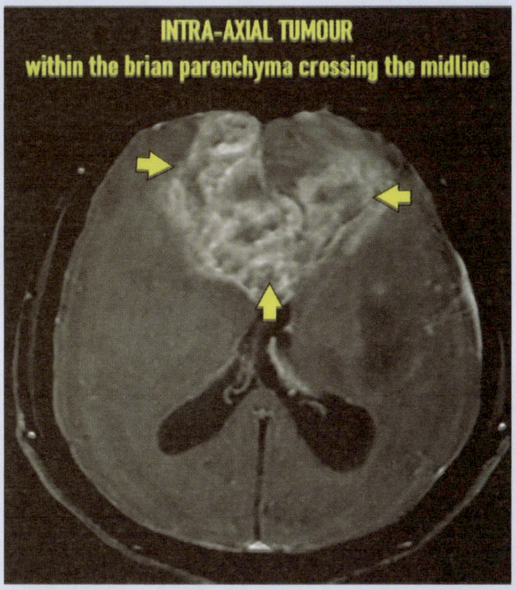

Glioblastoma multiforme (GBM)/WHO Grade IV Glioma:

- Most common primary intracranial neoplasm in adults[Q]
- Worst prognosis[Q]
- Tumor necrosis[Q]—hallmark finding of GBM
- Butterfly glioma[Q]—tumor spreading across the corpus callosum to involve the contralateral lobe

Contd...

Oligodendroglioma

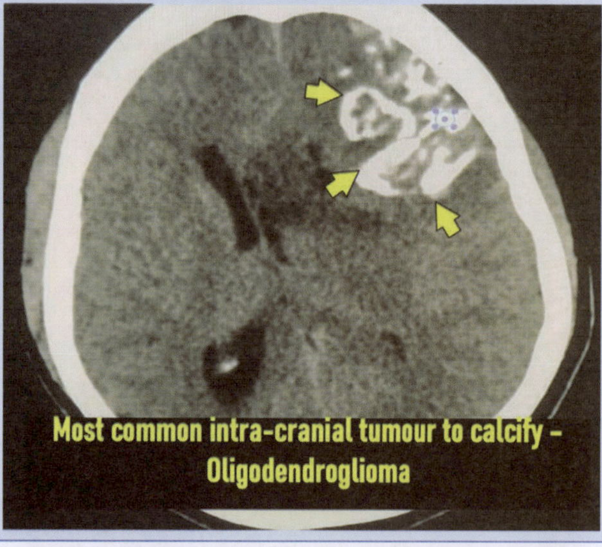

- Most commonly involves frontal lobe, involving the cortex[Q] and subcortical white matter
- Calcification[Q] in the tumor – important diagnostic feature – may be ribbon-like, central or peripheral

Miscellaneous tumors

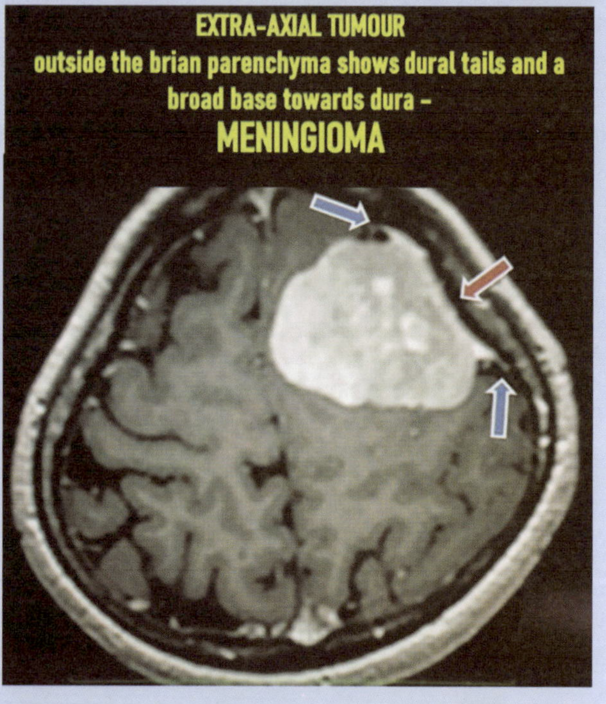

Meningioma:

- Most common primary nonglial tumor[Q]
- Dural-based intensely enhancing extra-axial mass lesion
- Hyperdense on NC-CT[Q]
- **Dural tails[Q]:** Tapered portion toward the dural surface – suggest a dural origin
- **Mother-in-law sign on angiography[Q]:** Enhancement is like a mother-in-law—comes early in life and stays put for a long time....hope you get it!!
- Associated with hyperostosis of skull[Q]
- **Pneumosinus dilatans[Q]:** Associated with enlargement of paranasal sinuses
- Sun-burst/spoke-wheel pattern of vessels[Q] on angiography
- Elevated Alanine[Q] on MR spectroscopy
- **May be associated with NF2[Q]:** MISME syndrome[Q]—multiple inherited schwannomas-meningiomas and ependymomas

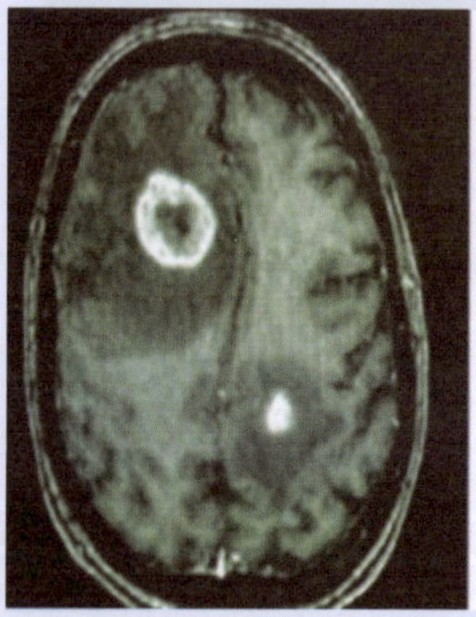
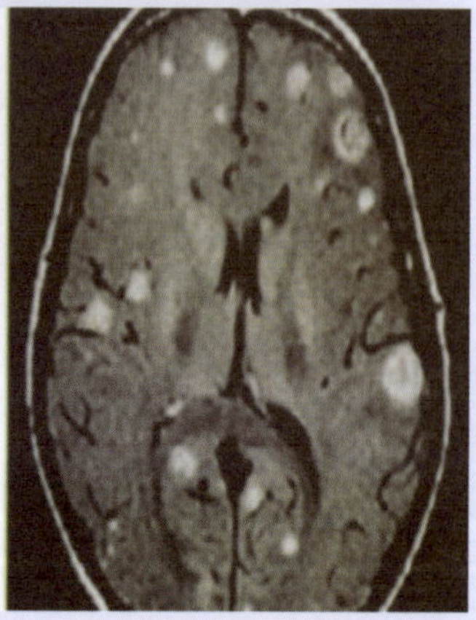

Brain metastases:

- Most common brain tumor in adults[Q]
- Most common Primary tumors — Lung[Q] > Breast > Melanoma
- Melanoma metastases – appear T1 hyperintense[Q]

Contd...

Miscellaneous tumors

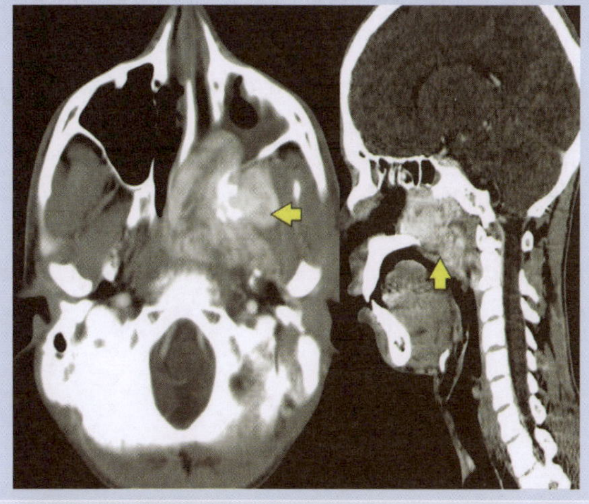

CLINICAL CLINCHER

Juvenile Nasopharyngeal Angiofibroma (JNAF)

- Adolescent male
- C/o epistaxis
- Intensely enhancing mass at Spheno-palatine foramen
- Seen exclusively in adolescent males^Q
- Hollman-Miller sign^Q Mass pushes the posterior wall of the maxillary sinus anteriorly
- MRI – salt and pepper appearance^Q due to flow voids of blood vessels

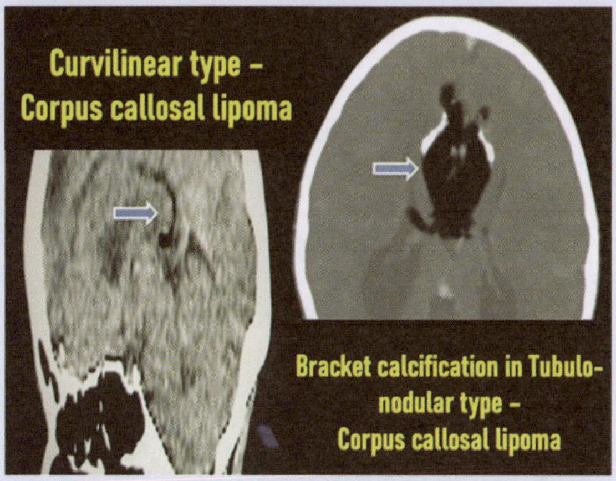

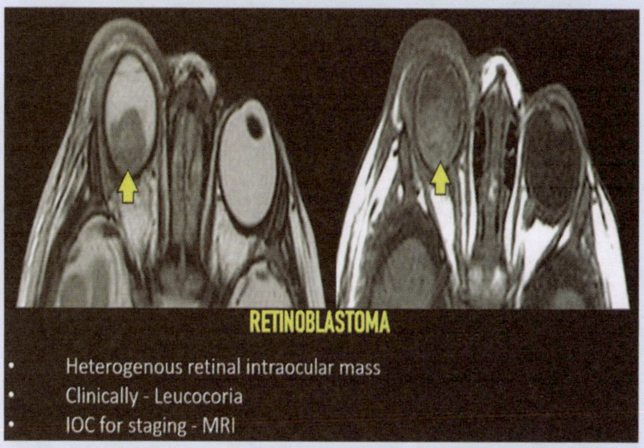

Familial brain tumor syndromes/phakomatoses

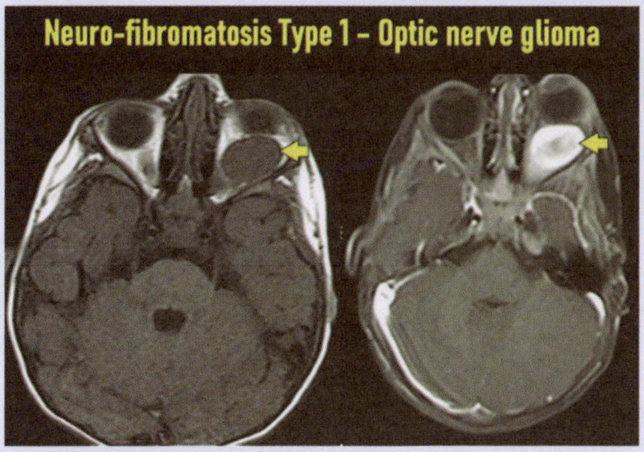

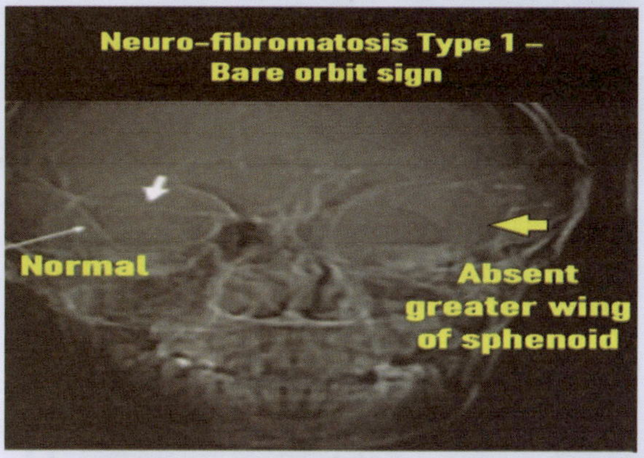

Neurofibromatosis type 1/Peripheral NF – Most common phakomatosis^Q

- Multiple variable sized Neurofibromas – all over body
- CNS features:
  - **Focal areas of signal intensity (FASI)**^Q: Areas of T2/FLAIR hyperintensity in deep white matter and basal ganglia or corpus callosum^Q, with no contrast enhancement^Q
  - **Optic nerve glioma**^Q: CT/MRI — central globular enlargement of the optic nerve^Q.
  - Sphenoid wing dysplasia^Q which gives the **Bare orbit sign**^Q – due to absent innominate line^Q – due to greater wing of sphenoid dysplasia^Q
  - Dural ectasia^Q
- Skeletal features – Kyphoscoliosis^Q + Posterior vertebral scalloping + Ribbon rib deformity^Q + Rib notching^Q + Tibial pseudoarthrosis^Q

Contd...

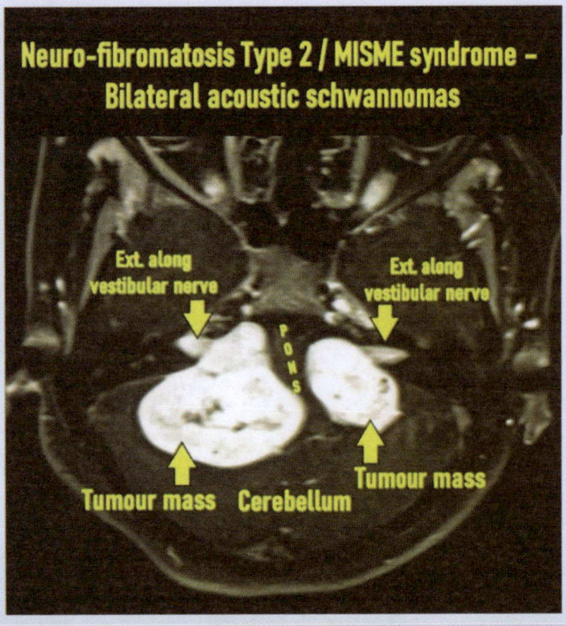

Neurofibromatosis type 2(NF2) Central multiple inherited schwannomas, meningiomas, and ependymomas (MISME)[Q]

- **Meningioma[Q]:** No specific location but they can be multiple.
- **Schwannomas[Q]:** Bilateral vestibular schwannoma[Q] – most common. Show ice-cream on a cone appearance[Q]
- **Ependymoma:** Most commonly spinal intramedullary location.

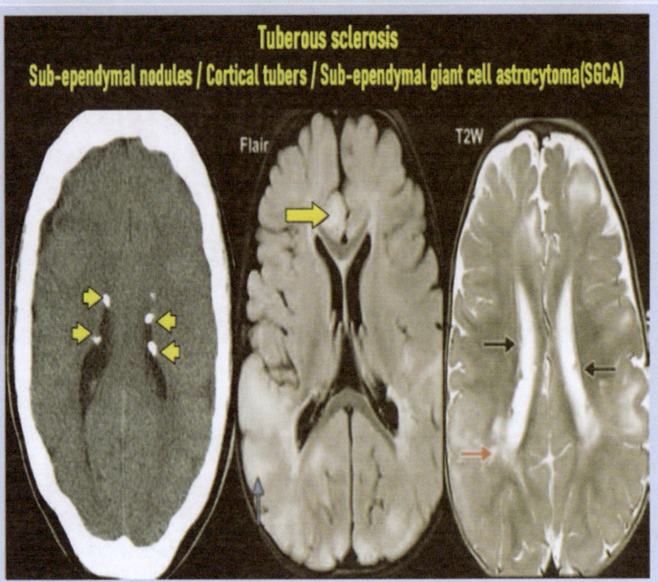

Tuberous sclerosis:

CNS

- Cortical/subcortical tubers[Q]: Most common in frontal lobe.
- White matter abnormalities[Q]
- Subependymal hamartomas[Q]
- Subependymal giant cell astrocytomas (SGCA)[Q] — Pathognomonic for TS[Q]
- Retinal phakomas

Abdomen

- Renal angiomyolipoma – Cysts – RCC – Oncocytomas.
- Retroperitoneal lymphangioleiomyomatosis
- Gastrointestinal polyps

Thorax

- **Lymphangioleiomyomatosis (LAM)[Q]:** Presents as cysts of uniform size involving lung parenchyma
- **Cardiac rhabdomyomas[Q]:** Seen in 40–80% of patients with TS

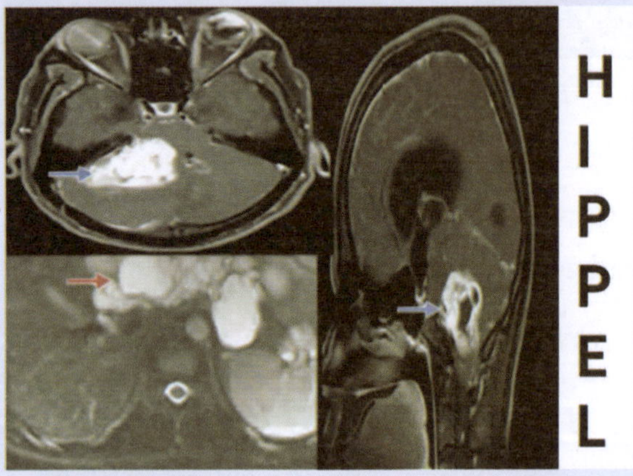

Von Hippel Lindau syndrome—remember using the Mnemonic HIPPEL

- H – Hemangioblastoma[Q] of retina/spine/cerebellum
- I – Increased risk of RCC[Q]
- P – Pneochromocytoma[Q]
- P – Pancreatic lesions[Q] – cysts/cancer cystadenomas
- E – Epididymal papillary cystadenoma[Q]
- L – Liver/renal/pancreatic cysts

Contd...

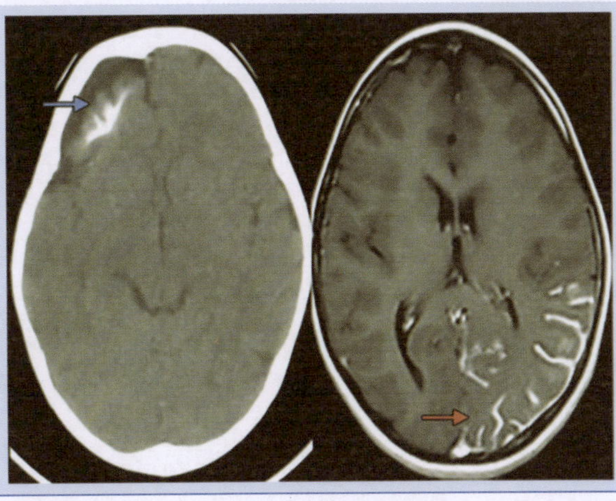

Sturge-Weber syndrome/Encephalotrigeminal Angiomatosis

- Facial port wine stains[Q] and pial angiomas
- X-ray—Gyriform cortical calcification
- CT Scan—Subcortical calcification—**Tram track sign**[Q]
- MRI—Intense Leptomeningeal/Gyriform enhancement[Q] in affected area.

CNS INFECTIONS

Parenchymal infections

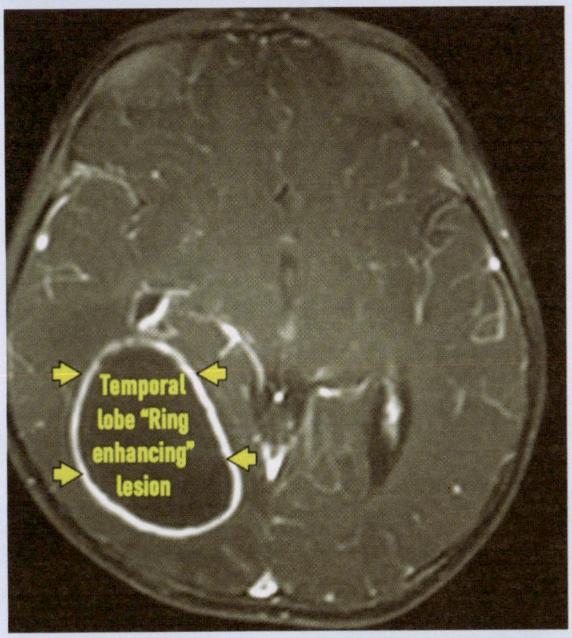

PYQ ALERT "NEET-PG 2021 PATTERN"

Brain abscess

- Site of abscess may point toward the cause:
  - Frontal lobe abscess – may result from frontal sinusitis[Q]
  - Temporal lobe/Cerebellar abscess – from Otitis media/Mastoiditis[Q]
  - Blood borne spread – usually involves middle cerebral artery territory – frontoparietal lobe
- Ring enhancing lesion[Q] on Contrast CT/MR
- Restricted diffusion on DWI[Q]
- MR Spectroscopy: Central area will show abundant lactate, acetate, alanine, succinate, etc.

CLINICAL CLINCHER

Clinical approach to ring-enhancing lesions

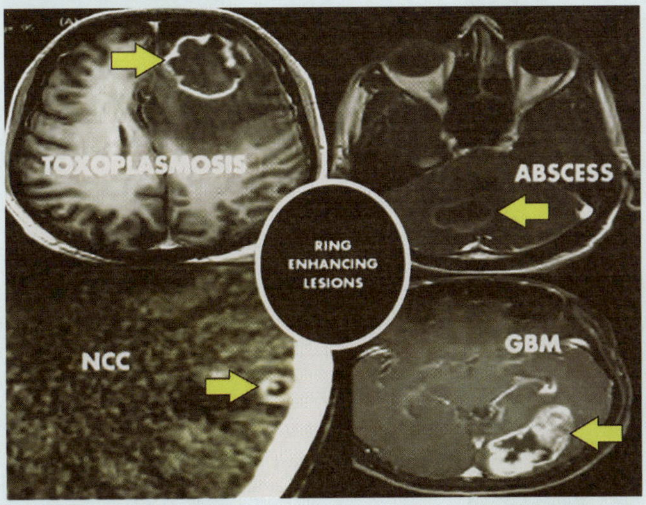

Let's try a clinical-integrated approach to ring lesions in brain

Clinical profile	Imaging findings	Diagnosis
• Fever, headache, seizures • K/c/o pulmonary TB • Signs of meningitis	• Diffuse basal enhancing exudates • Disc/Ring-enhancing lesions • Hydrocephalus	**Tuberculoma/TB meningitis**
• Headache • Seizures	Ring-enhancing lesion with an eccentric dot within – Cyst with a dot sign[Q]	**Neurocysticercosis**
• Young/middle-aged patient with CSOM/Chronic ear discharge • Fever, headache, altered sensorium	• Temporal lobe ring enhancing lesion • Signs of meningitis	**Brain abscess**
• HIV positive patient • Fever, malaise, headache	• Ring enhancing lesion in basal gangla/ Grey-white junction • Target sign/Concentric/Eccentric target sign	**Toxoplasmosis**
• Middle aged/Elderly • Focal deficits, Seizures	Irregular ring enhancing lesion with thick peripheral enhancing rim and central necrosis	**Glioblastoma multiforme (GBM)**
• Elderly patient • K/c/o Ca lung/Ca breast/ Melanoma • Seizure/Focal deficits	• Single/Multiple ring/diffusely enhancing lesions at GM-WM junction • Surrounding edema	**Metastases**

Other miscellaneous ring lesions:

- Sub-acute infarct (peripheral leucocyte infiltration central infarction)
- Cerebral Contusion
- AIDS
- Lymphoma in immunocompromised patient (in immunocompetent patient, it shows homogenous solid enhancement)
- Demyelination (peripheral inflammation)
- Radiation necrosis (peripheral inflammation, central necrosis)

Neurocysticercosis (NCC):

- Caused by infection due to the pork tapeworm Taenia solium[Q]
- Cerebral convexity subarachnoid spaces – most common site[Q]
- 4th ventricle—most common intraventricular site[Q]

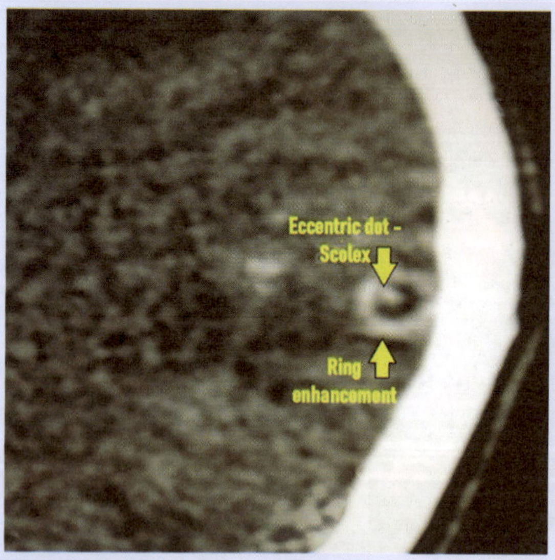

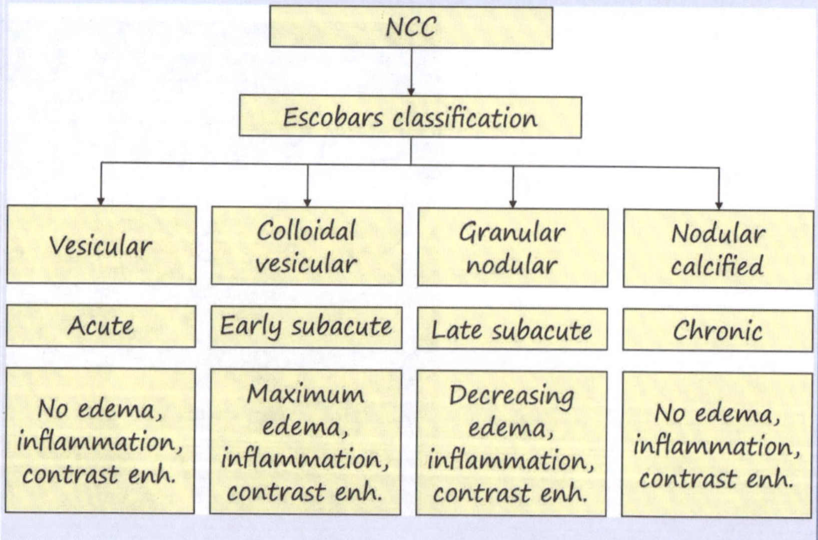

Miscellaneous infections

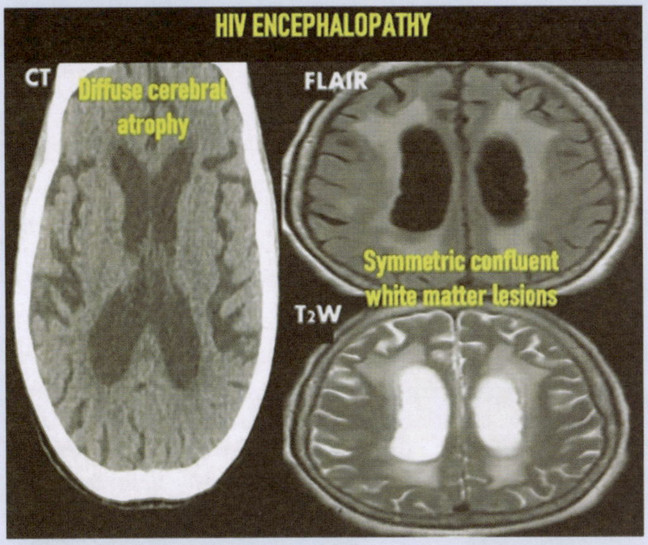

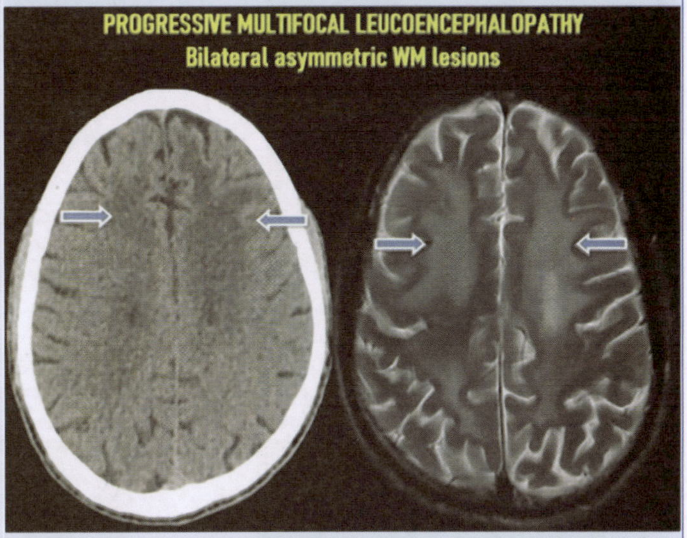

HIV Encephalopathy/HIV associated dementia

- Presents clinically as subcortical dementia with slowness, forgetfulness and apathy.
- MRI[Q] – is IOC
- Cerebral atrophy — most common imaging finding[Q].
- Symmetric confluent white matter lesions seen in the periventricular and centrum semiovale white matter[Q].

Progressive Multifocal Leukoencephalopathy (PML)

- Central demyelinating disease resulting from the reactivation of a latent infection of oligodendrocytes by John Cunningham (JC) polyomavirus[Q], seen in HIV patients
- MRI is best investigation[Q]
- Multifocal, asymmetric bilateral white matter lesions, most commonly in parieto-occipital regions, seen as high signal on T2W image and low signal on T1W image
- Scalloped appearance of lesions[Q] — due to extension up to subcortical U-fibers

Leukodystrophies—Dysmyelinating disorders which typically, although not invariably, affect children

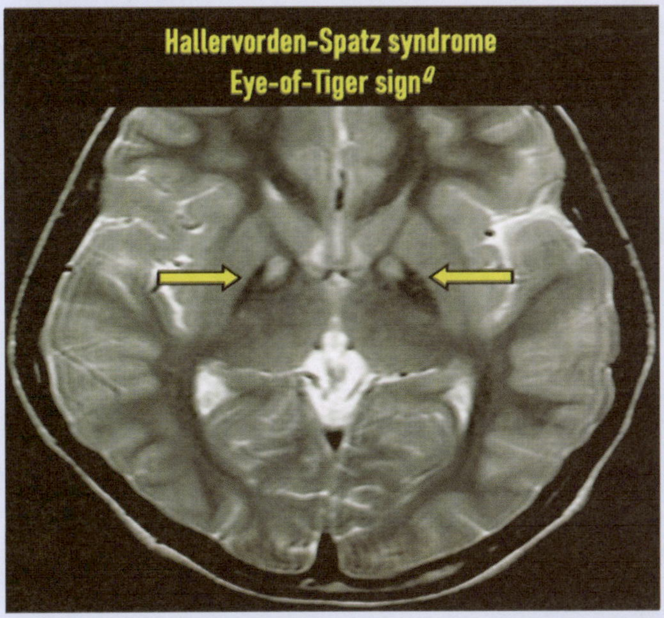

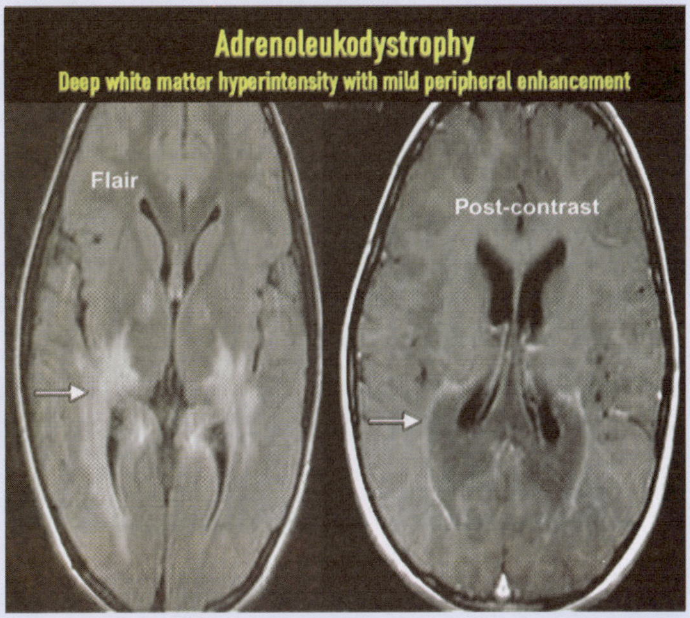

Multiple sclerosis acquired chronic relapsing demyelinating disease involving CNS

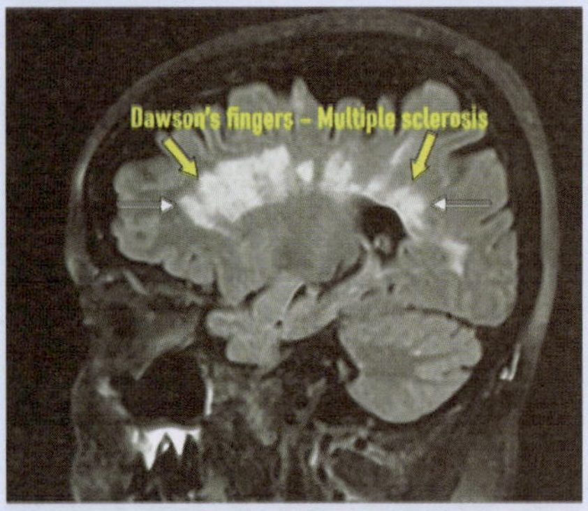

- IOC - MRI with contrast[Q]
- White matter lesions (WML)[Q] with involvement of corpus callosum[Q], U-fibers, temporal lobes, brainstem, cerebellum and spinal cord
- MRI: T1—Black holes[Q]
- Venus necklace[Q]: It is formed due to small holes at the callososeptal interface[Q]
- T2: Regions of high signal, with surrounding edema
- FLAIR: Dawson's fingers[Q] are the WML propagating centrifugally along the medullary venules and arranged perpendicular to the lateral ventricles in a triangular configuration
- Ependymal dot-dash sign[Q]

CNS Spotters

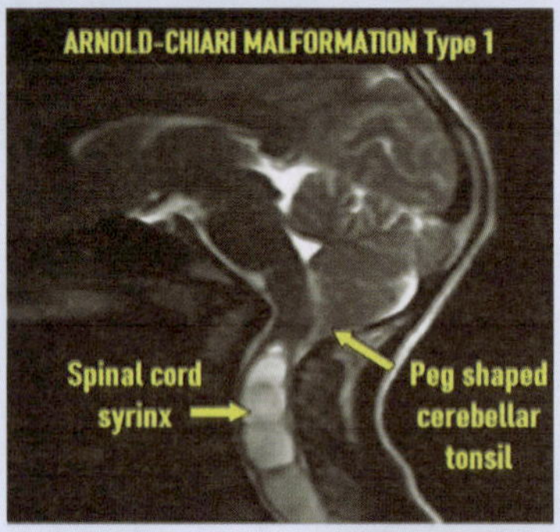

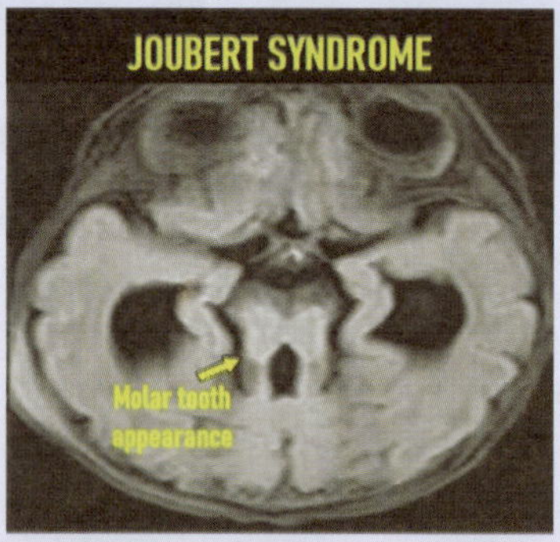

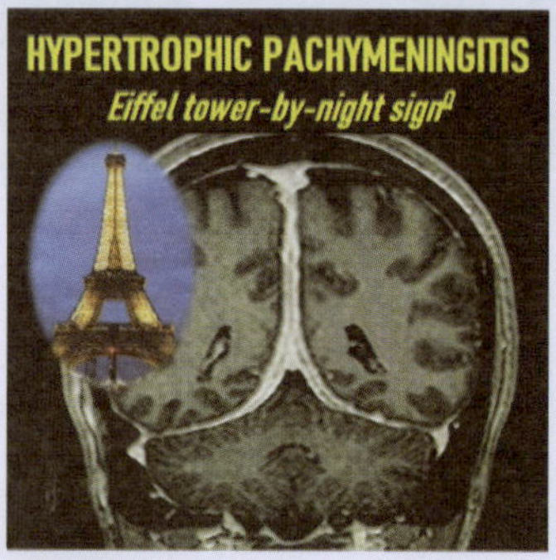

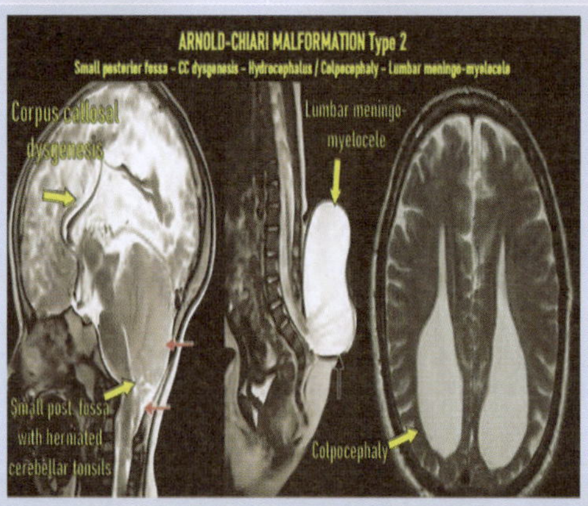

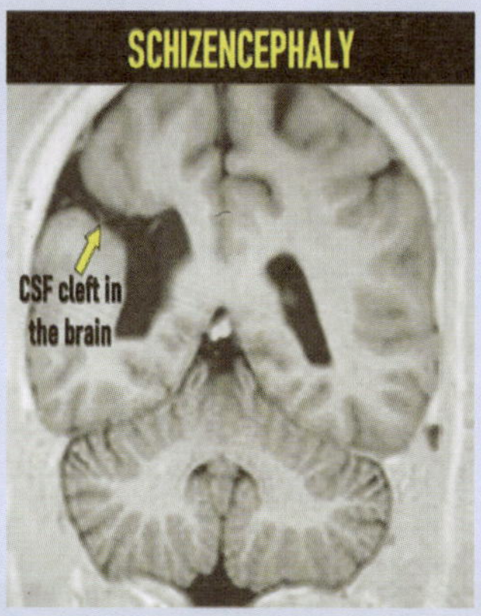

PYQ ALERT "FMGE JUNE 2022 PATTERN"

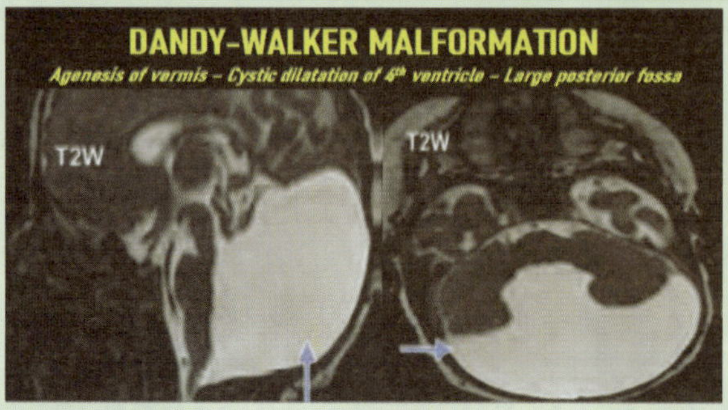

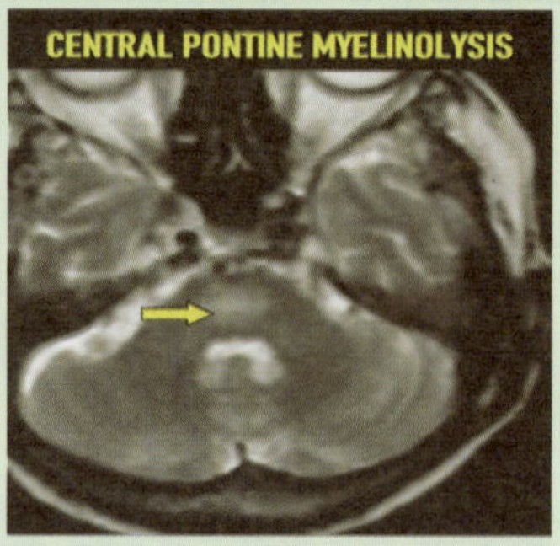

Signs of raised Intracranial tension (ICT)

- Sutural diastasis[Q]/Widening of sutures[Q]: Earliest finding[Q] of raised ICT
- Copper beaten[Q]/Silver beaten appearance[Q] of skull/Increased convolutional markings[Q]
- Widening and erosion of sella turcica[Q]/Truncation of dorsum sella
- Lacunar skull[Q]/Membranous transformation of skull[Q]
- Pineal gland displacement across midline – suggesting midline shift[Q]

8. WOMEN'S IMAGING

BREAST IMAGING

Mammography—IOC for Screening of Breast Cancer[Q]

- Uses characteristic spectrum[Q] radiation
- Anode in mammography X-ray tube is made of molybdenum[Q]
- Most common anode-filter combination is molybdenum-rhodium combination[Q]
- Mammography screening results in 15-20%[Q] reduction in mortality due to breast cancer
- Radiation exposure in bilateral mammography—3.7–4.7 μGy[Q]

Mammography – craniocaudal view (CC)

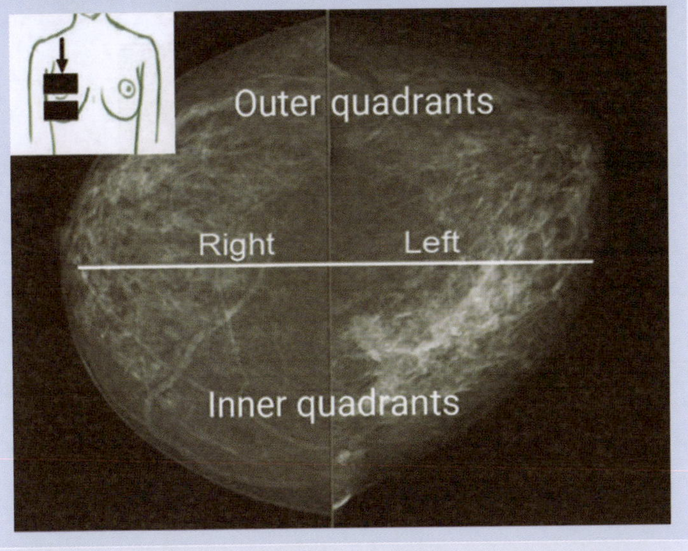

Mammography–mediolateral-oblique view (MLO)

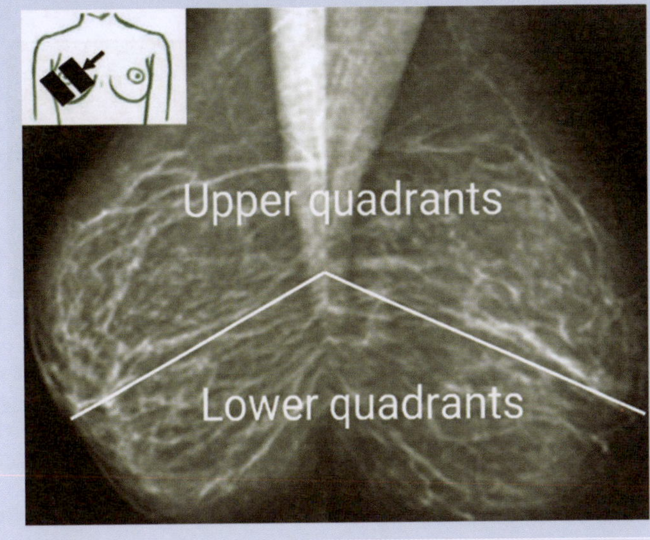

Timing of mammography screening—most recent guidelines

American Society of Breast Surgeons' Recommendations for Breast Cancer Screening—2019

Formal clinical risk assessment at – 25 years[Q]

Risk category	Risk factor	Recommendation
Women with higher than average risk	Hereditary susceptibility from pathogenic mutation carrier status Prior chest wall irradiation in age 10–30 years	Start screening at 25 years[Q] Start with MRI annually[Q] Shift to mammography screening at 30 years age[Q]
Women with higher than average risk	Predicted lifetime risk >20% by any model Strong family history – 1st degree relatives affected	Annual screening with mammography starting at 35 years[Q]
Women with average risk	None of the above risk factors	Women with Nondense breasts — Annual screening with mammography starting at 40 years[Q] Women with dense breasts—Consider supplemental imaging[Q]

BENIGN VERSUS MALIGNANY LESIONS

Feature	Benign lesions	Malignant lesions
Shape and margins	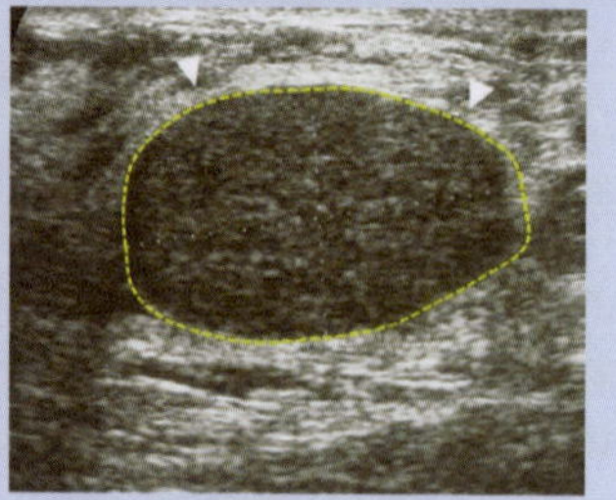 Oval—Wider than taller Smooth, No lobulations/ spiculations	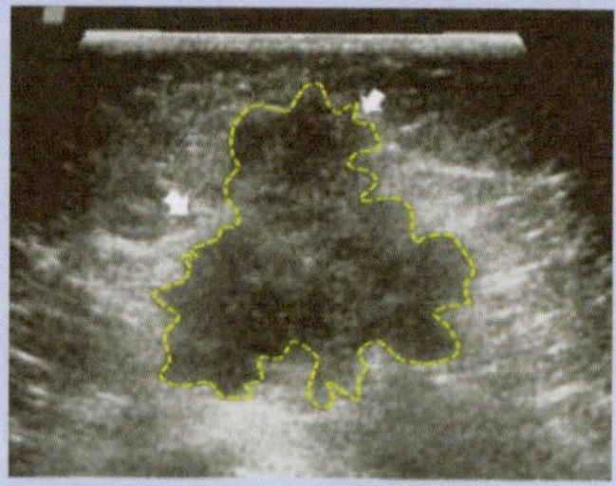 Irregular shape—taller than wider Irregular margins with lobulations and spiculations
Calcifications	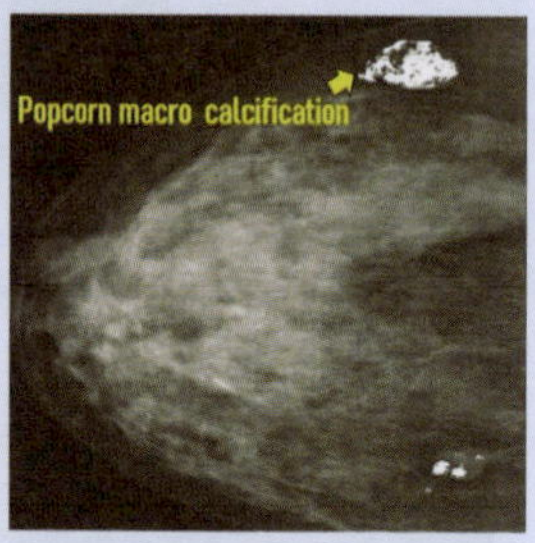 Macrocalcifications Typical popcorn calcifications are seen in involuting fibroadenoma[Q]	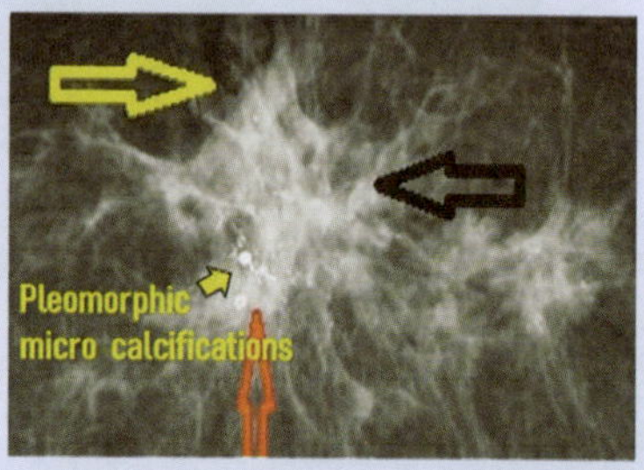 Pleomorphic microcalcifications
Architectural distortion	Absent	Present
Echogenic halo	Absent	Present

Breast Imaging Reporting and Data system (BI-RADS):

- Designed to standardize breast imaging reporting and to reduce confusion in breast imaging interpretations.
- It can be applied to mammography, ultrasound and MRI of the Breast.
- The latest version classifies lesions into the following seven categories:

Category		Management	Likelihood of cancer
0	Need additional imaging or prior examinations	Recall for additional imaging and/or await prior examinations	Not Applicable
1	Negative	Routine screening	0%
2	Benign	Routine screening	0%
3	Probably benign	Short interval-follow-up (6 months) or continued	>0% but <2%
4	Suspicious	Tissue diagnosis	4a. Low suspicion for malignancy (>2% to ≤10%) 4b. Moderate suspicion for malignancy (>10% to ≤50%) 4c. High suspicion for malignancy (>50% to <95%)
5	Highly suggestive of malignancy	Tissue diagnosis	≥95%
6	Know biopsy proven	Surgical excision when clinical appropriate	Not applicable

Breast MRI/dynamic contrast enhanced breast MRI:

- Overall best imaging technique for Ca breast
- Most sensitive investigation for ductal carcinoma in situ (DCIS)

Noncontrast MRI images → Gadolinium injected rapidly using a pressure injector → Rapid image acquisition done for 5–6 minutes → Dynamic enhancement curves are plotted

Type 1 curve – Benign lesions

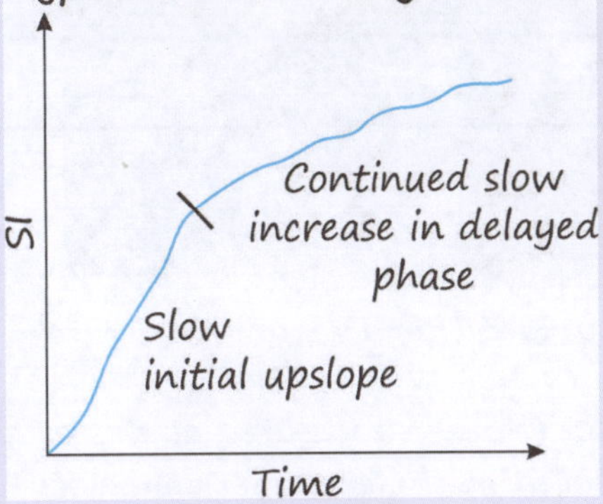

Type 2 curve – Indeterminate lesions

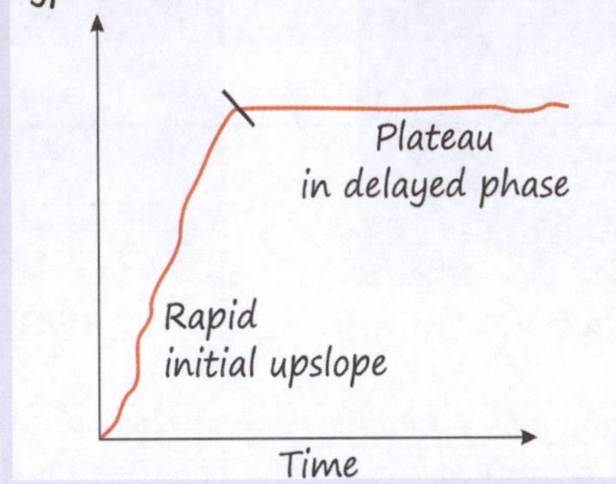

Type 3 curve – Malignant lesions

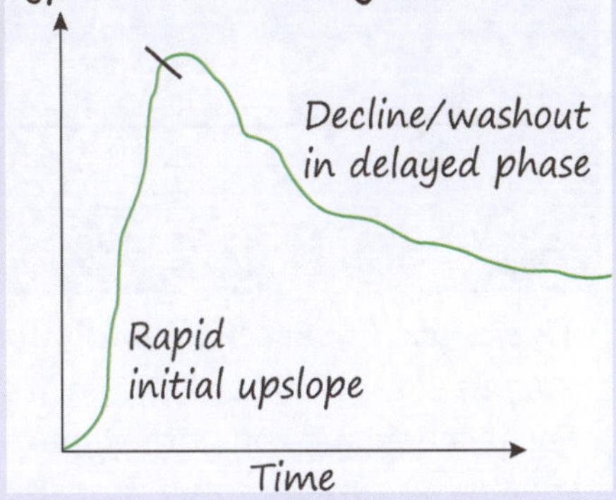

BREAST IMAGING SPECIFICS

Fibroadenolipoma/breast hamartoma

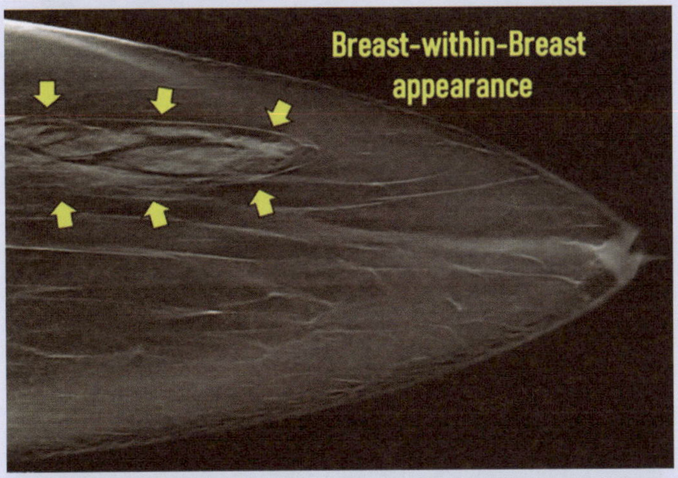

Breast implant – intracapsular rupture

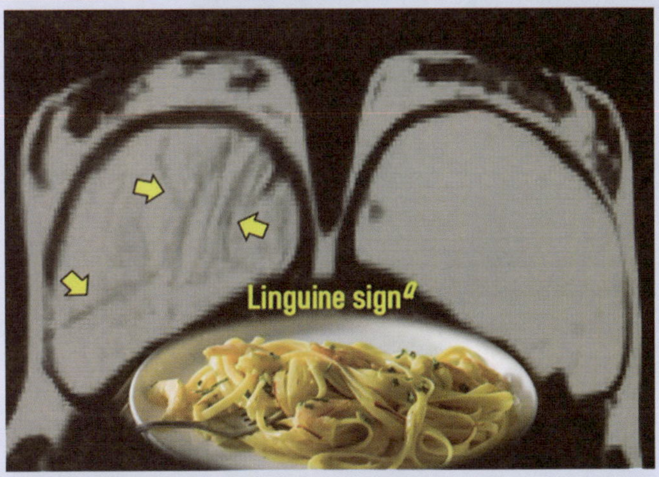

Digital breast tomosynthesis

Multiple 2D Projections

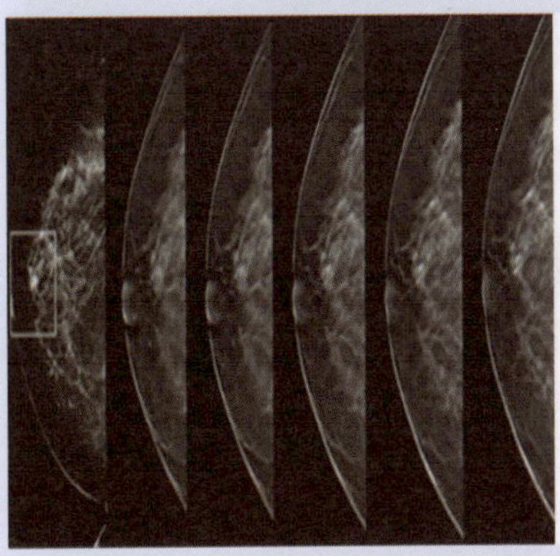

- Volumetric reconstruction of breast tissue
- Multiple slice images obtained
- Higher sensitivity for small breast lesions
- Similar radiation exposure

Breast Elastography

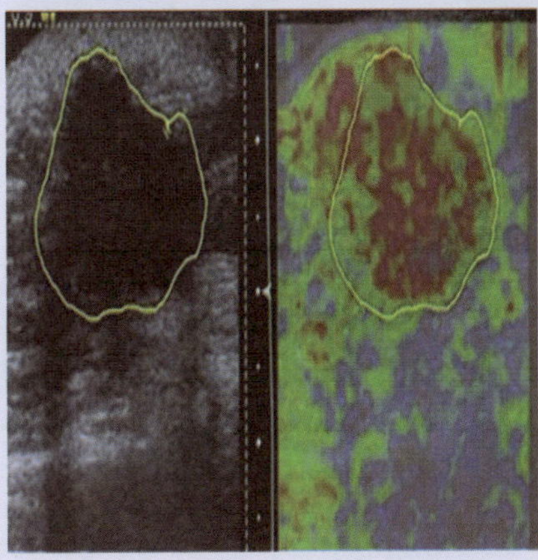

- Estimates hardness/ elasticity of tissues
- Strain elastography shear wave elastography
- Benign – more elastic Malignant – less elastic
- Breast/liver/thyroid

OBSTETRIC IMAGING

Early Pregnancy Imaging

Landmark findings in early pregnancy

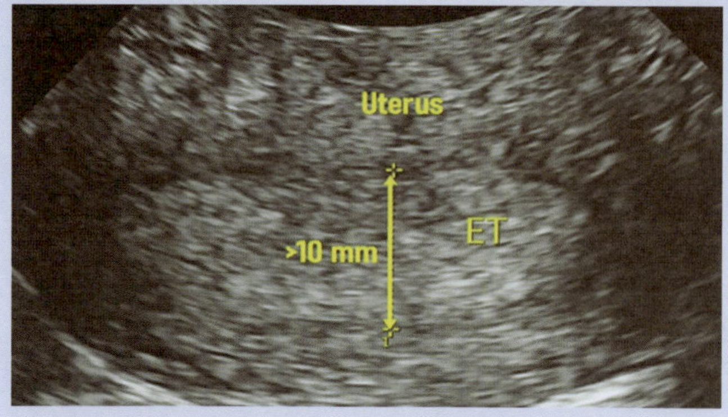

- Thickened hyperechoic endometrium >10 mm
- Corpus luteum in either ovaries
- Focal echogenic zone at implantation site – bright spot in endometrium – nonspecific finding
- Gestational sac not seen

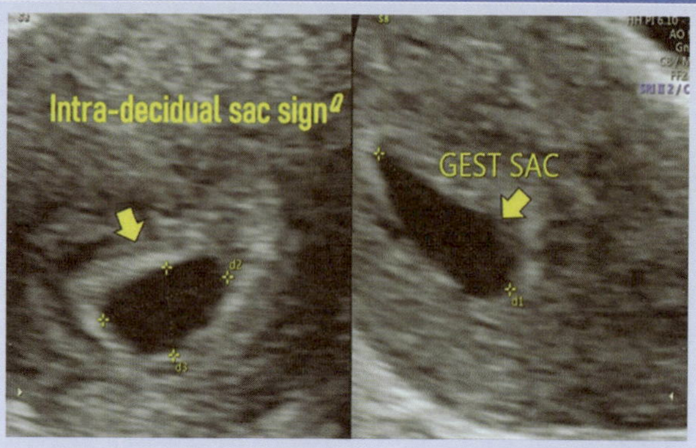

- Seen at 4w0d to 4w3d on TVS and at 5w0d on TAS
- Mean sac diameter (MSD) is measured at this stage
- Eccentrically located in the endometrial cavity
- Thin single hyperechoic rim of chorionic tissue around it
- No contents seen inside the sac

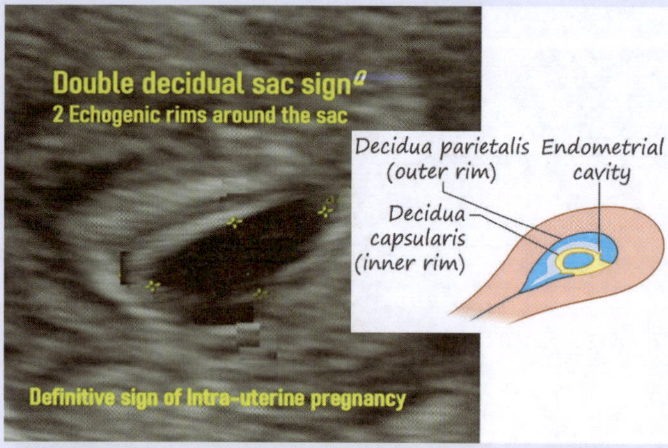

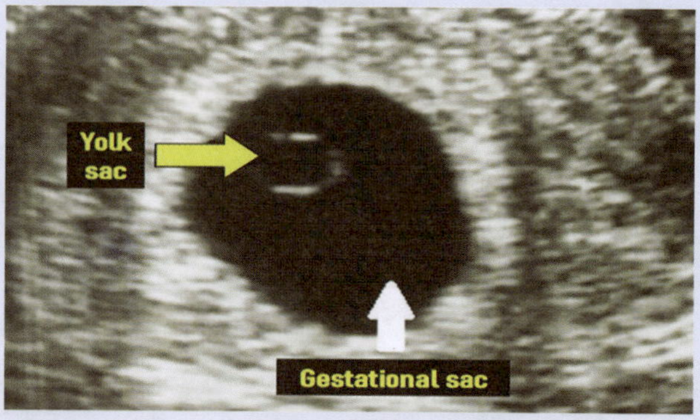

- Yolk sac – 1st structure seen within gestational sac
- Seen at 5w0d on TVS and at 5.5 weeks on TAS
- Yolk sac determines amnionicity of pregnancy[Q]

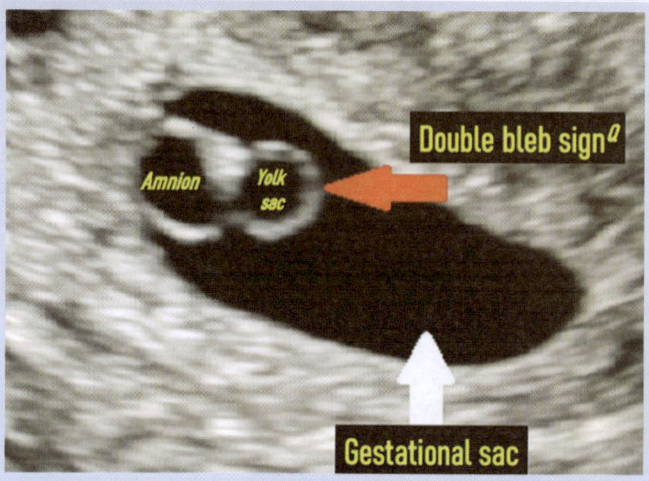

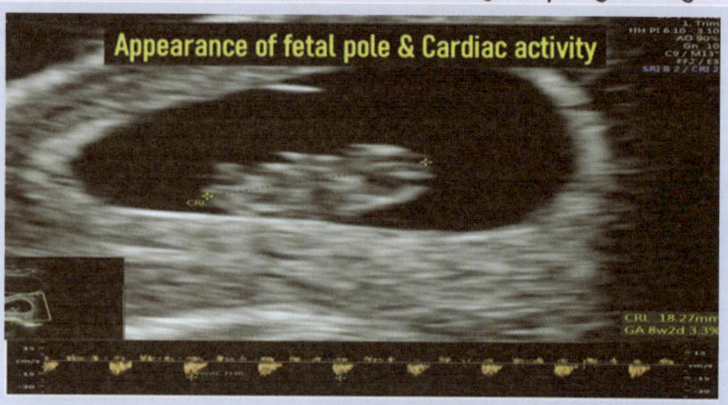

- Embryo and cardiac activity seen
- Crown rump length (CRL) is measured
- Seen at 5–6 weeks on TVS and at 6–7 weeks on TAS
- Fetal heart rate always >100 bpm

Contd...

Landmark findings in early pregnancy

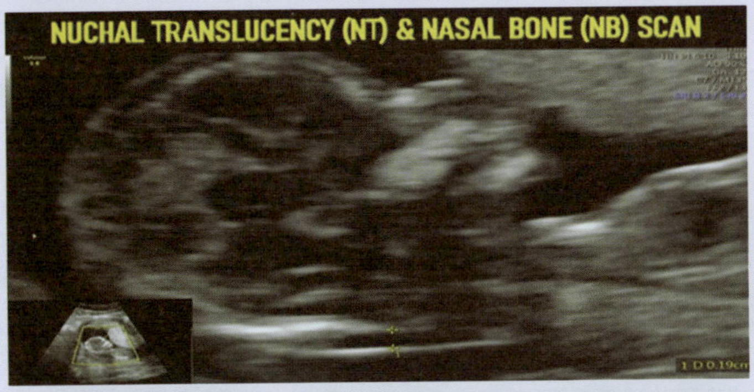

- To be done only when CRL is between 45 mm and 84 mm
- A translucency at nuchal region (back of neck) is measured
- Screening test for aneuplodies-trisomy 21/18/13
- If fetus has aneuploidy/turnor syndrome/ cardiac disease – NT is increased
- Combined test = NT scan + double marker blood test – has higher sensitivity

CLINICAL CLINCHER

Best parameter for Dating of gestation in 1st trimester	Crown rump length (CRL)[Q]
Best parameter for Dating of gestation in 2nd trimester	Biparietal diameter (BPD)[Q] > Head circumference (HC)[Q]
Best parameter for Dating of gestation in 3rd trimester	Femur length (FL)[Q]
Overall best time for dating of gestation	1st trimester[Q]
Overall best parameter for dating of gestation	Crown rump length (CRL)[Q]
Overall best parameter for estimation of birth weight (IUGR/macrosomia)	Abdominal circumference (AC)[Q]

OBSTETRIC IMAGING SPECIFICS

DIchorionic pregnancy

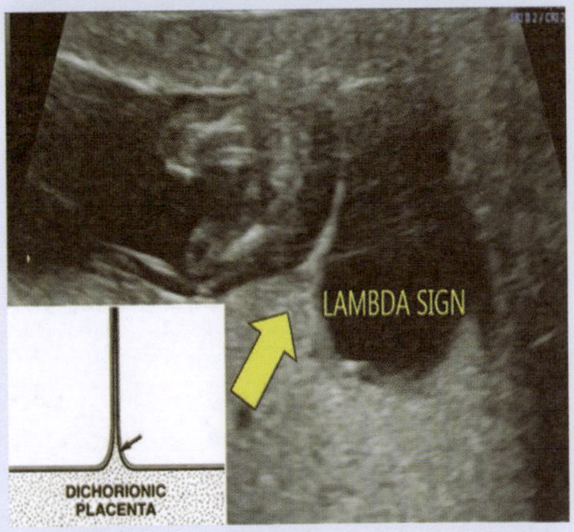

Twin peak sign[Q]/Lambda sign[Q]

Monochorionic pregnancy

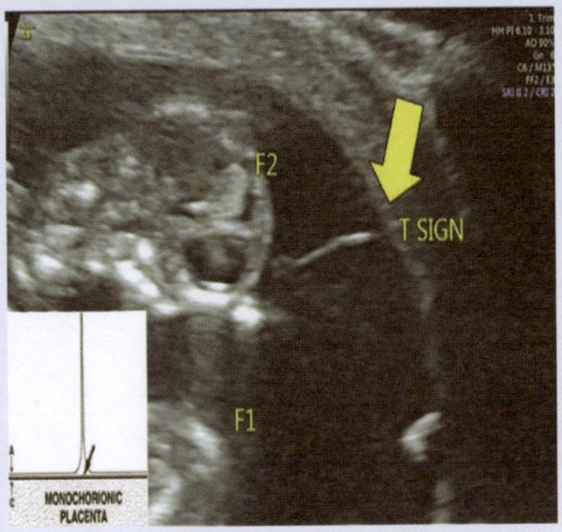

T sign[Q]

Anencephaly

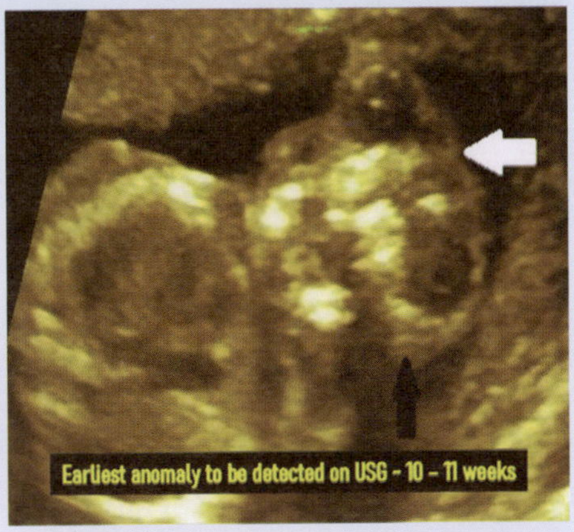

Mickey mouse sign[Q]/Frog eye appearance[Q]

GYNECOLOGY IMAGING

Hysterosalpingography (HSG) Spotters

Left sided cornual tubal block

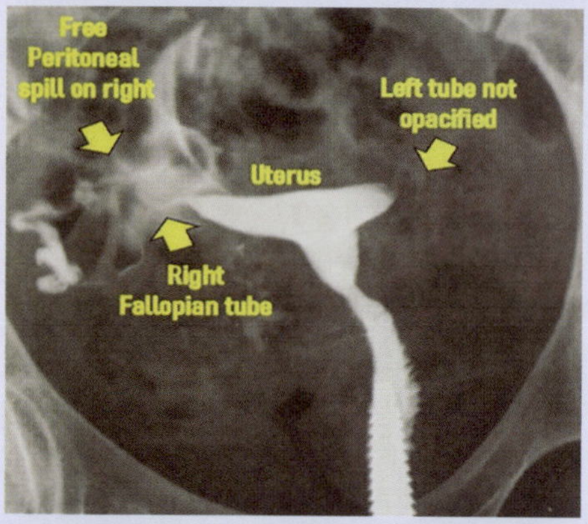

Unicornuate uterus

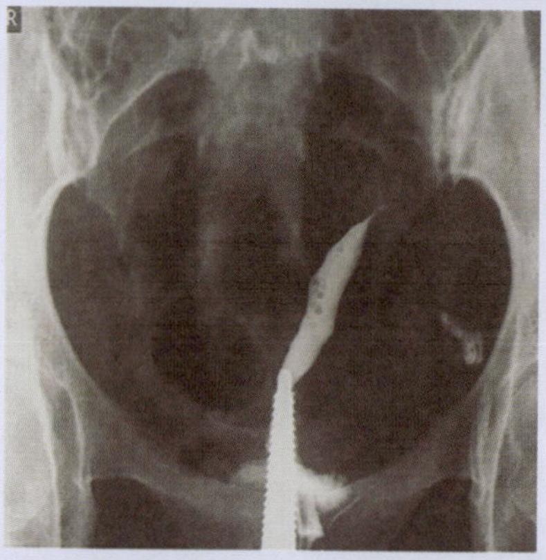

Bicornuate uterus

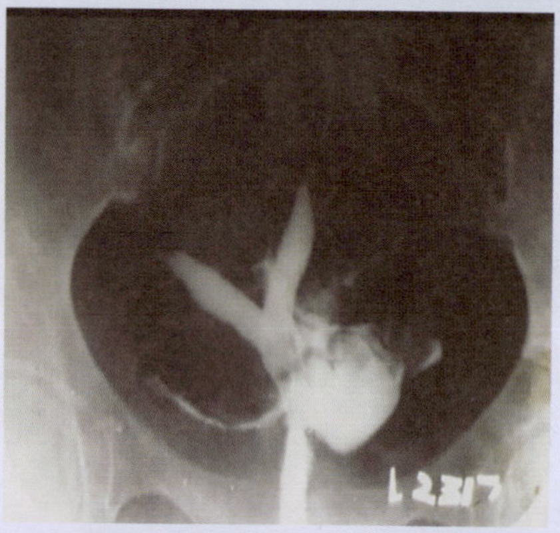

Bilateral hydrosalpinx

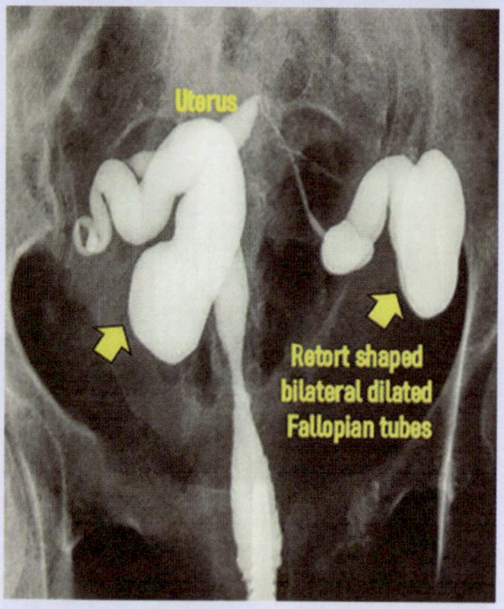

Arcuate uterus

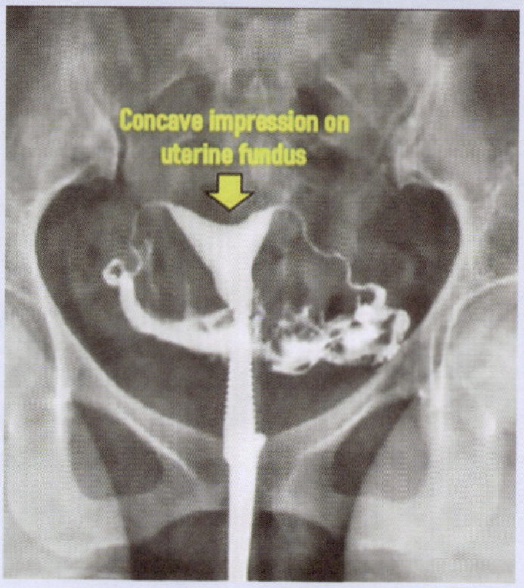

Uterine synecha/adhesion

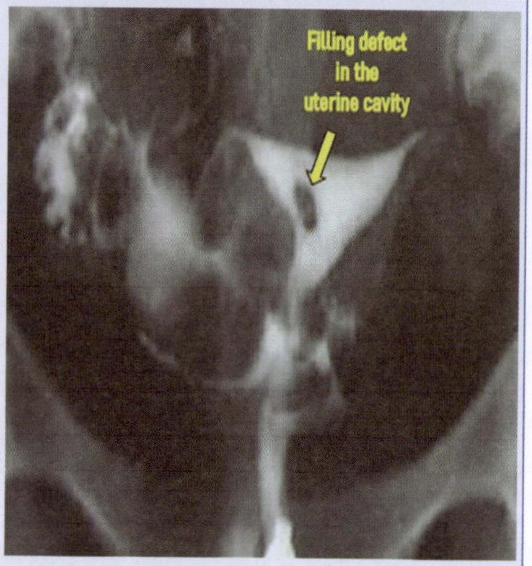

9. RADIONUCLIDE IMAGING AND RADIOTHERAPY

How do Radionuclide scans/Nuclear medicine scans work?

Specific radioactive agent injecting IV

↓

Gets localized to target organ and emits radiation

↓

This emitted information is read using a gamma camera

Radionucilde scan factuals

Planar Scintigraphy[Q]	• Signals emerging from patient's body are measured by using gamma cameras in ONE plane[Q] only. • Has limited sensitivity and resolution.
Single Photon Emission Computed Tomography[Q] (SPECT)	• Gamma cameras/detectors placed in a ring around the patient's body, so that a tomographic image acquisition is done like in CT • Better sensitivity and resolution
Standard-Uptake-Value (SUV)[Q]	• SUV[Q] = Activity per unit mass of tissue/ Injected Activity per unit body mass • The cut off between benign and malignant lesion/nodule is in the SUV range of 2.0-2.5[Q]. **Many infectious and inflammatory processes will also have high SUV**

Positron emission tomography (PET) scan: Used for diagnosis/staging/assessing response to treatment/ recurrence of Cancer

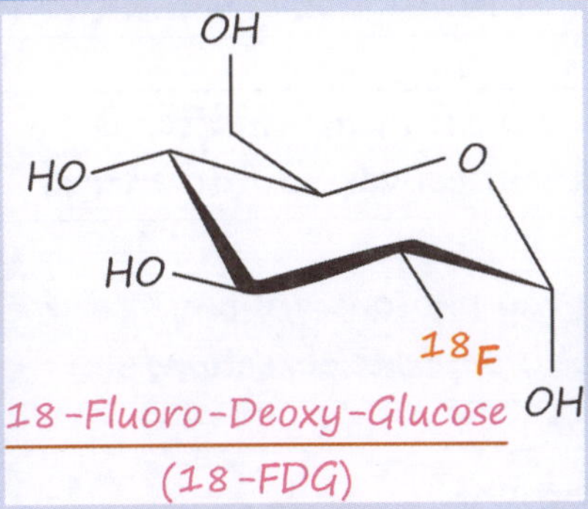

18-FDG: Fluorodeoxyglucose[Q] - Most common isotope used in PET scan

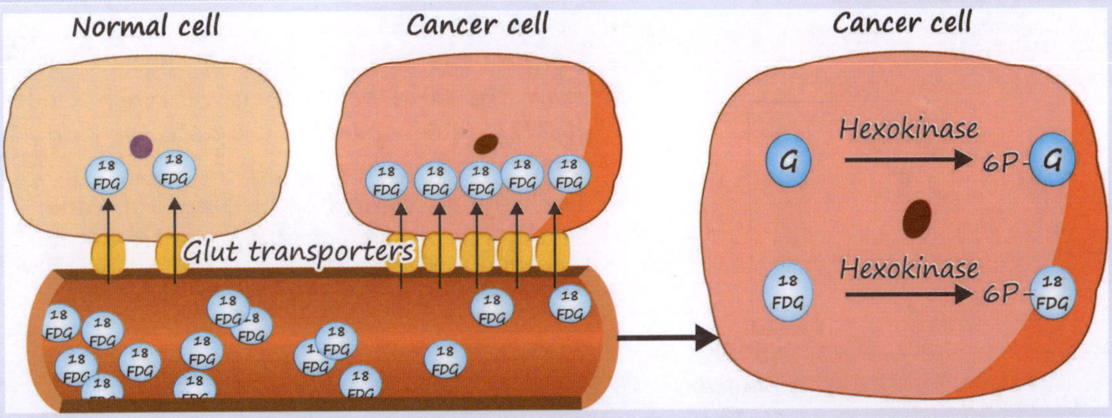

FDG–The Concept

As neoplastic cells require more ATP to divide rapidly – they will try and aplify every step of glucose metabolism – right from its uptake to its metabolism. So GLUT-1 transporters are over-expressed on neoplastic cells – so most of the glucose (and also FDG) in the blood-stream will be selectively be taken up by neoplastic cells. Hexokinase is over-expressed within cancer cells – so will jump on Glucose – and also on FDG – and phosphorylate it. Thus FDG gets trapped within the cancer cell.

Contd...

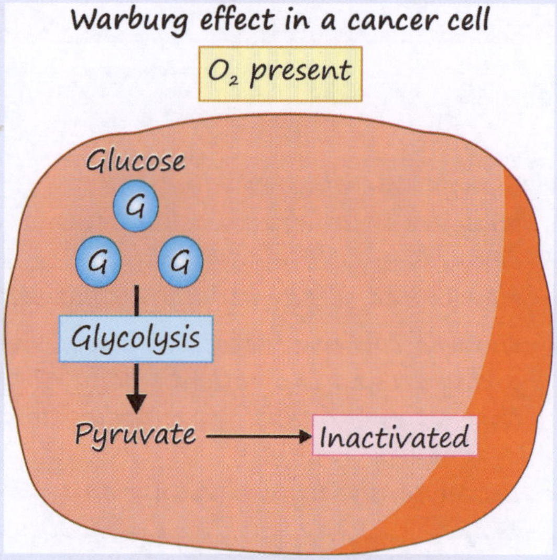

Warburg Effect[Q]

- Cancers cells use glucose in an inefficient manner
- Inside a cancer cell—even when oxygen is present – the TCA/Kreb's cycle and oxidative phosphorylation is inactivated. Thus, only 2 ATPs are produced from 1 glucose.
- This results in excess production of pyruvate and lactate – both are shunted off for production of cell division structural component prosuction – as these are required by a cancer cell for rapid cell division. This gives the cancer cell a distinct survival advantage[Q].
- However Glucose is being use inefficiently for ATP synthesis, this further aggravates the glucose hunger of a cancer cell.
- Inside a cancer cell - even in presence of O_2 – glucose is utilized by glycolysis - hence, this is termed as Aerobic Glycolysis[Q]

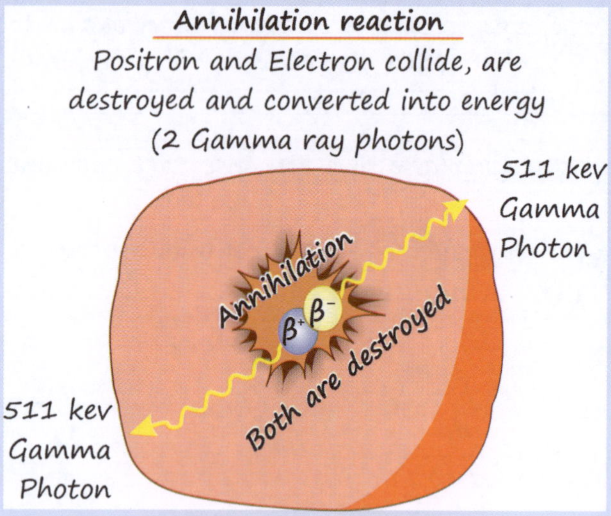

Annihilation reaction

18-FDG trapped inside the cancer cell emits a Positron (β+)

↓

This Positron (β+) collides with a tissue Electron (β–)

↓

Both are destroyed – Matter is destroyed and converted into energy

↓

2 gamma ray photons are emitted in exactly opposite directions

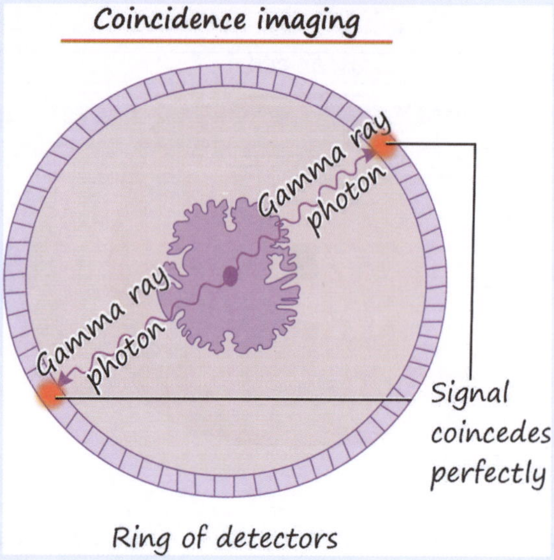

Coincidence phenomenon

- Specific for PET scan
- Because the above 2 Gamma photons have started from the same point, they will reach 2 detectors located 180° apart on the detector ring at the same time.
- Such signals coinciding in time and signal configuration are taken as true signals and are amplified. The other signals are suppressed.

Contd...

CLINICAL CLINCHER

False positive for malignancy on PET[Q]	False negative for malignancy on PET[Q]
• Sarcoidosis[Q]	• Bronchoalveolar carcinoma[Q]
• Tuberculoma[Q] and TB Lymphadenopathy[Q]	• Small sized lesions <1 cm size[Q]
• Cryptococcosis[Q]	• Lung metastasis from a Mucinous extrapulmonary tumor[Q]
• Paragonimiasis	• Tumor response after chemotherapy[Q]
• Pneumocystis infection[Q]	• Carcinoid tumor[Q]: Typical carcinoid
• Abscesses	
• Radiation fibrosis[Q]–due to secondary inflammation	
• Pneumoconiosis with Massive fibrosis[Q]	
• Sclerosing hemangioma of lung	
• Granulation tissue around tumors	

SYSTEMIC RADIONUCLIDE IMAGING

Technetium 99m
Most common radionuclide used in Nuclear medicine

Synthesized from

Molybdenum-99 → Tc-99m → Tc-99 → Degenerates into → Ruthenium 99

- Atomic number–43°
- Technetium means Artificial/Man-made
- m[Q]-in its name stands for-Metastable nuclear isomer[Q]
- Half-life–is 6 hours[Q]
- Emits:
  - Gamma rays[Q]-140.5 keV energy-Most commonly emitted
  - Beta rays/electrons-Small amount emitted

DIAGNOSTIC RADIONUCLIDE STUDIES

Infective/inflammatory pathology – Pyrexia of unknown origin	
Gallium scan (Ga67)[Q] – is a component of markers of inflammation	• Hot spots on Abscess, Sarcoidosis, Lymphoma • Highly sensitive but poor specificity – Positive also in Sarcoidosis/Lymphoma
Leukocyte tagging – Tc99m-WBCs, In111-WBCs	More specific than Gallium scan
Renal imaging	
Anatomic imaging	Tc99m-DMSA[Q] (S-A stands for Structure and Anatomy)
GFR Estimation	Tc99m-DTPA[Q] – Excreted exclusively by glomerular filtration
Functional evaluation	Tc99m - MAG3[Q] – Excreted by both glomerular filtration and tubular secretion
Renovascular hypertension – Renal artery stenosis	**Captopril-DTPA** scan[Q]: • Captopril (ACE inhibitor) is contraindicated in Renal artery stenosis – as it will suppress the glomerular filtration • Step 1 – Baseline DTPA scan = GFR1 • Step 2 – Small dose of Captopril given • Step 3 – Repeat DTPA scan = GFR2 • If GFR2 < GFR1 = Diagnosis is renal artery stenosis

Contd...

Cardiac imaging	
Cardiac perfusion scan (Perfusion = Capillary level blood flow)	• Thallium-201[Q] = behaves exactly like K+(Intra-cellular compartment) • Normal myocardium = Normal perfusion = Hot spot on Thallium scan • Infarcted myocardium = Absent perfusion = Cold spot on Thallium scan[Q] Best recent method – Rubidium 82 /13N Ammonia – PET scan
Infarct scintigraphy	• Tc99m – Stannous pyrophosphate • Infarct = Hot spot[Q]
Radionuclide ventriculography – Ventricular function assessment	• Tc99m – RBCs – helps us measure LV volume • EDV – ESV = SV x HR = Cardiac Output
Myocardial viability – Myocardial cells alive or dead?	• BEST – 18-FDG PET scan[Q] • Normal myocardium = Energy substrate is fatty acids[Q] = Cold spot on 18-FDG PET scan • Ischemic myocardium = Energy substrate is Glucose[Q] = Hot spot on 18-FDG PET scan
Pulmonary imaging	
Pulmonary Ventilation (V) – Perfusion (Q) scan – Pulmonary embolism	• Ventilation (V) – Airway patency - Xe133, Kr81, Technegas – Tc99m labeled aerosols • Perfusion (Q) – Capillary level blood flow – Tc99m-Macro-aggregated albumin (MAA) • Normal lung: V = Q • Infarcted lung in Pulmonary Embolism: V (Normal) – Q(Absent) – Mismatched defect[Q]
Solitary pulmonary nodule (SPN) – Single nodule <3cm in size	• 18FDG PET scan – to rule out malignancy • IOC for SPN – CE-CT[Q]
Gastrointestinal imaging	
GI Bleeding	

Angiography	Radionuclide scans
• Invasive technique • Only active bleeding detected • Low sensitivity • Threshold rate of bleeding – 0.5 mL/min[Q]	• Non invasive • High sensitivity • Threshold rate of bleeding 0.05 – 0.1 mL/min[Q] • Radio-isotopes used – ▪ Tc99m - Sulfur colloid[Q] –Active GI bleed only ▪ Tc99m – RBCs[Q] – Active and Intermittent GI bleed ▪ Tc99m – Pertechnetate[Q] – Specific for bleed from Meckels diverticulum.

Ectopic splenic tissue (White pulp in spleen removes damaged RBCs)	Tc99m – Heat damaged RBCs[Q]
Hepatobiliary imaging	
Liver hemangioma	Tc99m – RBCs – RBCs get pooled/accumulated inside a Hemangioma
Tc99m - Imino-diacetic acid derivatives HIDA/IODIDA/DISIDA scan	• Nonvisualization of GB on HIDA scan – Acute cholecystitis[Q] • Imino-di-acetic acid compound injected IV – Liver cells – Secreted into bile – entire biliary tree visualized • Acute cholecystitis due to impacted calculus – IDA compound does not enter GB • Also used in - **Biliary atresia, Biliary. Dyskinesia, Post-op biliary leak**

Contd...

Musculoskeletal imaging	
Tc labeled Bisphosphonate drug Methyl diphosphonate (MDP)	
Bone tumor/Fracture/Metabolic disease/ AVN	Tc99m – MDP (Bisphosphonate) scan
Osteomyelit (Vs Cellulitis)	Tc99m – MDP Triphasic bone scan
Lymphedema	Tc99m – Nanocolloid lymphoscintigraphy
99mTc – MDP SUPER-SCAN – Excessive skeletal radioisotope uptake in relation to soft tissues along with absent or faint activity in the genitourinary tract on bone scintigraphy is known as a 'superscan.' Seen in: • Renal failure • Paget's disease • Fibrous dysplasia • HPT • Widespread metastatic disease • Metabolic bone disease • Hyperthyroidism	
Adrenal imaging	
Adrenal cortical tumor	I123- Iodocholesterol
Adrenal medullary tumor	I123 - MIBG scan
CNS Imaging	
CVA/Stroke	Tc99m –HMPAO SPECT
CSF rhinorrhea/Hydrocephalus	Intrathecal In111 – DTPA
Encephalitis	Tc99m –HMPAO SPECT
Adrenal imaging	
Dementia	Tc99m –HMPAO SPECT, 18FDG PET scan
Epilepsy – Ictal SPECT	Tc99m –HMPAO SPECT
Epilepsy – Inter-ictal PET	18FDG PET scan
Neck imaging	
Thyrotoxicosis	I123 – Na iodide scan
Thyroid nodule/Ectopic thyroid nodule	Tc99m - Pertechnetate
Hyperparathyroidism/Parathyroid localization	SestaMIBI scan/Tetrofosmin scan – FMGE Jan 2023 pattern
Dry mouth/Connective tissue disorders	Tc99m – Pertechnetate.
I123 MIBG scan is used for	Neuroblastoma – Pheochromocytoma – Ganglioneuroma - Paraganglioma

RADIOTHERAPY

Radiotherapy Basics

Radiation components			
Alpha particles	**Beta particles**	**X-rays**	**Gamma rays**
• MAX Ionizing power[Q] • MAX Damaging power[Q] • MIN Penetrating power[Q]	• Beta particles are electrons used in • Intra-operative radiotherapy	Most common component used in RadioRx[Q]	• MIN Ionizing power[Q] • MIN Damaging power[Q] • MAX Penetrating power[Q]
--→ Ionizing/Damaging power decreases and Penetrating power increases in this order ---→			

Contd...

Bragg's peak[Q] – is seen with Alpha particles and Protons

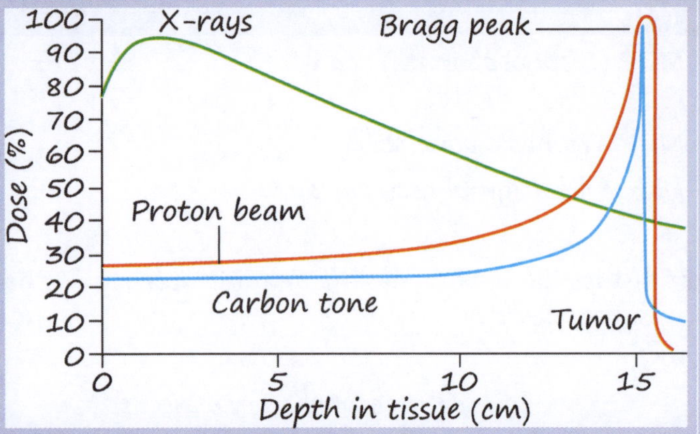

- The curve denotes the dose delivered (Y-axis) with increasing depth in the patient's body (X-axis)
- The dose delivered in case of protons and alpha particles is inversely proportional to their velocity in tissues.
- At a certain depth when the velocity is minimum, the dose deposited is MAXIMUM – forming a sudden sharp peak of exposure – Bragg's peak
- Thus if the tumor is localized at this depth – precise dose delivery to the tumor can be achieved. The normal tissues beyond this point is also not exposed.

Sources of radiation exposure occurring to humans	
Natural sources – 0.1 Rad / yr[Q]	Artificial sources
• Cosmic rays – from space • Ground related sources	• X-ray/CT/Radio Rx/Nuclear medicine equipment
• Background radiation exposure: Radiation exposure occurring constantly from natural sources- MAX in Kerala[Q]	

Radiosensitivity of tumors	
Maximum radiosensitivity – "WELMS"	Minimum radiosensitivity – "MOP"
• Wilm's tumor • Ewings sarcoma • Lymphoma • Multiple myeloma • Seminoma	• Melanoma • Osteosarcoma • Pancreatic cancer

Radiation damage to tissues

Indirect damage – Through free radical generation

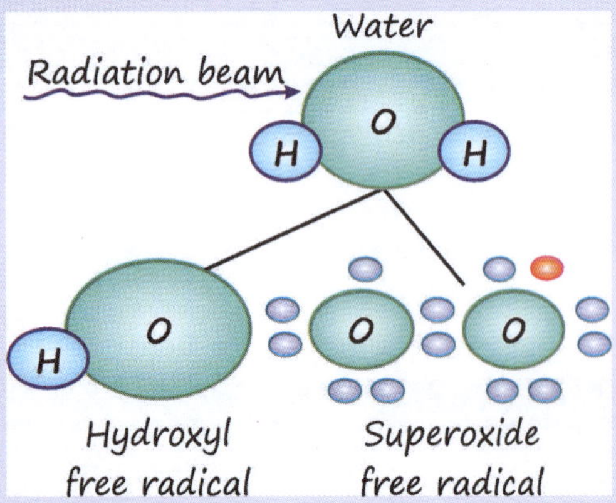

Direct damage – Direct DNA damage – Double stranded DNA breaks

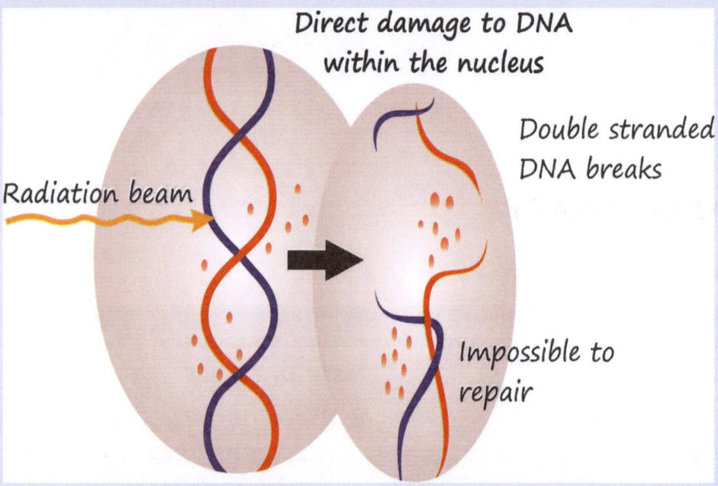

- 1st Step of radiation induced cell damage – Ionization[Q]
- Mechanism of cell death - DNA double stranded breaks[Q]

Radio-sensitivity of cells:

- Maximum at: G2M junction[Q]/M-phase[Q]
- Least at: S phase[Q]

Fractionated radioRx

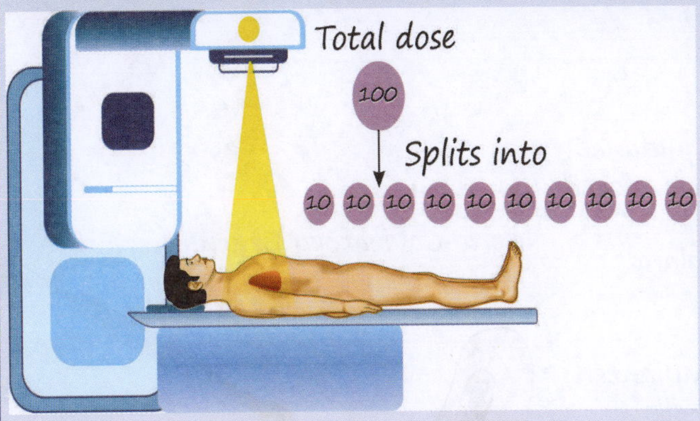

- Conventional fraction[Q]:
  - 1 Fraction per day[Q] from Monday-to-Friday
  - Weekend holiday[Q] (Saturday and Sunday)
  - The holiday allows body to process the metabolic by-products of cell death and excrete them out.
- Hyperfractionation[Q]/Accelerated fractionation[Q]:
  - >1 fraction administered per day[Q]
  - Used for Cerebral gliomas[Q], small cell carcinoma lung[Q], Head and neck cancers[Q]
- Hypofractionation[Q]:
  - <5 fractions[Q] administered per week
  - May be associated with higher local recurrence/ treatment failure
  - Used for Melanomas[Q], soft tissue sarcomas[Q] and in Palliative radiotherapy[Q]

Fractionated radiorx

Five Rs of Fractionated Radiotherapy

1. Repopulation[Q]:
2. Repair/Recovery[Q]:
3. Reassortment/Redistribution[Q]:
4. Reoxygenation[Q]:
5. Radiosensitivity[Q]:
   - SF2[Q] = Surviving cell fraction after a 2 Gy radiation dose[Q]. As SF2 increases, radiosensitivity decreases[Q].

Types of Radiotherapy: Based on method of administration

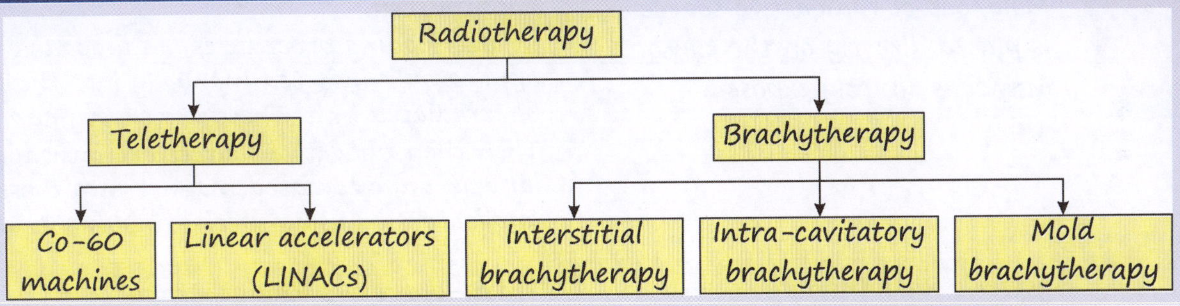

External Beam Radiotherapy (EBRT)/Teletherapy

Cobalt 60 machines

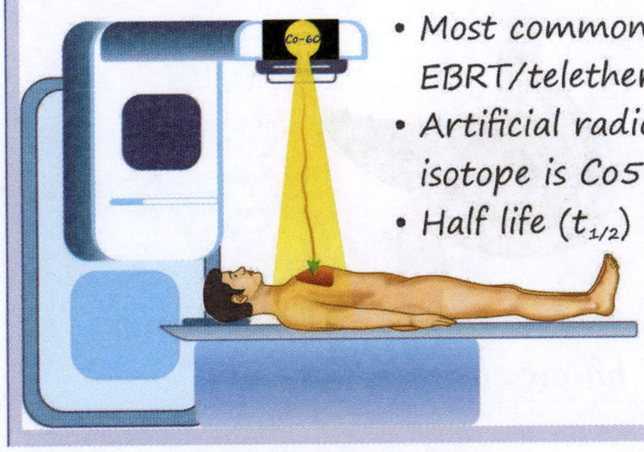

Disadvantages of Co-60 machines:

1. Radiation exposure to department personnel[Q]
2. Inefficient functioning[Q]

- Most common isotope used in EBRT/teletherapy[Q]
- Artificial radio-isotope[Q] (Natural isotope is Co59-Non-radioactive)
- Half life ($t_{1/2}$) = 5.2 years[Q]

Linacs-Linear accelarators

Linacs are modified, heavy duty X-ray tubes

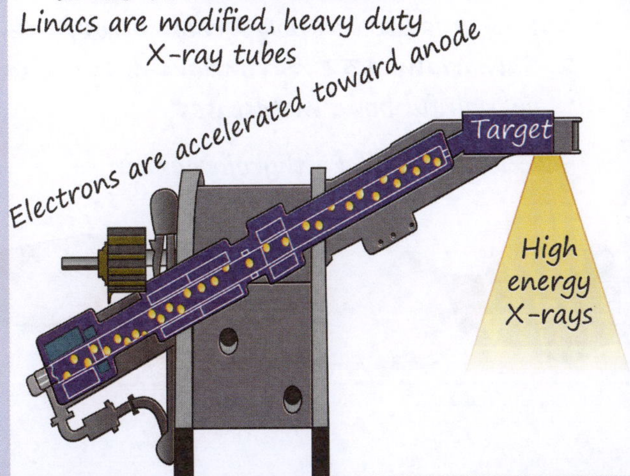

Contd...

Types of Radiotherapy: Based on method of administration

Brachytherapy
Interstitial Brachytherapy:

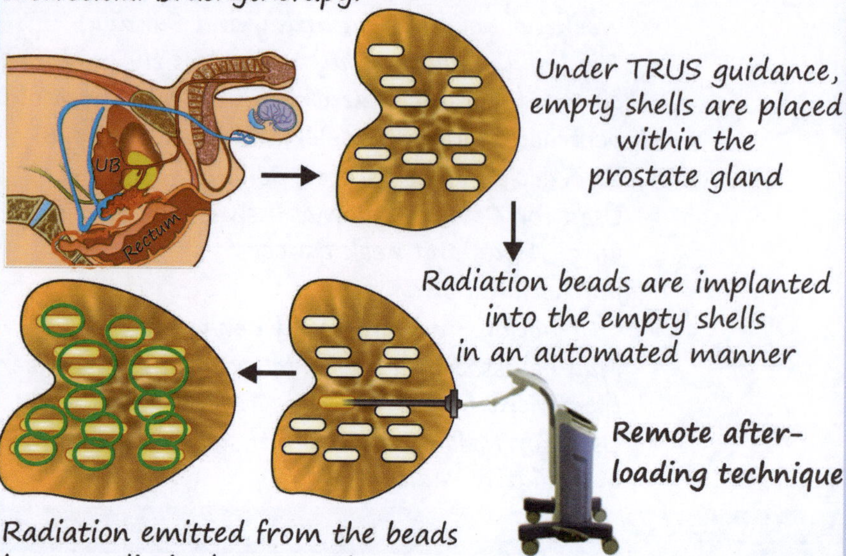

Radiation emitted from the beads has very limited penetrating power

Brachytherapy
Intra-Cavitatory Brachytherapy

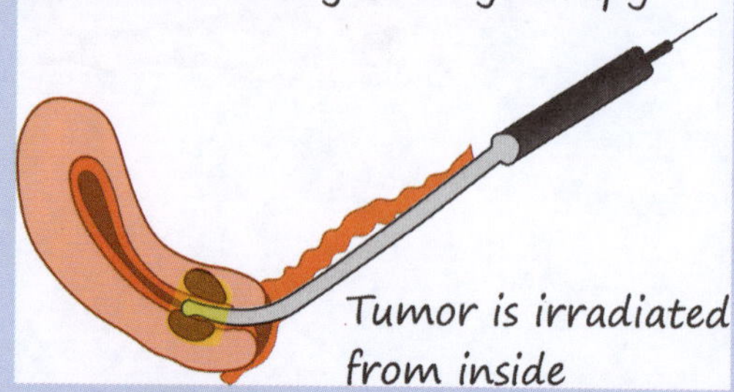

Brachytherapy
Mold brachytherapy

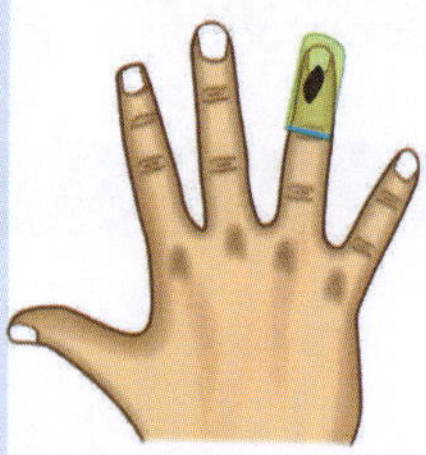

Used for treating superficial tumors- penile cancer,[Q] Sq. cell cancer at nail bed[Q]

Mold/cap of radioactive source is placed directly on the tumor. Tumor is directly exposed.

Remote afterloading in Brachytherapy (NEET 2020 Pattern)

- These systems automatically administer a radioisotope directly to cancerous tissue, thereby minimizing the radiation dose to surrounding tissue and eliminating the radiation exposure to hospital staff.
- In afterloading procedures, an unloaded applicator is inserted manually into the tissue to be irradiated first. These are empty applicators.
- Then the radioactive sources are introduced later in an automated manner into these empty applicators by using special equipment.

Systemic Radiotherapy

Other applications:

1. P-32[Q] is used in polycythemia rubra vera[Q]
2. Samarium-132[Q]/Strontium-89[Q] are used in painful bone metastases[Q]

I-131 for Papillary thyroid cancer

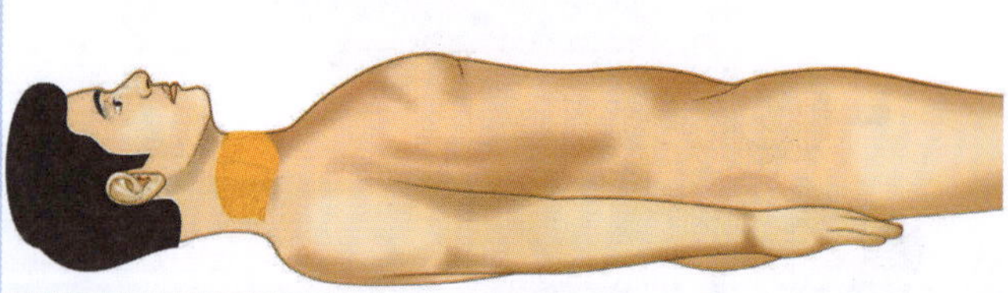

Intra-operative Radiotherapy

Most commonly used radiation component:

1. Electron beam (Stationary megavoltage electron beam)
2. X-rays - occasionally used

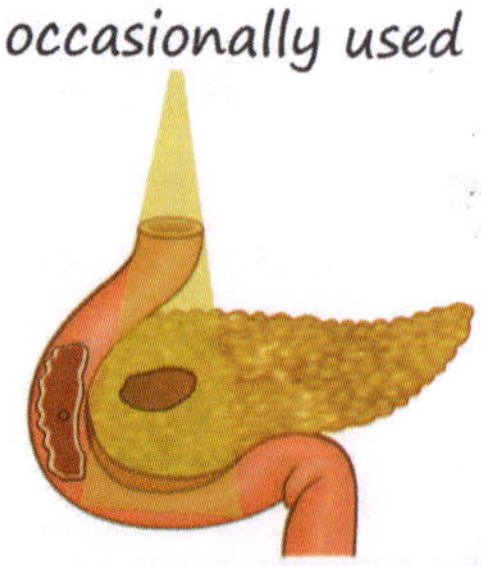

Intra-operative irradiation of the tumor bed by an electron beam[Q]

Contd...

Stereotactic Radiotherapy

Stereotactic – Accurate localization

MC used for brain tumors

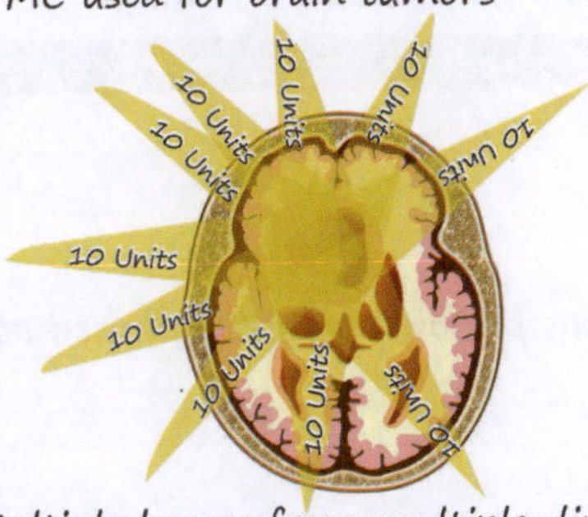

Multiple beams from multiple directions are used – all focused on the tumor

Intensity Modulated Radiotherapy (IMRT)

Used for Ca prostate

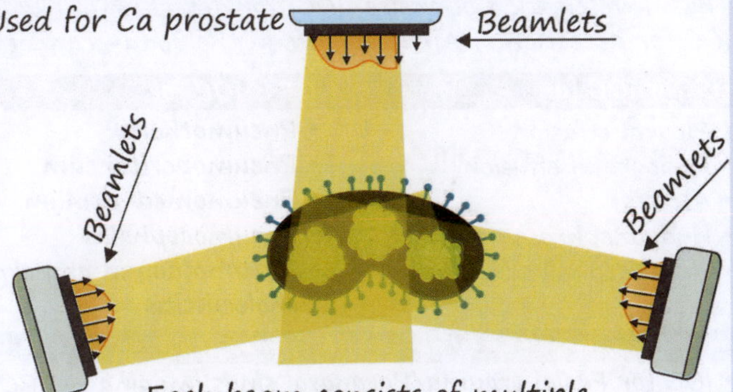

Each beam consists of multiple beamlets

CHEMICAL MODIFIERS OF RADIOTHERAPY

Radiosensitizers[Q]

They play a role of fixation of free radicals generated in the tissues as a result of radiation exposure, thus minimizing tissue repair.

- Hypoxic cell sensitizers[Q]: Enhance the tissue response to standard radiation, by mimicking the effects of oxygen, which induces the formation and stabilization of toxic DNA radicals. These include:
  - Nitroimidazones–Metronidazole[Q], Misonidazole, etc.
  - Hyperbaric oxygen[Q]—Most potent radiosensitizer
  - Antineoplastic drugs–Actinomycin D, 5-FU, Hydroxyurea, Bleomycin, Cisplatin, etc.
- Nonhypoxic cell sensitizers: Exact mechanism of action is not known. Include Halogenated pyrimidines— BUdR[Q], IUdR[Q]
- Caffeine[Q]–also increases the damaging effect of radiation

Radioprotectors[Q]

- These are compounds that trap free electrons in tissues, thus making them unavailable for further chemical reactions that may lead to cellular damage.
- They increase the therapeutic ratio by promoting repair of irradiated normal tissues.
- Examples include:
  - Thiophosphate compounds containing sulfydryl groups–Cysteine, Cysteamine
  - Amifostine—has no effect on CNS as it does not cross blood-brain barrier
  - GM-CSF, IL-1, Pentoxifylline, Zinc oxide, Melatonin, etc.

USES OF RADIOTHERAPY

Emergency Radiotherapy[Q] is used in

- SVC compression[Q]
- Acute metastatic spinal cord compression[Q]
- Cardiac tamponade due to tumor invasion[Q]
- Severe hypercalcemia[Q]
- Tumor lysis syndrome[Q]
- Raised ICT due to brain metastasis[Q]

Radiotherapy in Carcinoma Cervix

- It is usually a combination of Teletherapy (to treat the regional nodes and shrink the primary tumor) and Intracavitary Brachytherapy (for the central tumor core).
- Intracavitary Brachytherapy—may be used in early cases when the probability of lymph nodal metastasis is negligible.

Points	Dose	Location
Point A[Q]	8000 Rad[Q]	• Approximately at point in pelvis where the uterine artery and ureter cross • Located 2 cm above and lateral to base of radium tube in cervical canal
Point B[Q]	3000 Rad[Q]	• Corresponds to location of obturator nodes • 3 cm lateral to point A

Radiation induced cancers	
Neck irradiation in childhood for benign neck conditions	Thyroid cancer
Brush licking by Radium dial painters in watch factories	Bone sarcomas
Uranium mining	Lung cancer
In utero radiation exposure	Leukemia
Breast irradiation for post-partum mastitis	Breast cancer

INVESTIGATION OF CHOICE CLINICAL CONCEPTS

GOLDEN CONCEPT 1

Fluid is Friend of Ultrasound. Air is Enemy of Ultrasound

Thus, Investigation of choice (IOC) for detection of Fluid anywhere in the body is USG[Q]

IOC for detection of Air anywhere in the body—cannot be USG—hence, it is the next best modality - CT[Q]

USG is IOC for	CT is IOC for
• Pleural effusion • Pericardial effusion • Ascites • Hydronephrosis • Hydrocephalus in an infant	• Pneumothorax • Pneumoperitoneum • Pneumomediastinum • Pneumocephalus • Pneumo(air) in any organ—Emphysematous pyelonephritis/emphysematous cholecystitis

ENT IMAGING

- IOC for Facial trauma/Paranasal sinus imaging – HRCT/3D – CT
- Gold standard for Paranasal sinus conditions – Functional endoscopy
- IOC for middle and inner ear imaging – HRCT Temporal bone
- IOC for CSF rhinorrhea - CT Cisternography
- Best for Parathyroid imaging – 99mTc Sestamibi scan

BREAST IMAGING

- Screening IOC for Breast cancer – Mammography
- Overall best imaging investigation for breast cancer/DCIS – Dynamic contrast enhanced (DCE) – MRI
- Overall, best/IOC for staging of breast cancer – PET-CT
- IOC for fluid containing breast lesions (Abscess/cyst/galactocele)/Pregnant patient with breast lump/Young patient with a dense breast – USG
- IOC for patients with breast implants – MRI

THORAX IMAGING AND CARDIAC IMAGING

Thorax imaging

- IOC for all lung parenchymal abnormalities (Consolidation/Interstitial lung diseases/ COVID-19/TB). contrast enhanced CT done in Infections/Lung on tumors — HRCT
- IOC for Rib fractures — NC-CT Lung tumors: IOC for all lung tumors is CE — CT (except 1)
- IOC for Pancoast tumous is CE-MRI — to look for neural invasion of tumor into brachial plexus/cervical sympathetic ganglia
- IOC for all Mediastinal pathologies (such as Tumors/Mediastinitis) — CE-CT
- IOC for pleural effusion/Pericardial effusion - USG

Cardiac imaging

- IOC for cardiac function assessment – Echocardiography
- Gold standard for cardiac function assessment – Invasive catheter angiography
- Coronary artery imaging –
  - CT coronary angiography – Best noninvasive technique
  - Invasive catheter angiography – Overall IOC
  - Cardiac tumor assessment – CE-MRI is IOC
- Best noninvasive technique to assess myocardial viability – FDG – PET-CT

KUB IMAGING

- USG – 1st in renal colic/IOC for Hydronephrosis
- NC-CT – IOC for renal/ureteric calculi
- Dual source CT – IOC for detecting calculus composition
- CE-CT – IOC for Renal tumors (RCC/Oncocytoma)/Pyelonephritis/UB tumors/Renal TB
- IVU – Earliest investigation to detect Renal TB
  - IOC in adults — CE-CT
  - IOC in children — USG

Adrenal imaging:

- IOC for Adrenal pheochromocytoma — CE-MRI
- IOC for Extra-adrenal pheochromocytoma — MIBG scan/DOTA-PET
- IOC for Neuroendocrine tumors/Carcinoid tumors — Serotonin receptor/Somatostatin receptor scintigraphy/SPECT

VASCULAR IMAGING

- CE-CT (CT Angiography) > MR Angiography: IOC for almost all vascular conditions (Berry aneurysm/ Aortic aneurysm/Aortic dissection/Pulmonary embolism/Renal artery stenosis/Mesenteric artery thrombosis/ Fibromuscular dysplasia/Peripheral vascular disease)
- Invasive catheter angiography: Gold standard for all vascular abnormalities
- Duplex USG/Doppler USG: IOC for Varicose veins/Deep venous thrombosis
- Aortic dissection:
  - IOC in stable patient – CT angiography
  - IOC in unstable patient – Transesophageal echocardiography (TEE)

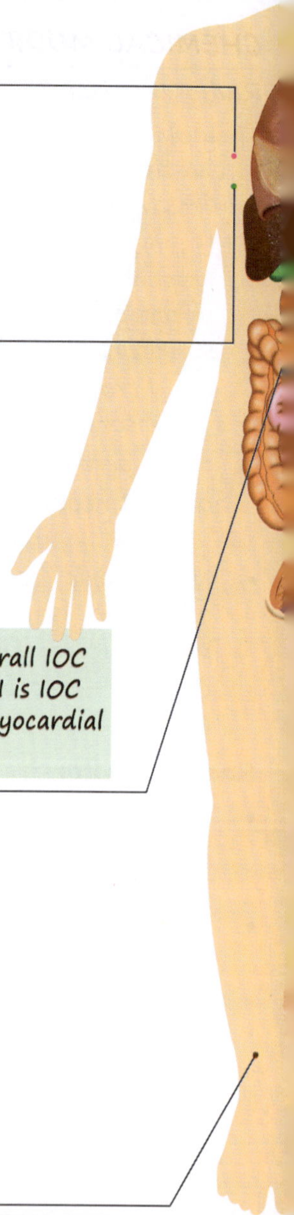

GOLDEN CONCEPT 2

In Neuroimaging ask yourself "Is TIME a crucial factor for diagnosis/treatment?" If Yes – Then CT is IOC, If No – Then MRI is IOC

Thus,

CT is preferred for	MRI is preferred for
• Head trauma • Status epilepticus • Acute stroke (CT is 1st Investigation, DWI-MRI is IOC)	• Brain tumors • CNS infections • Demyelinating disorders • Epilepsy/Seizure disorder • Developmental delay/Mental retardation • Metabolic disorders • Leukodystrophies

CNS IMAGING

- CT–IOC for conditions in which time is a crucial factor - Head trauma/Status epilepticus
- MRI–IOC for almost all other conditions
- Acute stroke:
  - CT–First investigation to rule out hemorrhage
  - MRI with Diffusion Weighted Imaging (DWI) – Overall best investigation
- CT is IOC for Head trauma except for Diffuse Axonal Injury (DAI). MRI is IOC for DAI

SPINE IMAGING

- IOC for Spinal trauma/Pott's spine/Spondylosis/Spinal cord abnormalities (Transverse myelitis/Syrinx/Tethered cord, etc.) – MRI
- CT – May be used in vertebral bone tumors

ABDOMINAL IMAGING

Multiphasic/Triphasic CE-CT – IOC for almost all Abdominal tumors. Liver and Pancreatic Imaging:

- IOC for all Focal liver lesions (Abscess/Hemangioma/Hydatid cyst/Tumors/Mets) - Multiphasic/Triphasic CE-CT
- IOC for Cholelithiasis (GB calculus) - USG
- Best noninvasive technique for biliary system abnormalities/Choledochal cyst/Choledocholithiasis (CBD calculus)/Pancreatic duct abnormalities—MRCP
  - Overall, best/IOC/Gold standard test for all Biliary tree abnormalities – ERCP
  - IOC for Acute pancreatitis/Pancreatic pseudocyst – CE-CT
  - IOC for Chronic pancreatitis – MRCP with secretin stimulation

Bowel Imaging:

- IOC for Peptic ulcer/GI polyps/Intraluminal lesions—Endoscopy
- IOC for Ca esophagus/Ca stomach/Small bowel intraluminal tumors - Endoscopy and Biopsy
- IOC for staging of GIT malignancies/to detect distant metastases – PET-CT
- IOC for T-N staging of Esophageal/Gastric cancer – Endoscopic Ultrasound (EUS)
- IOC for Diverticulitis — CE-CT
- IOC for Hiatus hernia — CT with oral contrast
- IOC for GERD — Upper GI endoscopy
- IOC for Infantile pyloric stenosis – USG

- **Bowel obstruction:**
  - Initial investigation — X-ray Abdomen — Erect and supine
  - Overall IOC in adults — CE-CT
  - Overall IOC in children — USG

- **Acute appendicitis/Intussuception:**
  - IOC in adults — CE-CT
  - IOC in children — USG
- IOC for Meckel's diverticulum – 99mTc-pertechnate scan
- IOC for perianal fistula/fistula-in-ano – MR fistulogram

Peritoneum and mesenteric vascular:

- IOC for Ascites/Hemoperitoneum/1st Investigation in abdominal trauma—USG/FAST
- IOC for Solid abdominal organ injury – CE-CT
- IOC for Pneumoperitoneum — CT
- IOC for Pseudomyxoma peritonei — CE-CT
- IOC for Mesenteric artery thrombosis/Mesenteric ischemia — CE-CT
- IOC for Abdominal lymphoma — CE-CT

MISCELLENEOUS IMAGING

- IOC for Joint imaging – MRI
- IOC for Mullerian/Uterine anomalies – 3D USG > MRI
- Gold standard test for Mullerian/Uterine anomalies – Hysteroscopy and Laparoscopy

Notes

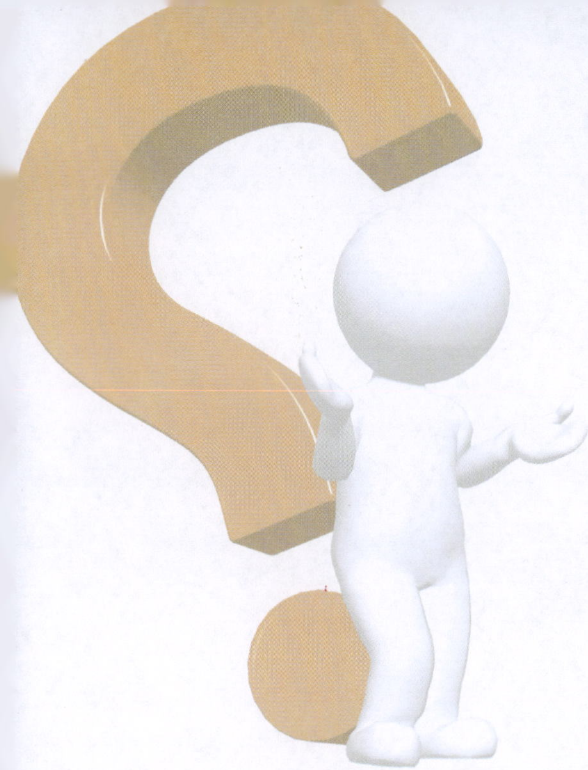

Latest Question Papers

- → NEET PG 2023
- → NEET PG 2022
- → NEET PG 2021
- → NEET PG 2020
- → INI-CET NOVEMBER 2023
- → INI-CET MAY 2023
- → INI-CET NOVEMBER 2022
- → FMGE JANUARY 2024
- → FMGE JANUARY 2023
- → FMGE JULY 2023
- → FMGE JUNE 2021
- → FMGE DECEMBER 2021
- → FMGE AUGUST 2020
- → FMGE DECEMBER 2020

NEET PG 2023

1. **A 2-month-old infant is brought to the OPD with parietal swelling present since birth. The X-ray image is given as follows. What could be the most likely diagnosis?**

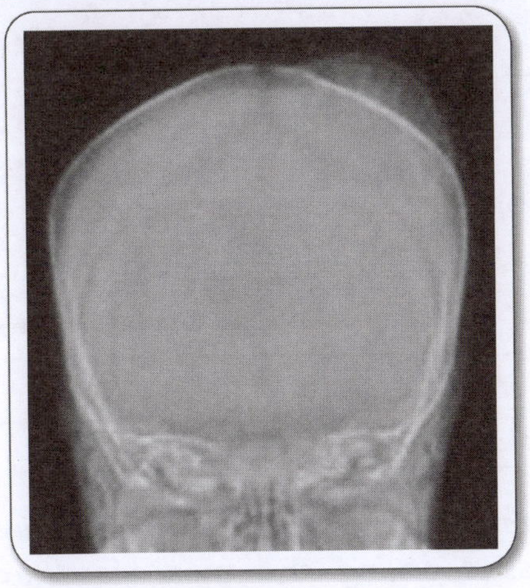

   a. Subgaleal hematoma
   b. Cephalohematoma
   c. Caput succedaneum
   d. Encephalocele

Ans: b. Cephalohematoma

2. **A patient presented with abdominal pain and sterile pyuria – X-ray done is in the given image. What is the most likely diagnosis?**

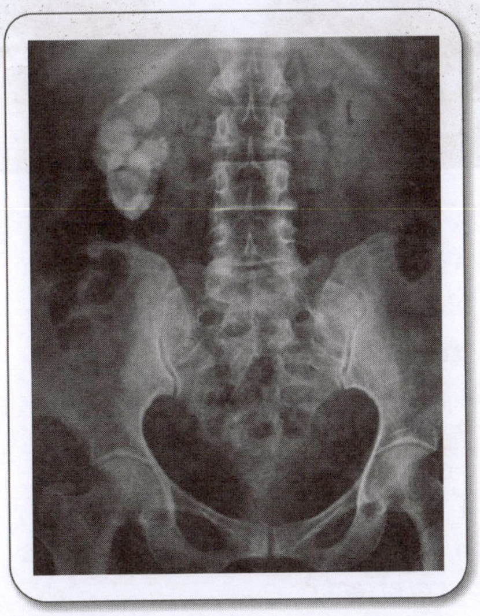

   a. Putty kidney
   b. Nephrocalcinosis
   c. Staghorn calculus
   d. Psoas muscle calcification

Ans: a. Putty kidney

3. **A woman diagnosed with endometrial cancer is undergoing radiotherapy. Which of the following is true?**
   a. Intensity of radiation is inversely proportional to the square of distance from the source
   b. Small blood vessels are most radioresistant
   c. Rapidly proliferating cells are most radioresistant
   d. Small intestinal mucosa is most radioresistant

Ans: a. Intensity of radiation is inversely proportional to the square of distance from the source

4. **A patient with fever and cough for last 5 days has chest crepitations on auscultations. CXR is given as follows. What is the most likely diagnosis?**

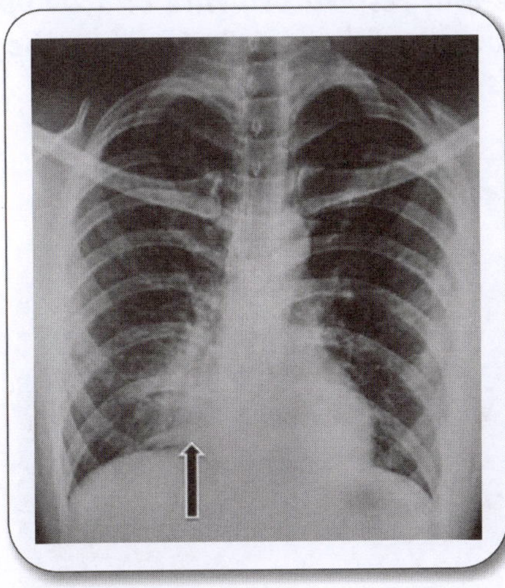

   a. Superior segment of right lower lobe consolidation
   b. RML consolidation
   c. Posterobasal segment of right lower lobe consolidation
   d. Loculated pleural effusion

Ans: b. RML consolidation

NEET PG 2022

5. **Identify the following imaging modality.**
   a. Cerebral blood flow scan
   b. PET-CT
   c. Sestamibi scan
   d. Full body MDCT

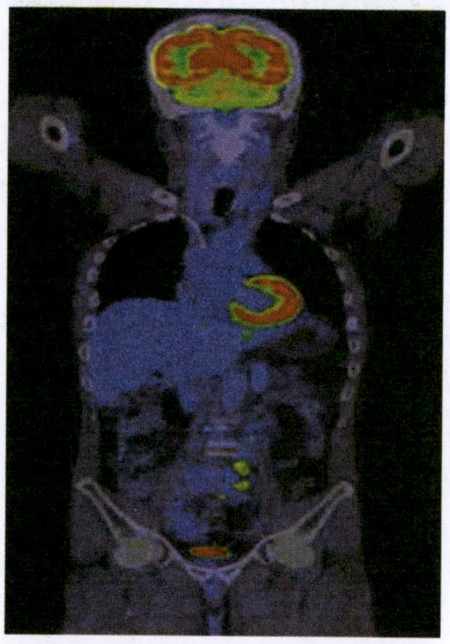

Ans: b. PET-CT

6. **A road traffic accident victim is brought to the casualty with BP 90/60 mm Hg, conscious state and respiratory rate of 120 bpm. X-ray is shown as follows. What will be the next step in his management?**

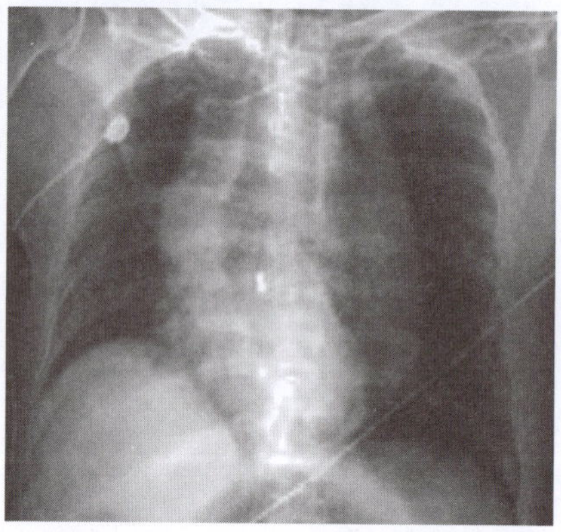

a. Chest tube insertion
b. Pericardiocentesis
c. Needle thoracotomy
d. Pleurodesis

Ans: c. Needle thoracotomy

7. **A patient presents with pain in abdomen. A delayed phase IVU image is shown as follows. What will be the most likely diagnosis?**

a. Staghorn calculus
b. Renal cyst
c. Putty kidney
d. PUJ obstruction

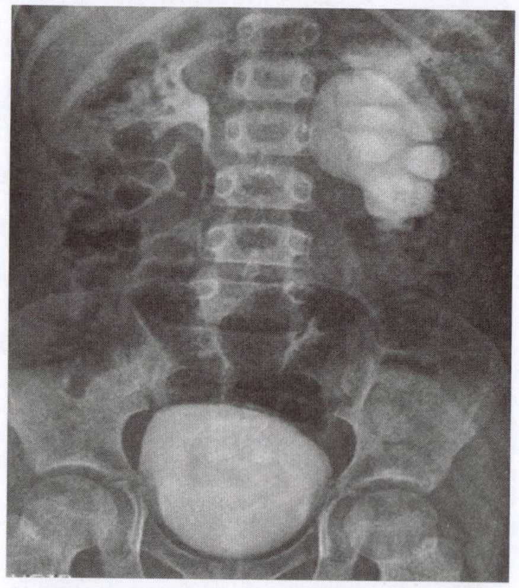

Ans: d. PUJ obstruction

8. **A baby presents with severe pain in abdomen excessive crying and mild blood in stools. A Barium enema is done and shown as follows. What will be the diagnosis?**

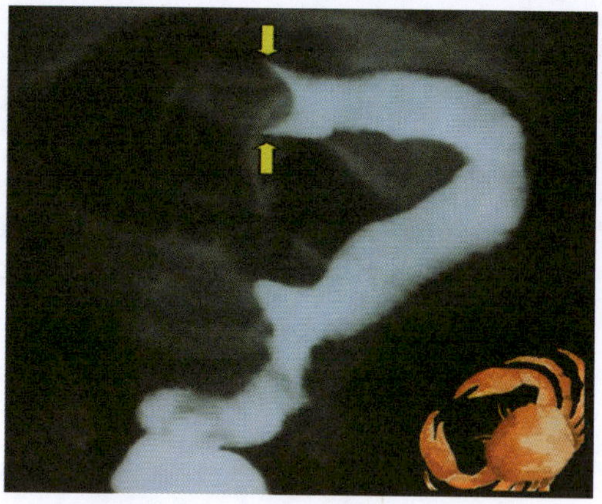

a. Intestinal obstruction
b. Volvulus
c. Intussusception
d. Duodenal atresia

Ans: c. Intussusception

9. **Which of the fillowing is true regarding Warburg effect?**

a. Tumor cells use less glucose
b. More ATP generated
c. Cell gets metabolites for cellular components
d. Helps tumor cell to be immortal

Ans: c. Cell gets metabolites for cellular components

NEET PG 2021

10. A 16-year-old patient who is a known case of spinal TB presents with low grade fever, dull backache and persistent hip flexion. Hip joint movement is painful and limited. Which of the following muscles, as marked in the following figure from A to D, is abnormal?

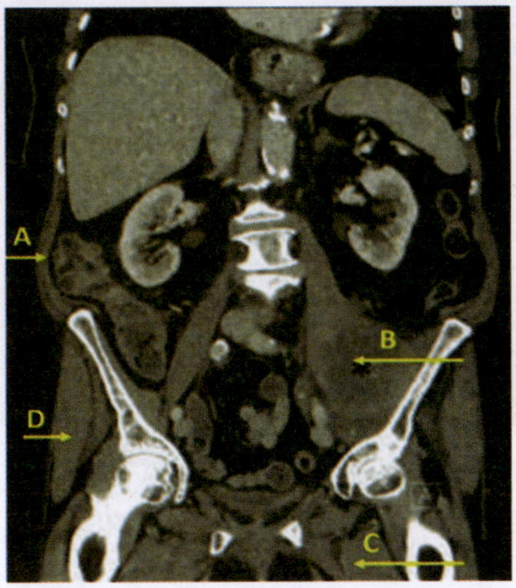

a. A b. B
c. C d. D

Ans: b. B

11. A 10-year-old child presented with limb pain with normal bone mineralization. His knee radiograph is shown as follows. What is the most likely diagnosis?

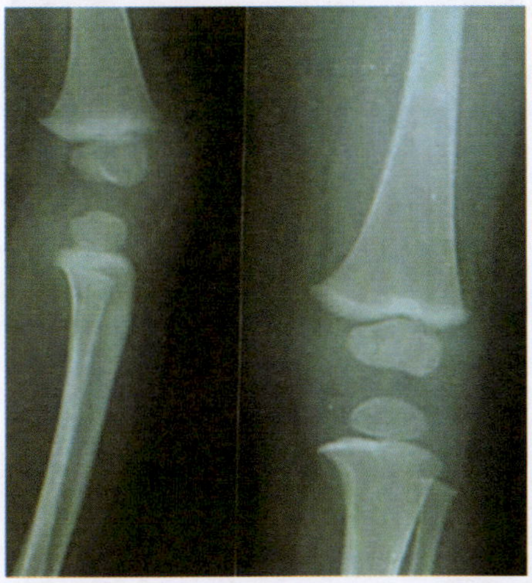

a. Scurvy b. Rickets
c. Pyknodysostosis d. Hemophilia

Ans: a. Scurvy

12. A patient presented to the emergency department with severe abdominal pain and tachycardia. An erect radiograph was done and is shown as follows. What is the diagnosis?

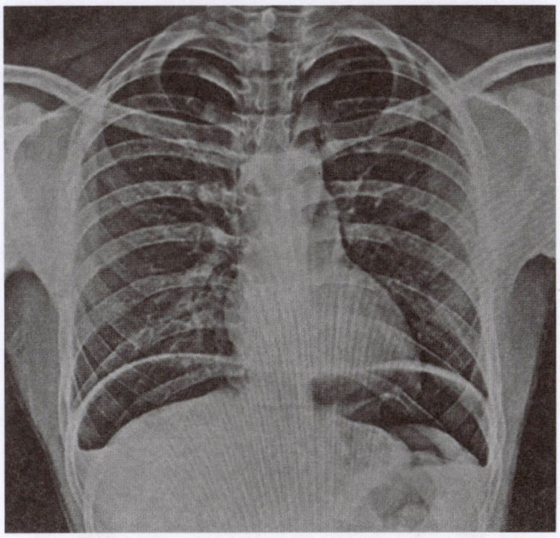

a. Intestinal obstruction b. Sigmoid volvulus
c. Perforation d. Hiatus hernia

Ans: c. Perforation

13. A 12-month-old child presented with fever, cyanosis and fatigue. His chest X-ray is shown as follows. What is the most likely diagnosis?

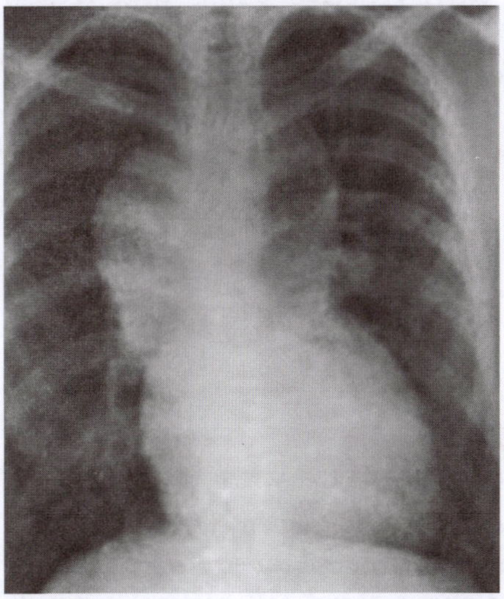

a. TAPVC
b. TOF
c. TGA
d. Pericardial effusion

Ans: a. TAPVC

14. A patient presents with abdominal pain and distension. An X-ray was taken which showed dilated bowel loops as given in the image. Identify the segment involved/marked by the arrow.

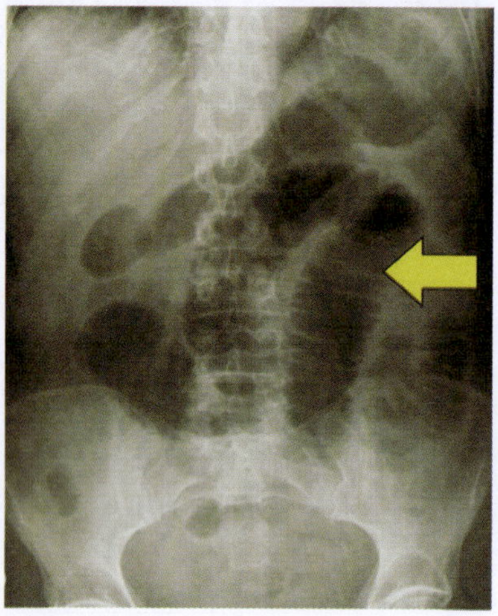

a. Jejunum
b. Ileum
c. Duodenum
d. Transverse colon

Ans: a. Jejunum

15. A patient following a skid injury resulting in an accident was brought to the emergency 2 hours later. He was stable with GCS 15/15 with reactive pupils and tenderness and bruising over the left lower chest wall and petechiae. Severe tenderness was present in the left hypochondriac region. BP was 90/60 mm Hg. The Best investigation used in the ER will be:

a. FAST
b. X-ray
c. Diagnostic peritoneal lavage
d. CT

Ans: a. FAST

16. A child with acute lymphoblastic leukemia undergoes prophylactic irradiation prior to autologous stem cell transplant. Which of the following will be the least affected?

a. Spermatogonia
b. Intestinal epithelial cells
c. Neurons
d. Bone marrow/Erythroid precursor cells

Ans: c. Neurons

17. A 35-year-old male presented with pain at wrist and swelling. His radiograph is shown as follows. What is the most likely diagnosis?

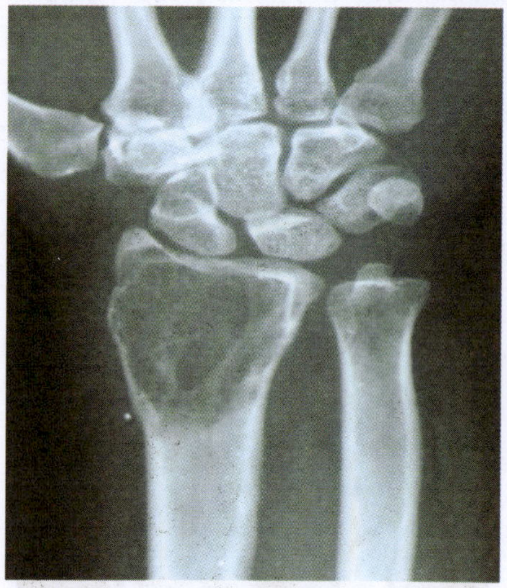

a. ABC
b. GCT
c. SBC
d. Enchondroma

Ans: b. GCT

18. A 13-year-old child who has a history of chronic right ear discharge presents with headache, fever and altered sensorium. A CE-MRI was done. What is the diagnosis?

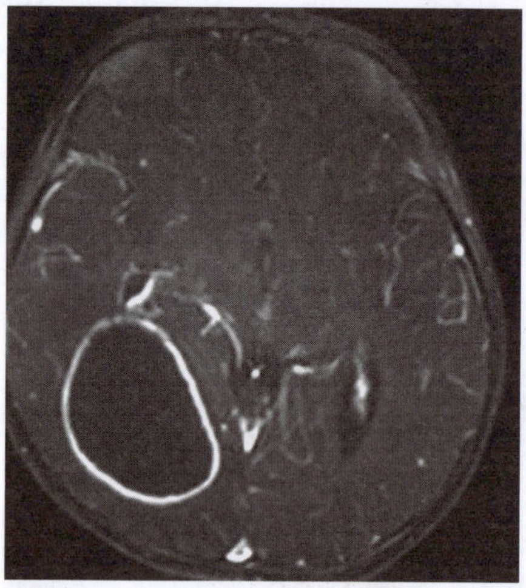

a. Cerebellar abscess
b. Extradural abscess
c. Brain abscess
d. Meningitis

Ans: c. Brain abscess

19. A laborer was working at his site with a Chisel and a hammer. He suddenly felt an impact when he hit his hammer and had an eye injury due to a flying fragment. He was brought to the hospital. Which of the following investigations would be detrimental if done in his case?
 a. B-scan
 b. CT
 c. MRI
 d. X-ray orbit

Ans: c. MRI

NEET PG 2020

20. A 56-year-old female patient presented with progressive dysphagia for solids, loss of weight and loss of appetite. A barium swallow test was done. What will be the most likely diagnosis?

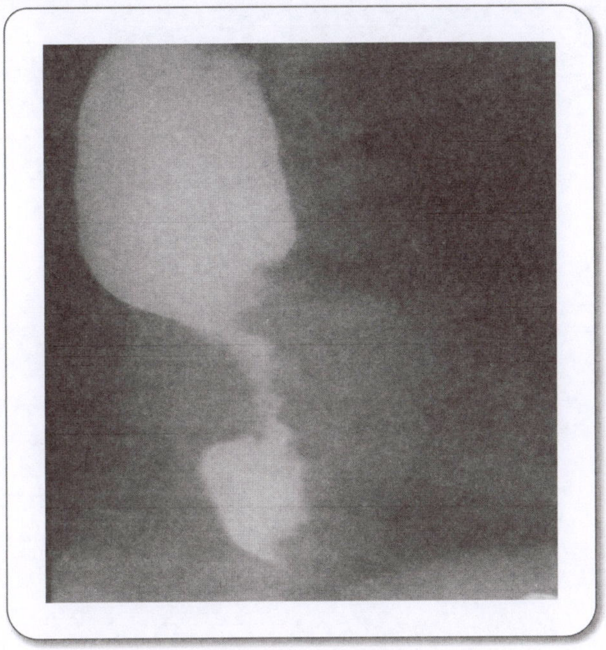

 a. Achalasia cardia
 b. Diffuse esophageal spasm
 c. Esophageal leiomyoma
 d. Esophageal cancer

Ans: d. Esophageal cancer

21. Identify the diagnosis in the given X-ray with protracted barking cough.
 a. Epiglottitis
 b. Acute laryngotracheobronchitis
 c. Retropharyngeal abscess
 d. Adenoid enlargement

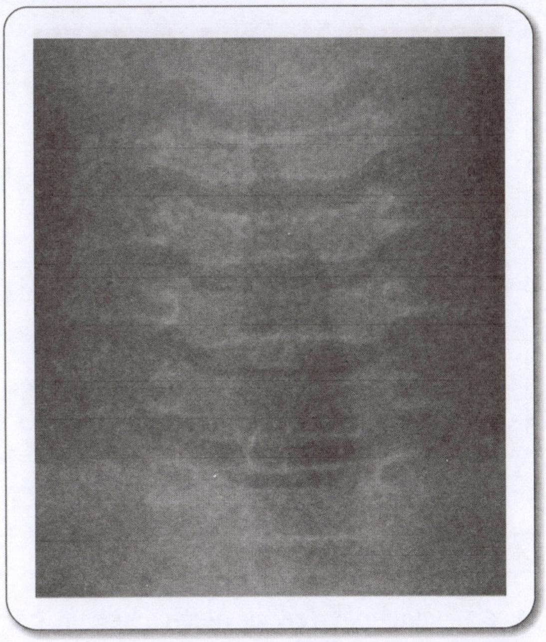

Ans: b. Acute laryngotracheobronchitis

INI-CET NOVEMBER 2023

22. Identify the diagnosis in the 6-month-old child. Whose X-ray is as follows:

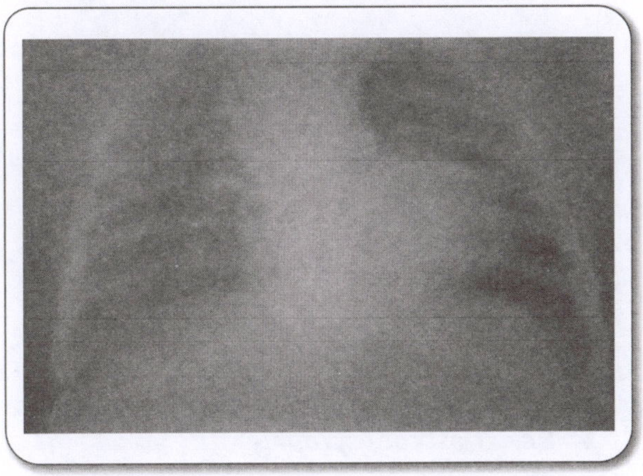

a. TGA	b. TAPVC
c. Ebstein anomaly	d. TOF

Ans: d. TOF

23. A child with a known skeletal deformity was being evaluated and an angle was measured as shown. Can you name the measurement being made here?
 a. Cobb angle
 b. Pauwel's angle
 c. Pott's angle
 d. Bohler's angle

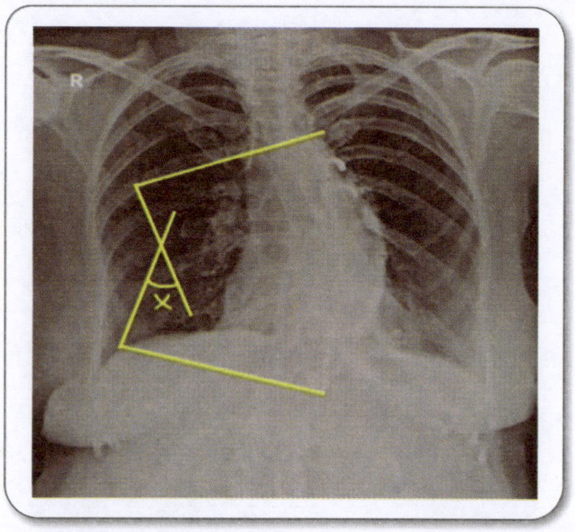

Ans: a. Cobb angle

24. A 65-year-old female with chronic backache revealed the following appearance on a lumbar radiograph. What is the most likely cause?

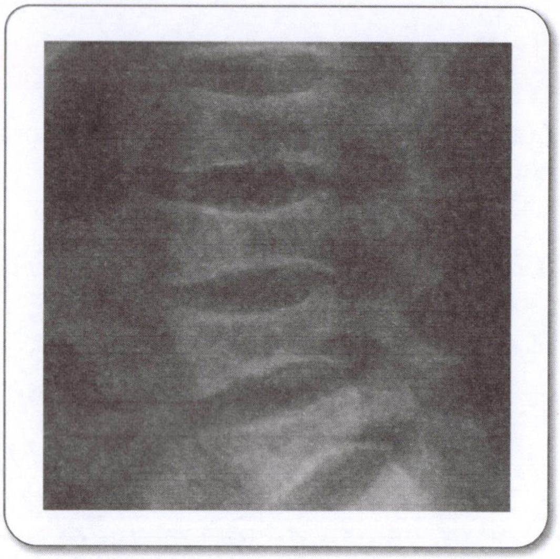

a. Paget's disease
b. Renal osteodystrophy
c. Osteoporosis
d. Ankylosing spondylitis

Ans: c. Osteoporosis

25. A 10-month-old girl child presented with pain in abdomen, blood in stool and lump felt over abdomen. A barium enema was done and revealed this image. What is the most likely diagnosis?
a. Meckel's diverticulum
b. Volvulus
c. Intussusception
d. Diverticulitis

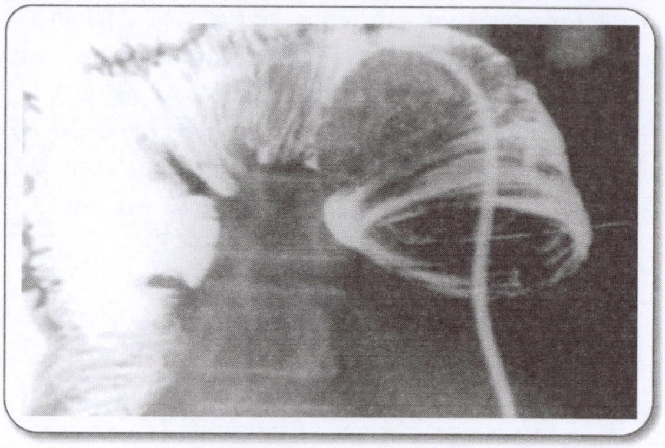

Ans: c. Intussusception

26. A 42-year-old patient with sudden onset headache, neck rigidity without any obvious history of trauma. What is the most likely diagnosis based on this CT image?

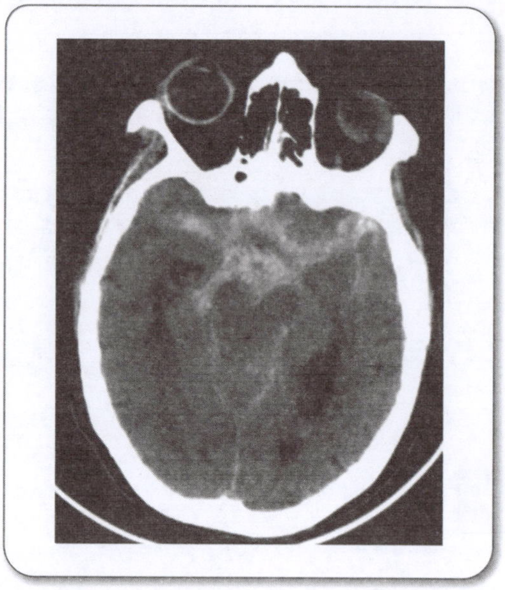

a. EDH
b. Aneurysmal SAH
c. Subdural bleed
d. Hypertensive bleed

Ans: b. Aneurysmal SAH

27. Patient presented with neck swelling and regurgitation with gurgling sound when pressed over the neck. A barium swallow was performed and is revealed here. Most likely diagnosis will be:
a. Esophageal stricture
b. Zenker's diverticulum
c. Esophageal web
d. Ca esophagus

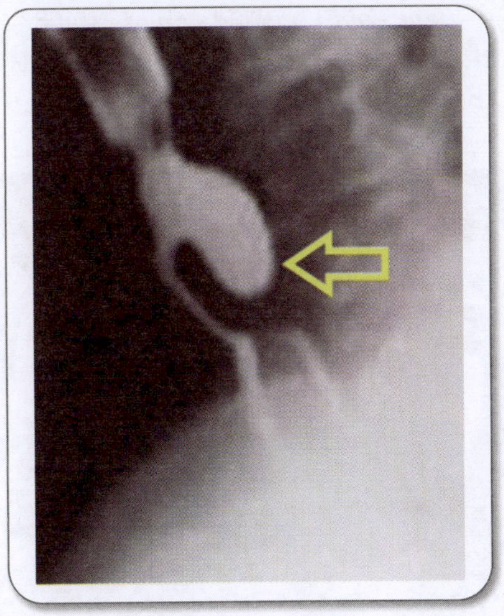

Ans: b. Zenker's diverticulum

28. A patient complains of incomplete evacuation of urine and frequent micturition. Identify the diagnosis in the following image?

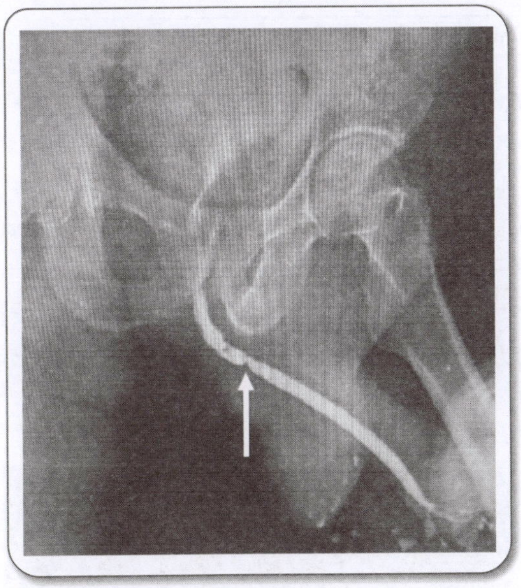

a. Urethral stricture
b. Urethral diverticulum
c. Urethral rupture
d. Urethritis

Ans: a. Urethral stricture

29. A USG was done for infertility evaluation in a patient. Most likely diagnosis is:

a. Arcuate uterus
b. Bicornuate uterus
c. Hydrosalpinx
d. Uterine synechia

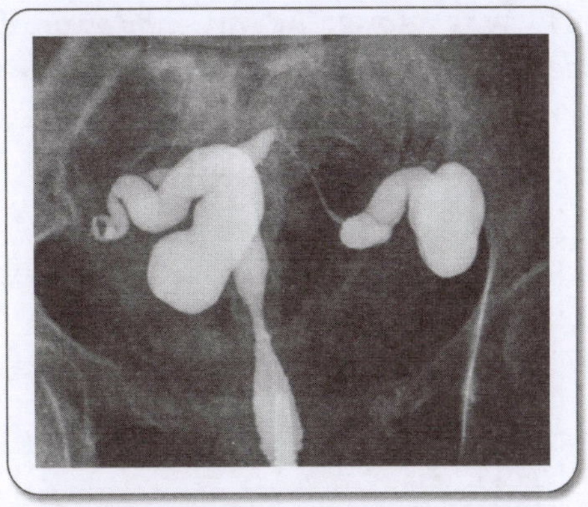

Ans: c. Hydrosalpinx

30. A patient being treated for infertility was treated with injection HMG following which she presented with abdominal distension and vomiting. Most likely diagnosis based on this USG image is:

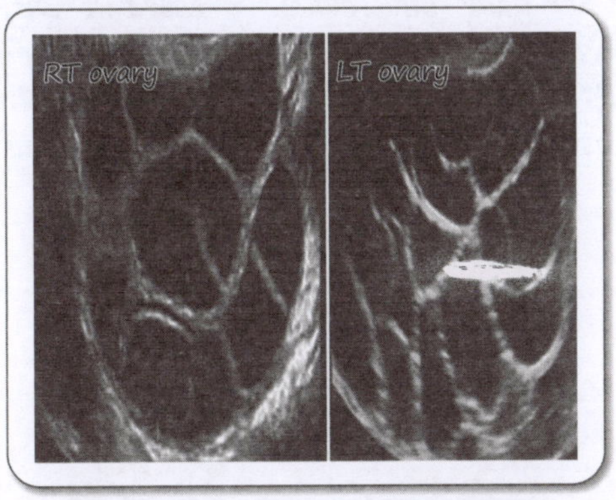

a. OHSS
b. PCOS
c. Theca lutein cyst
d. Ovarian torsion

Ans: a. OHSS

31. The appearance seen in M-mode USG thorax is suggestive of:

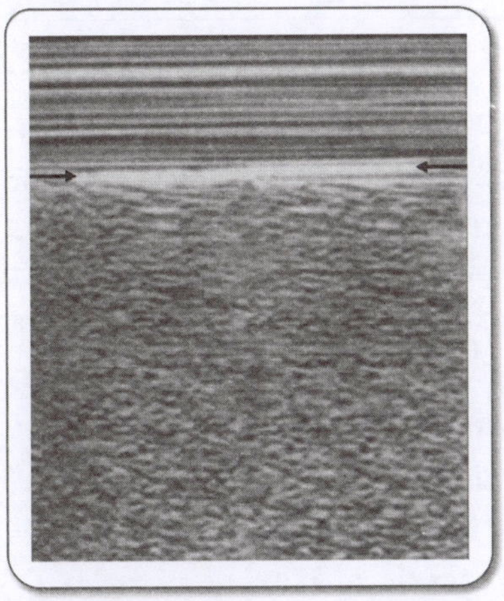

a. Stratosphere sign
b. Barcode sign
c. Seashore sign
d. A-line sign

Ans: c. Seashore sign

32. FAST was done in an abdominal trauma patient and reveals this finding. What will be the most likely diagnosis?

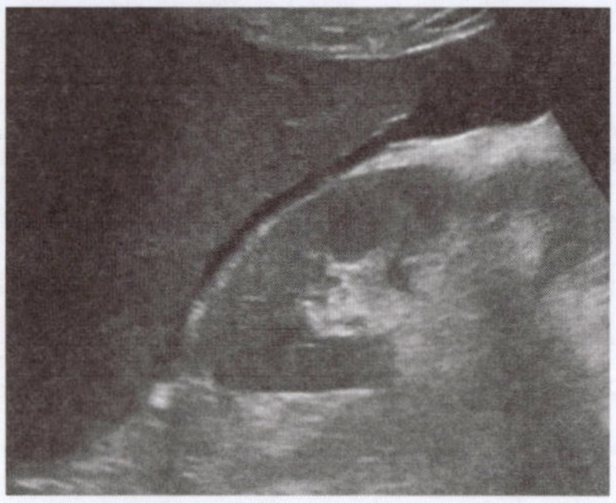

a. FAST negative
b. FAST positive
c. FAST inconclusive
d. None of these

Ans: b. FAST positive

33. A 30-year-old female presented with hypertension, chest pain and cramping of legs. A CXR was done and is shown as follows. What is the most likely cause of hypertension in this patient?

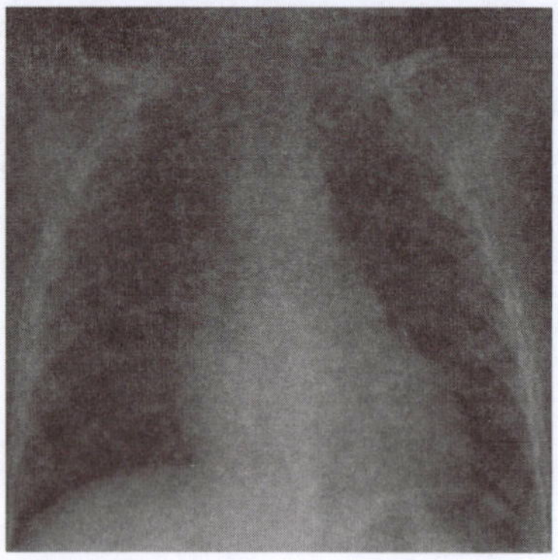

a. Aortic aneurysm
b. Aortic dissection
c. Coarctation of aorta
d. Mitral stenosis

Ans: c. Coarctation of aorta

34. A 32-year-old female undergoes a CXR for fitness. Later that day her UPT comes as positive. USG reveals a 6 weeks pregnancy. Extremely anxious, she comes to docter for consultation. Best advice given her is:

a. Immediate termination of pregnancy
b. Mandatory invasive testing for genetic defects
c. Counseling, reassuring advice to continue with the pregnancy
d. Obstetric MRI

Ans: c. Counseling, reassuring advice to continue with the pregnancy

35. A 9-year-old female child with history of headache and visual disturbance. What could be the possible diagnosis?

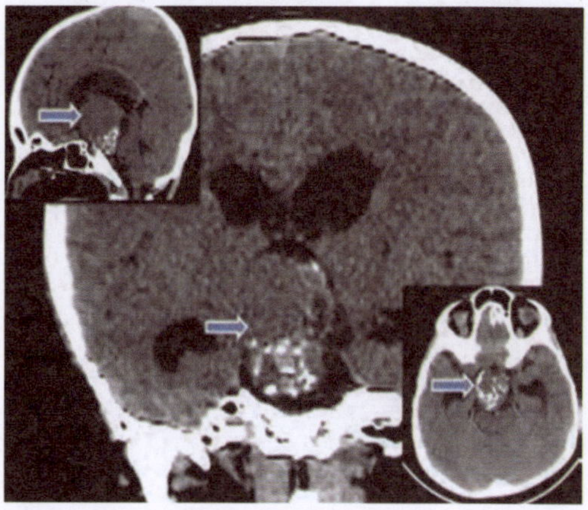

a. Craniopharyngioma
b. Optic nerve glioma
c. Hypothalamic hamartoma
d. Pituitary macroadenoma

Ans: a. Craniopharyngioma

36. Radiology department personnel radiation exposure monitoring is done by using:

a. TLD badge
b. Collimators
c. Linear accelerators
d. Gamma cameras

Ans: a. TLD badge

37. Identify the structure marked in the following image:

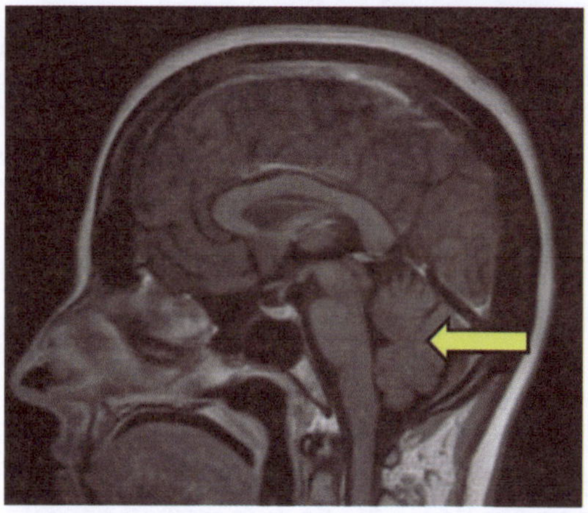

a. Cerebrum
b. Cerebellum
c. Brainstem
d. Corpus callosum

Ans: b. Cerebellum

38. A patient presented with recurrent abdominal pain. Identify the investigation in the following image:

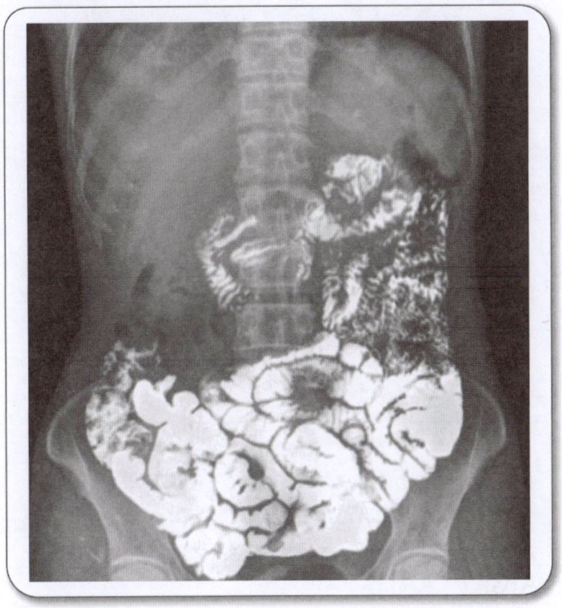

a. Barium swallow
b. Barium meal
c. Barium meal follow through
d. Barium enema

Ans: c. Barium meal follow through

39. A 67-year-old hypertensive and diabetic male presents with left-sided hemiplegia. Diagnosis based on the following CT is:

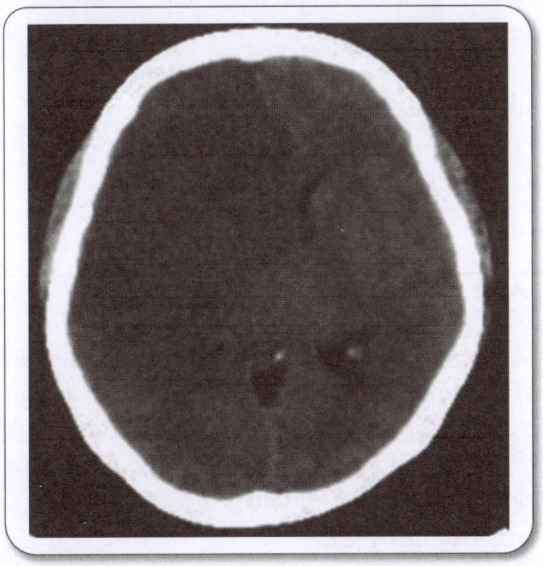

a. Hypertensive bleed
b. Ischemia
c. SAH
d. EDH

Ans: b. Ischemia

40. Diagnosis based on the following CT image is:

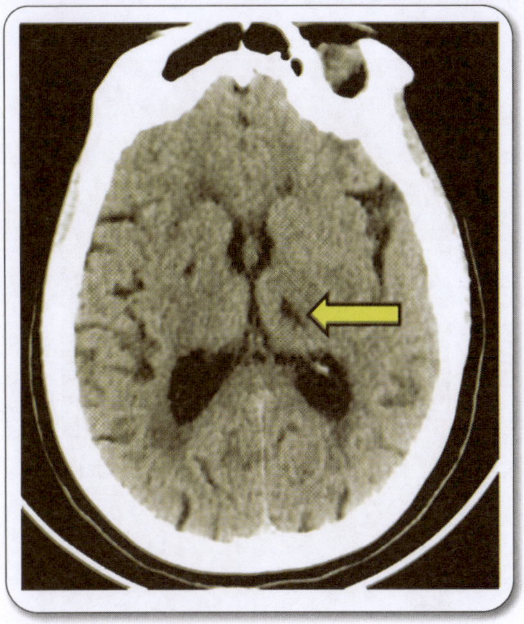

a. MCA territory infarct
b. Lacunar infarct
c. Hypertensive bleed
d. SAH

Ans: b. Lacunar infarct

41. A patient presented with history of trauma followed by periorbital swelling and diplopia. Diagnosis based on the following CT image is:

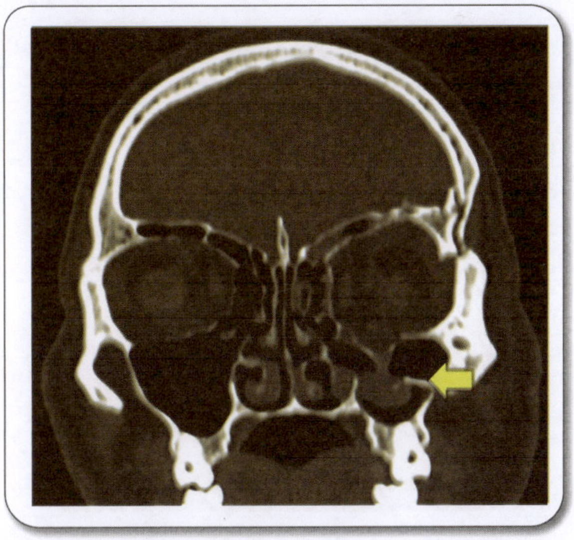

a. Zygomatic fracture
b. Blowout fractures
c. Tripod fracture
d. Frontal fracture

Ans: b. Blowout fractures

42. Incorrect statement regarding the condition given in the following image is:

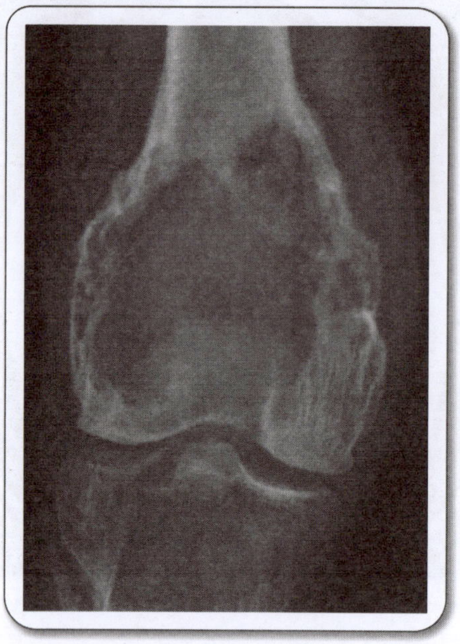

a. Epi-metaphyseal location
b. Has well-defined margins
c. Eccentric in location
d. Chemotherapy is treatment of choice

Ans: d. Chemotherapy is treatment of choice

43. Most likely diagnosis in the following IVU image is:

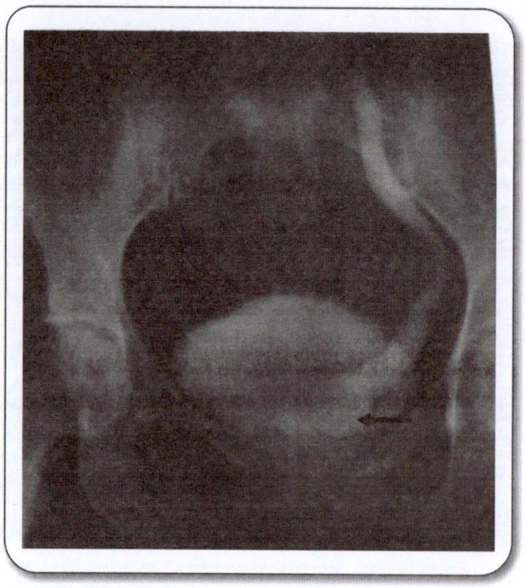

a. VU reflux
b. Ureterocele
c. Ureteric stricture
d. UB diverticulum

Ans: b. Ureterocele

44. A known case of pancreatitis presents on day 4 with breathlessness, basal crepitations. Diagnosis is:

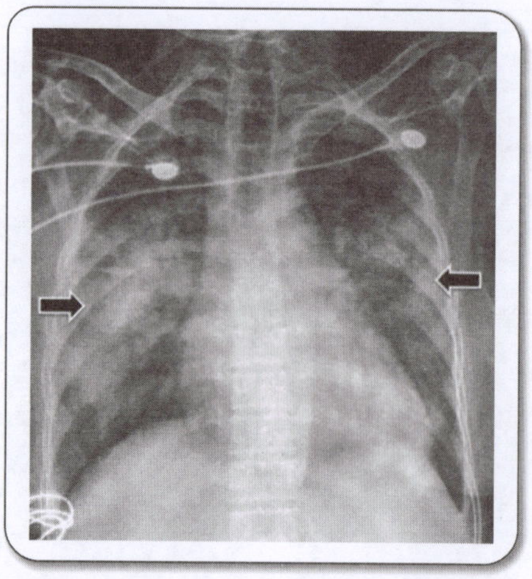

a. Lung collapse
b. ARDS
c. Pleural effusion
d. Bronchiectasis

Ans: b. ARDS

45. A patient presents with low-grade fever and mild cough. Diagnosis is:

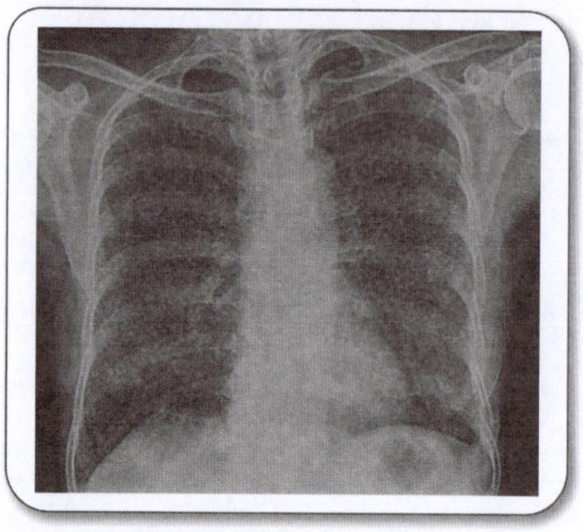

a. RUL consolidation
b. Miliary TB
c. Cannon-ball lung metastasis
d. Interstitial lung disease

Ans: b. Miliary TB

46. A patient has recently suffered a MI and has been diagnosed to have ischemic cardiomyopathy. Angiography reveals multiple vessel disease. Prior to CABG, the cardiologist wants to assess the myocardial viability. Best test to be done is:

a. Thallium scan
b. 18-FDG PET scan
c. 99m Tc-Stannous pyrophosphate scan
d. MUGA scan

Ans: b. 18-FDG PET scan

47. A 55-year-old nonsmoker lady presented with on and off hemoptysis and productive cough for 1 year. There was no fever or constitutional symptoms. Physical examination showed clubbing of fingers and coarse crepitations over the lung base. Blood tests were essentially normal and an initial CXR was performed. CT scan was also performed, which is shown as follows. What is the radiological diagnosis?

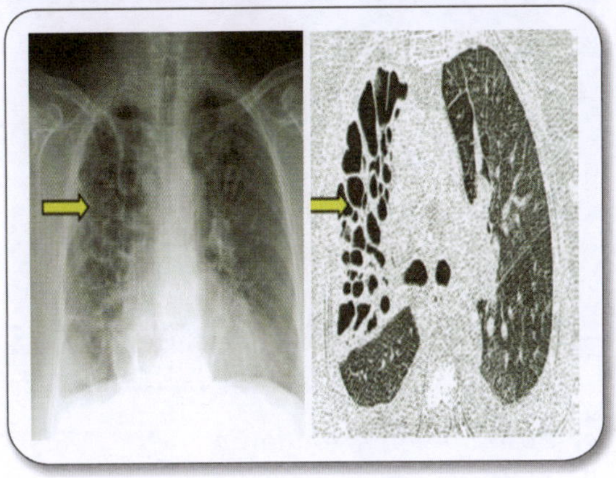

a. Interstitial lung disease
b. Bronchiectasis
c. Emphysema
d. Chronic bronchitis

Ans: b. Bronchiectasis

48. A 35-year-old male with history of 4 weeks of immobilization for fracture femur developed sudden onset of chest pain and hemoptysis. ECG shows S1 Q3 T3 pattern. Diagnosis is:

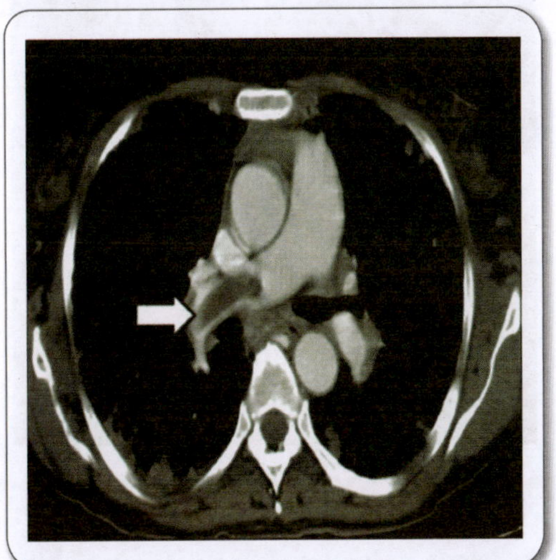

a. Pulmonary embolism b. Cor pulmonale
c. Aortic dissection d. Aortic aneurysm

Ans: a. Pulmonary embolism

49. A 20-year-old man presents with mild abdominal discomfort. A CE-CT is shown as follows. Diagnosis is:

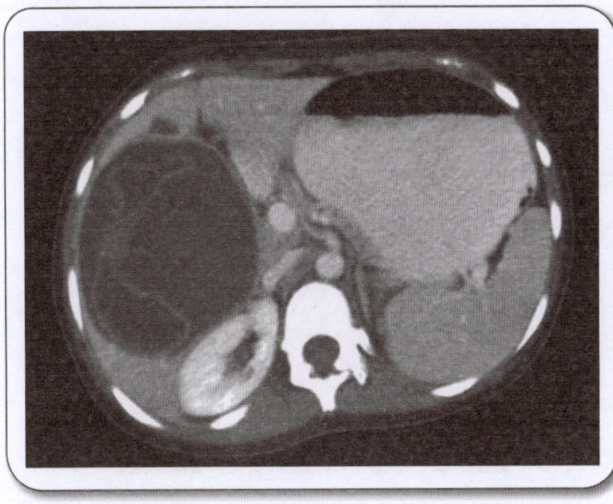

a. Liver abscess
b. Liver simple cyst
c. Hydatid cyst
d. HCC

Ans: c. Hydatid cyst

50. A patient suffering from morning stiffness >1 hour, presents with the following abnormality in the X-ray. What can be the most possible diagnosis?

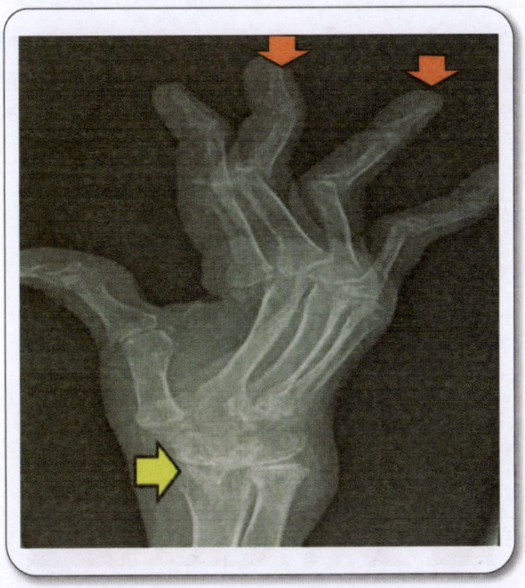

a. Rheumatoid arthritis
b. Psoriatic arthritis
c. Osteoarthritis
d. Erosive osteoarthritis

Ans: a. Rheumatoid arthritis

51. A young man had a fall on outstretched hand with pain on radial aspect of wrist and tenderness at anatomic snuff box. Diagnosis based on the following image is:

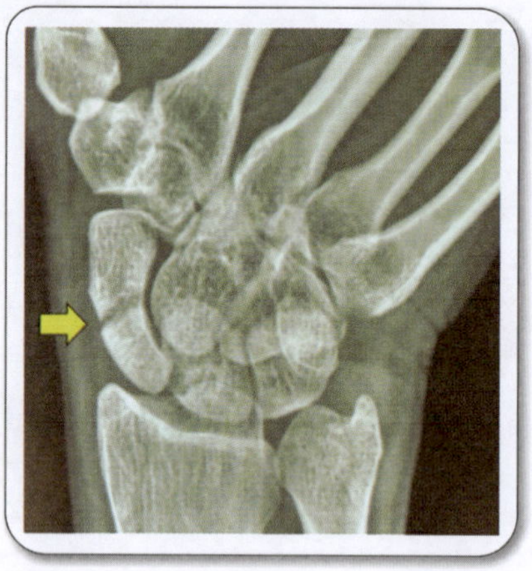

a. Colles fracture
b. Barton fracture
c. Bennett's fracture
d. Scaphoid fracture

Ans: d. Scaphoid fracture

52. Best time to detect chorionicity and amnionicity of pregnancy is:

a. First trimester
b. Second trimester
c. Third trimester
d. Peripartum

Ans: a. First trimester

53. A new-born male baby presented with congestive heart failure. On examination enlarged fontanels, a loud cranial bruit and the following radiological finding was noted—the most likely diagnosis is:

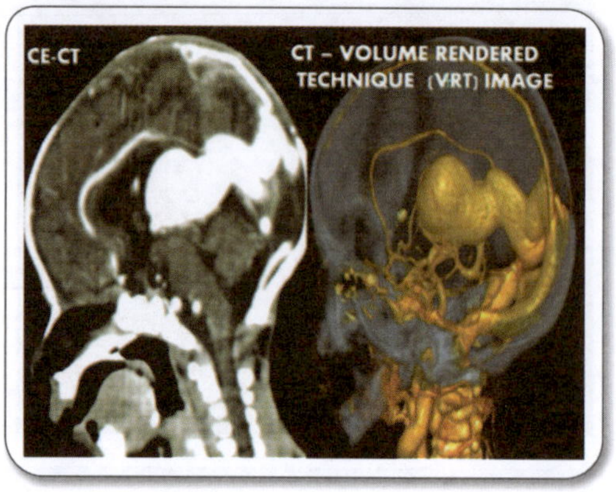

a. Sinus pericranii
b. Arachnoid cyst
c. Vein of Galen malformation
d. Dandy-Walker malformation

Ans: c. Vein of Galen malformation

54. A 65-year-old patient presented with weight loss and generalized weakness. Along with a basic blood work-up a skeletal survey was done and is shown as follows. Most likely diagnosis is:

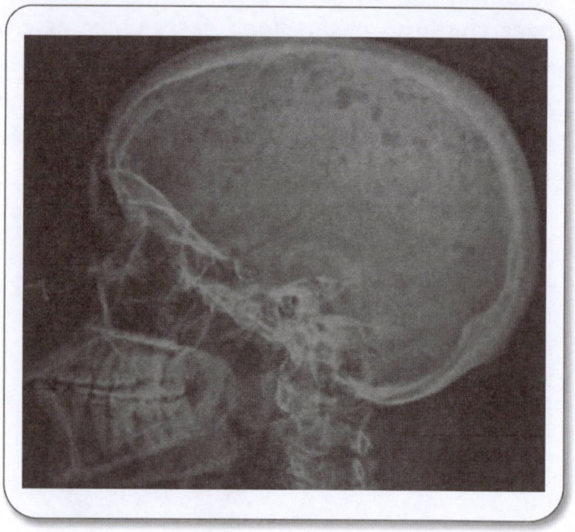

a. Eosinophilic granuloma
b. Multiple myeloma
c. Metastasis
d. Hyperparathyroidism

Ans: b. Multiple myeloma

55. Identify the structure marked in this image?

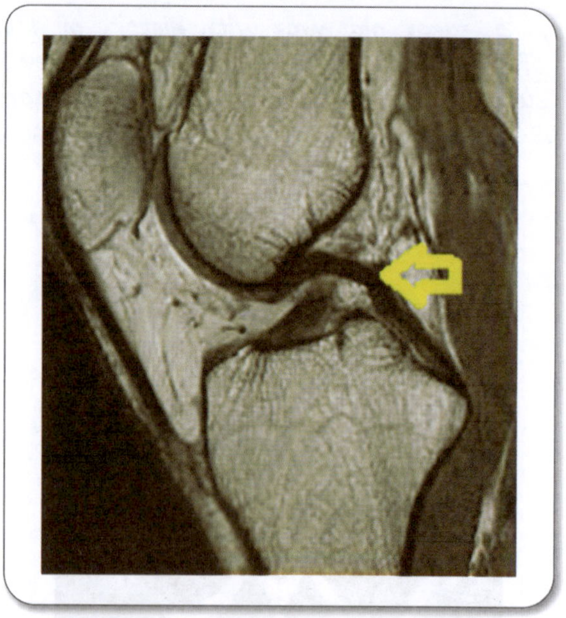

a. ACL
b. PCL
c. Medial meniscus
d. Lateral meniscus

Ans: b. PCL

INI-CET MAY 2023

56. Which of the following is not an advantage of USG over Mammography?

a. Useful in young females with dense breast
b. Differentiates between solid and cystic lesions in the breast
c. Guided biopsy can be done
d. Can be used for mammographically undetectable clinically nonpalpable breast mass

Ans: d. Can be used for mammographically undetectable clinically nonpalpable breast mass

57. Identify the abnormality found in the ultrasound image shown as follows:

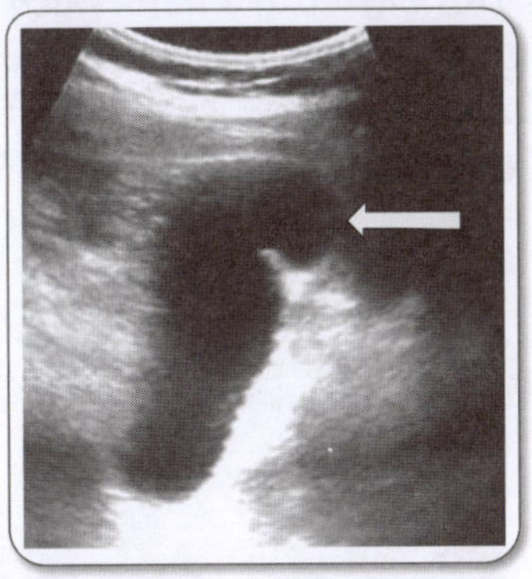

a. Phrygian cap
b. Mercedes-Benz sign
c. Gallbladder polyp
d. Gallbladder cancer

Ans: a. Phrygian cap

58. An MRCP image is shown as follows. Which among the following is the most likely diagnosis?

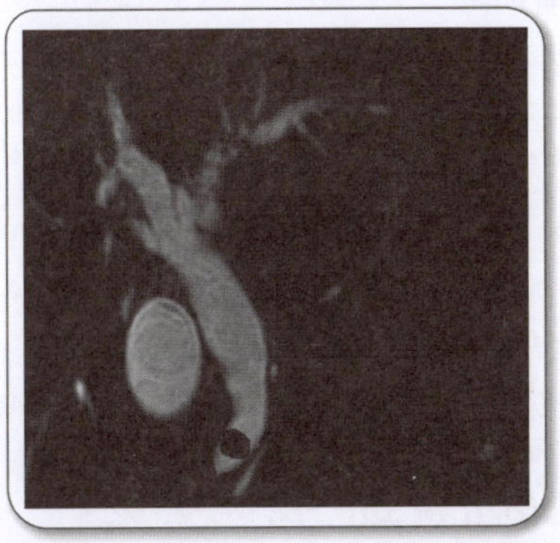

a. Choledocholithiasis b. Cholecystitis
c. Pancreatic duct stricture
d. Malignancy

Ans: a. Choledocholithiasis

59. Identify the fracture site in the X-ray shown as follows:

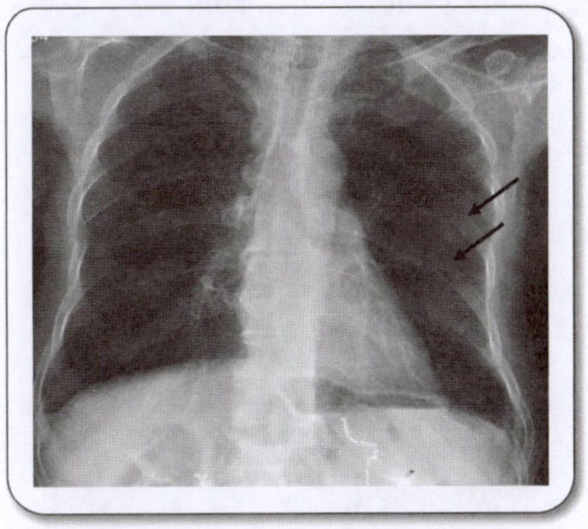

a. 5th and 6th rib
b. 6th and 7th rib
c. 5th, 6th and 7th rib
d. 7th and 8th rib

Ans: b. 6th and 7th rib

60. A patient presented with dysuria and pain in the back. His lumbar spine X-ray shows the below finding. What is the diagnosis?

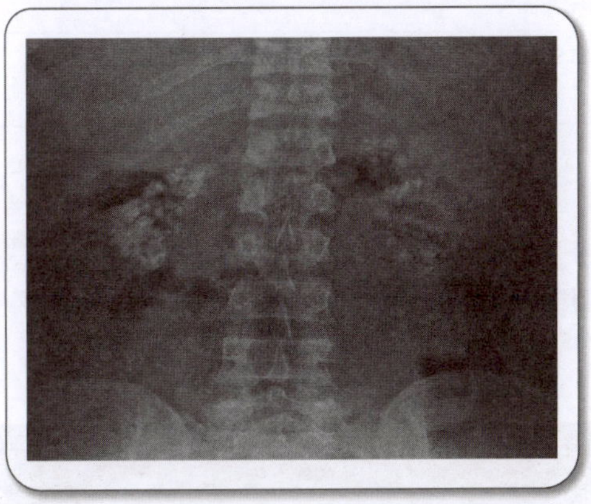

a. Wilson's disease
b. Hyperparathyroidism
c. Addison's disease
d. Cystic fibrosis

Ans: b. Hyperparathyroidism

61. Banana sign on USG is associated with which of the following conditions?

a. Spina bifida
b. Down syndrome
c. Omphalocele
d. Klinefelter's syndrome

Ans: a. Spina bifida

62. A 25-year-old male who sustained a shoulder injury presented with swelling of shoulder. X-ray is shown as follows, Which of the following ligament(s) is/are injured?

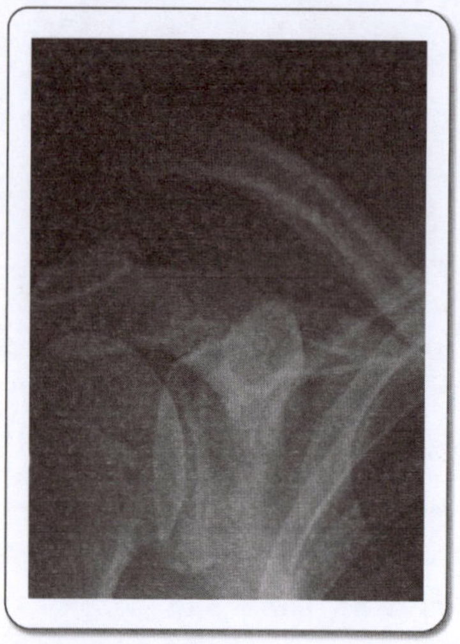

a. Acromioclavicular ligament
b. Coracoacromial ligament
c. Coracohumeral ligament
d. Both Acromioclavicular and Coracoclavicular ligament

Ans: d. Both Acromioclavicular and Coracoclavicular ligament

INI-CET NOVEMBER 2022

63. A patient underwent a NC-CT abdomen with this finding. Most likely diagnosis is:

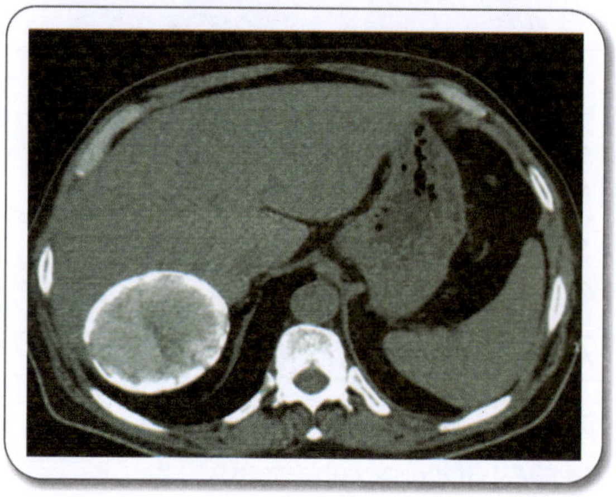

a. HCC
b. Hydatid cyst
c. Focal nodular hyperplasia
d. Liver abscess

Ans: b. Hydatid cyst

64. Match the following:

Football sign String sign Rat tail sign Inverted umbrella sign	Hypertrophic pyloric stenosis Achalasia cardia Ileocecal TB Pneumoperitoneum

a. A-4 B-1 C-2 D-3
b. A-2 B-3 C-4 D-1
c. A-3 B-2 C-1 D-4
d. A-4 B-3 C-1 D-2

Ans: a. A-4 B-1 C-2 D-3

65. An elderly female with curvature of the spine presents with abdominal pain and distension. She has this curvature deformity of spine since childhood and this has been progressive since then. Based on the imaging findings, most likely diagnosis is:

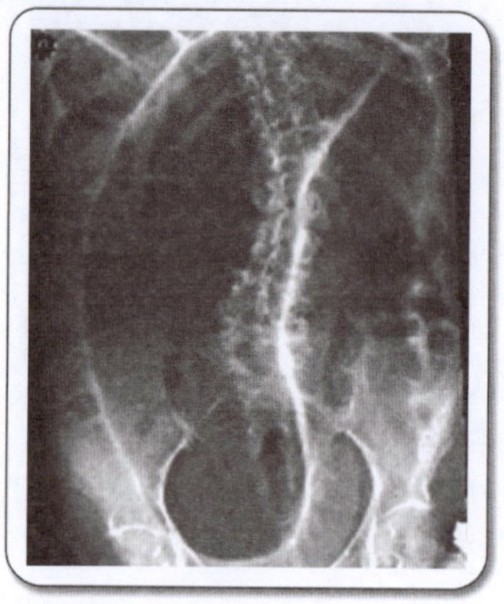

a. Cecal volvulus
b. Large bowel obstruction due to fecolith
c. Large bowel obstruction due to sigmoid volvulus
d. Small bowel obstruction

Ans: c. Large bowel obstruction due to sigmoid volvulus

66. A 28-year-old female with severe headache comes for a CT scan. What specific history should Doctor definitely ask before commencement of the CT study?

a. History of fall
b. Cochlear implant surgery
c. Last menstrual period
d. History of hypertension

Ans: c. Last menstrual period

67. Egg-shell calcification is seen in all of the following except:

a. Silicosis
b. Sarcoidosis
c. Metastatic lymph nodes
d. Postradiation therapy lymph nodes

Ans: c. Metastatic lymph nodes

68. A 55-year-old man presents with painless hematuria and CE-CT revealed a mass lesion in the right kidney. Most likely diagnosis is:

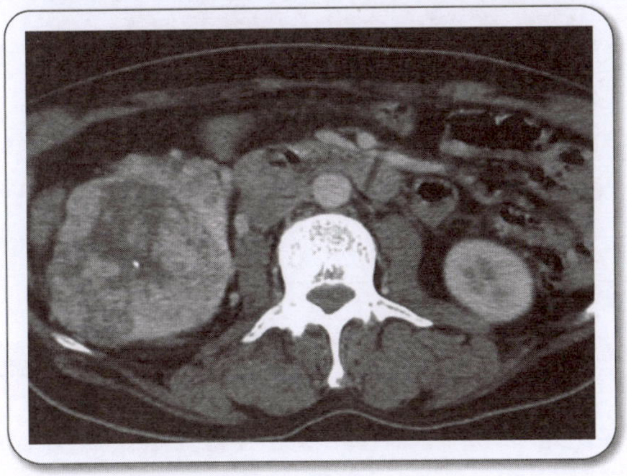

a. Angiomyolipoma
b. RCC
c. Simple cyst
d. Oncocytoma

Ans: b. RCC

69. A whole body CT scan done for trauma includes all except:

a. Cervical spine
b. Limbs
c. Head
d. Abdomen

Ans: b. Limbs

70. A 34-week primigravida is detected to have intra-uterine fetal demise on USG. The finding of hyperechoic air specks within the blood vessels is known as:

a. Hydrops appearance
b. Spalding sign
c. Robert sign
d. Maceration

Ans: c. Robert sign

71. The 99m-MDP Bone scan done in a known patient of prostate cancer with elevated Sr PSA is due to:

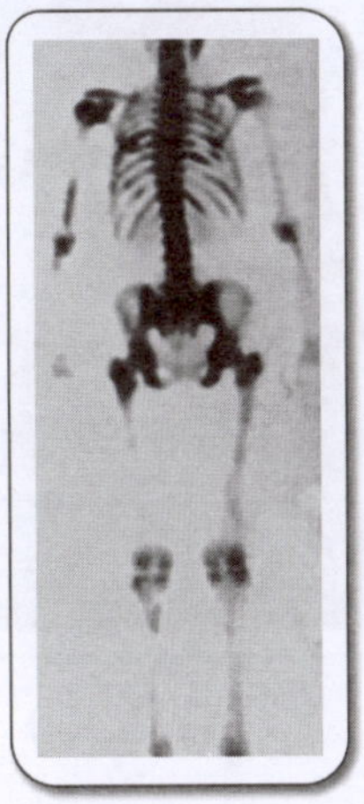

a. Superscan—due to diffusely increased uptake of MDP in the skeletal metastases
b. Superscan—due to increased uptake of MDP in adrenal glands and kidneys
c. Superscan—due to increased uptake of MDP in the short tubular bones
d. Superscan—due to increased uptake in the central nervous system

Ans: a. Superscan—due to diffusely increased uptake of MDP in the skeletal metastases

72. A 30-year-old patient presents with progressive difficulty in swallowing more for a liquids than solids for 8 months. A barium swallow was done and is shown in the following image. What other investigations should be done to confirm the diagnosis in this patient?

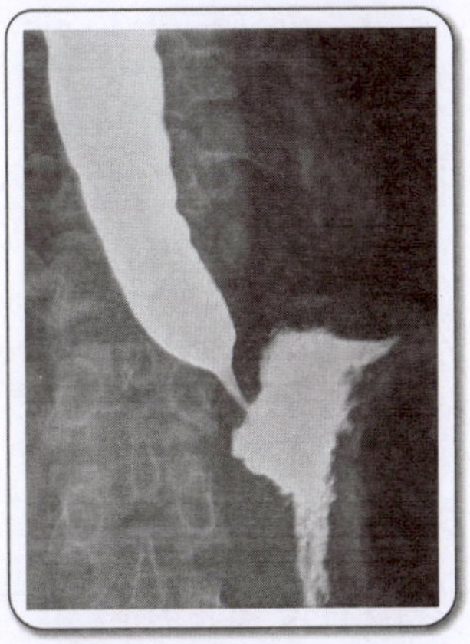

a. UGIE + manometry
b. UGIE + CECT
c. UGIE + PET
d. UGIE + 24 hr pH monitoring

Ans: a. UGIE + manometry

73. Identify the Imaging modality shown as follows:

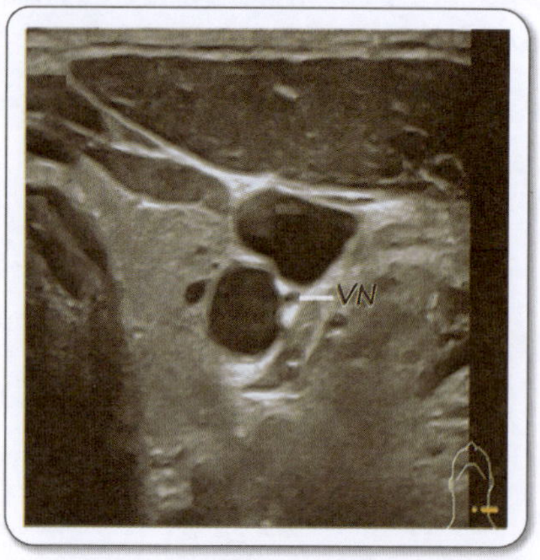

a. USG b. X-ray
c. MRI d. Fluoroscopy

Ans: a. USG

74. The following "Double bleb sign" seen in early pregnancy is due to:

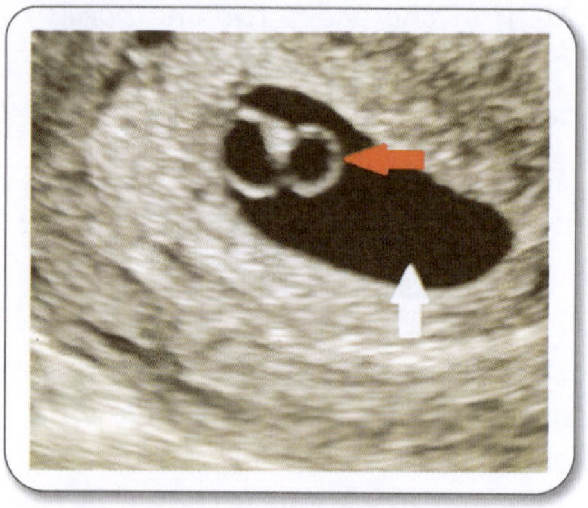

a. Heterotopic pregnancy
b. The amnion and yolk sac
c. Two uterine gestational sacs
d. Amnion and Chorion

Ans: b. The amnion and yolk sac

75. True regarding CO-RADS is:
a. CO-RADS 0 is a normal lung
b. CO-RADS 5 is typical of COVID
c. Pleural thickening is typical of COVID
d. COVID can present with lobar consolidation

Ans: b. CO-RADS 5 is typical of COVID

76. Most radioresistant phase of cell cycle is:
a. G1 phase b. G2 phase
c. M phase d. S phase

Ans: d. S phase

77. A 45-year-old patient presents with vague abdominal pain. USG revealed a Bosniak Grade 3 cystic lesion. A CE-CT was done and is revealed here. Most likely diagnosis is:

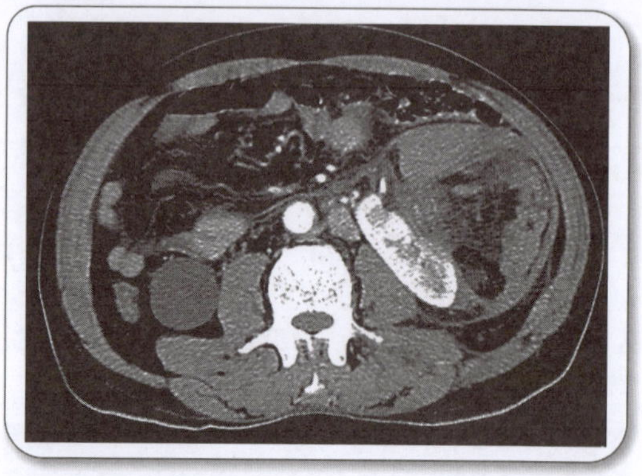

a. Renal colic b. RCC
c. Renal angiomyolipoma
d. Renal cysts

Ans: c. Renal angiomyolipoma

FMGE JANUARY 2024

78. Patient of head trauma presents with altered sensorium. Diagnosis is?

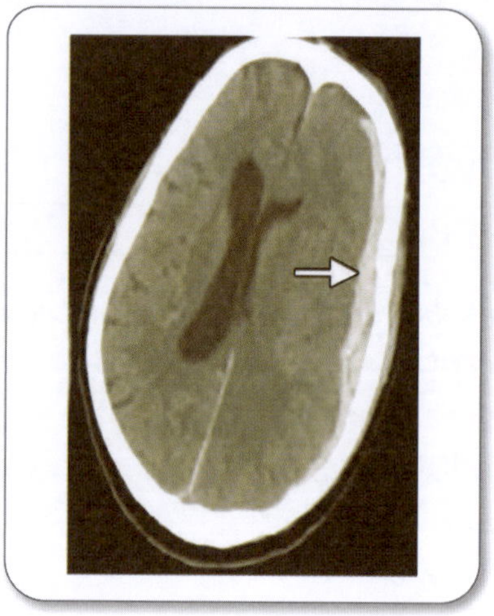

a. EDH
b. SDH
c. Hemorrhagic contusion
d. Diffuse axonal injury

Ans: b. SDH

79. Radio-isotope used in PET scan is?
a. Tc-99m b. Co60
c. 18-FDG d. Ra226

Ans: c. 18-FDG

80. Diagnosis based on this image?

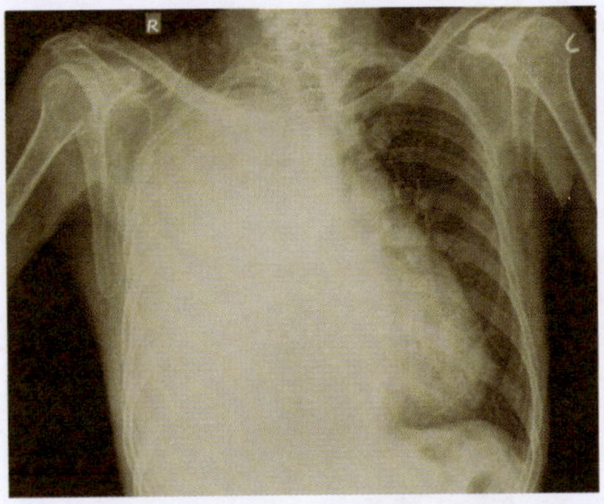

a. Pleural effusion
b. Collapse
c. Consolidation
d. Pneumothorax

Ans: a. Pleural effusion

81. Most radio-resistant phase of cell cycle is?

a. M phase
b. G1 phase
c. G2 phase
d. S phase

Ans: d. S phase

82. Identify this investigation?

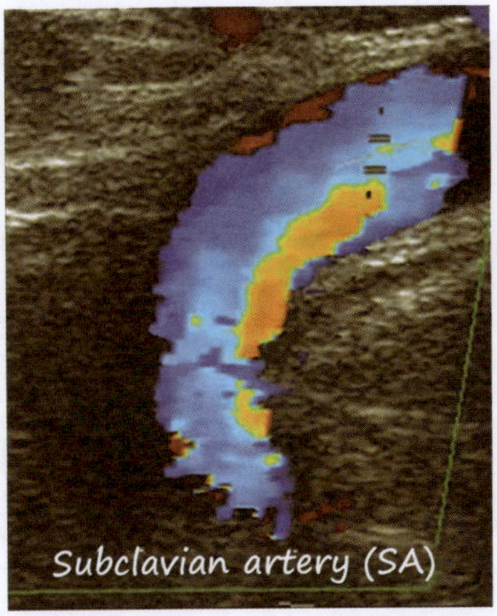

a. B mode USG
b. Duplex USG scan (B mode + Doppler)
c. Spectral Doppler
d. Elastography

Ans: b. Duplex USG scan (B mode + Doppler)

FMGE JANUARY 2023

83. A 2-year-old male child presents with difficulty in breathing and speaking. Following a basic clinical examination, which of the following is the best next step in the management of this child?

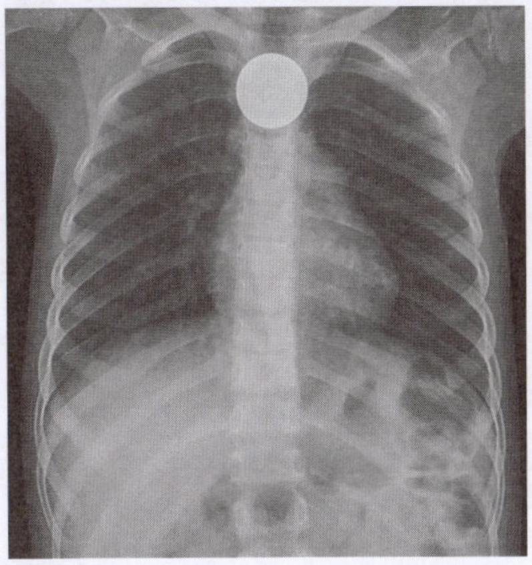

a. Bronchoscopy
b. Esophagoscopy
c. Tracheostomy
d. NGT insertion

Ans: b. Esophagoscopy

84. Diagnosis of the following CT scan is:

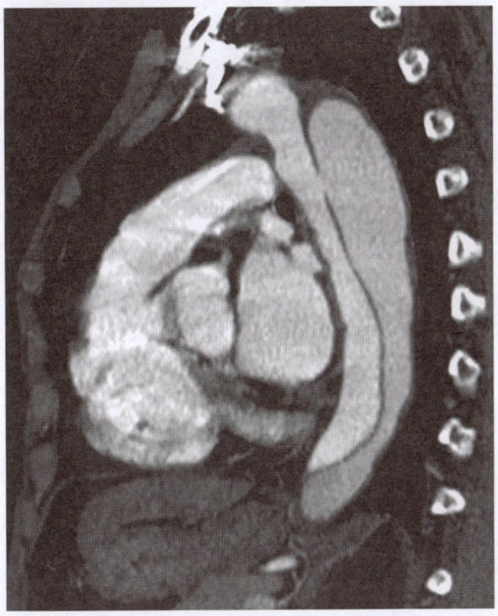

a. Aortic aneurysm
b. Aortic dissection
c. Aortic thrombosis
d. Coronary artery fistula

Ans: b. Aortic dissection

85. A 65-year-old female had a history of fall at home. CT revealed this finding. Diagnosis is:

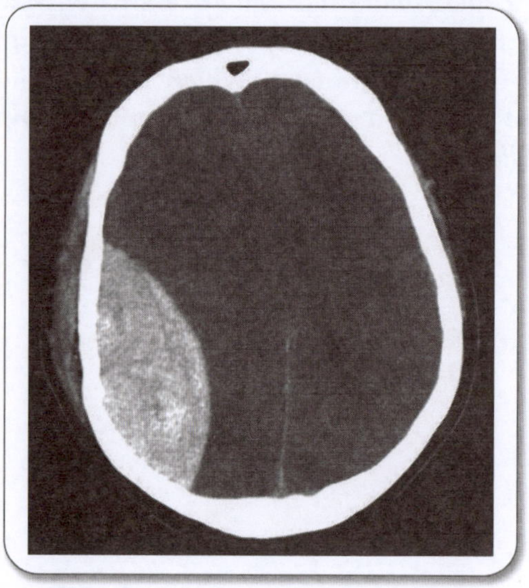

a. EDH
b. SDH
c. SAH
d. DAI

Ans: a. EDH

86. The following radiographic projection is:

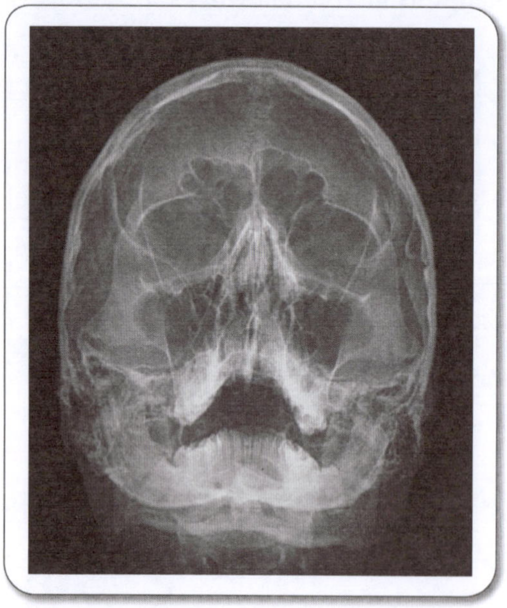

a. Water's view
b. Caldwell's view
c. Rhese view
d. Lateral sinus view

Ans: a. Water's view

87. A newborn has an abnormal lump in the lower back. An MRI was done. What will be the diagnosis?

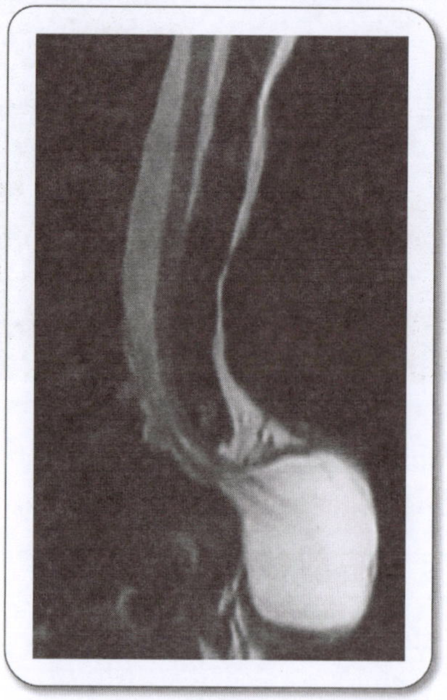

a. Spina bifida occulta
b. Meningocele
c. Meningomyelocele
d. Sacral fracture

Ans: c. Meningomyelocele

88. A 45-year-old female presents with back pain and stiffness. Most likely diagnosis based on this radiograph is?

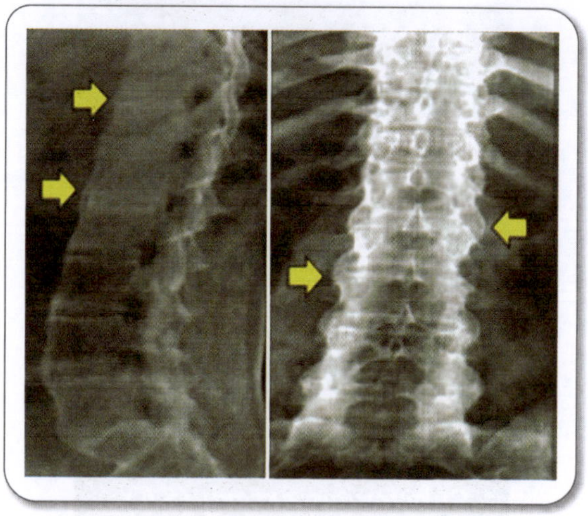

a. Degenerative disk disease
b. Ankylosing spondylitis
c. Pott's spine
d. Spinal cord syrinx

Ans: b. Ankylosing spondylitis

89. A 35-year-old male comes with cough and breathlessness. What is your diagnosis based on this X-ray?

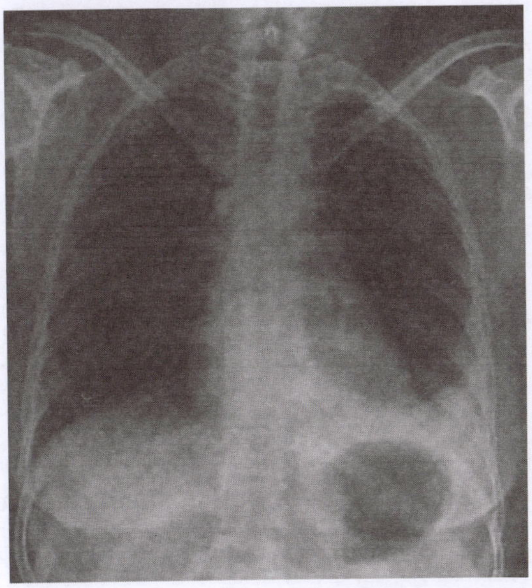

a. Pleural effusion
b. Pneumothorax
c. LLL consolidation
d. Left lung collapse

Ans: a. Pleural effusion

FMGE JULY 2023

90. Patient presents with high grade fever with chills, and pain in flank. He is a diabetic. Most likely diagnosis on the following X-ray image is:

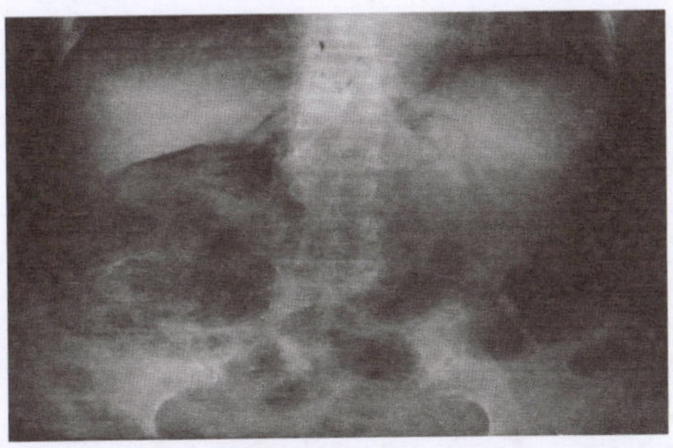

a. Staghorn calculus
b. Emphysematous pyelonephritis
c. Renal TB
d. Emphysematous pyelonephritis

Ans: b. Emphysematous pyelonephritis

91. A 45-year-old female presents with intermittent pain in abdomen. Diagnosis on the following CT image is

(FMGE July and Jan 2023 Pattern)

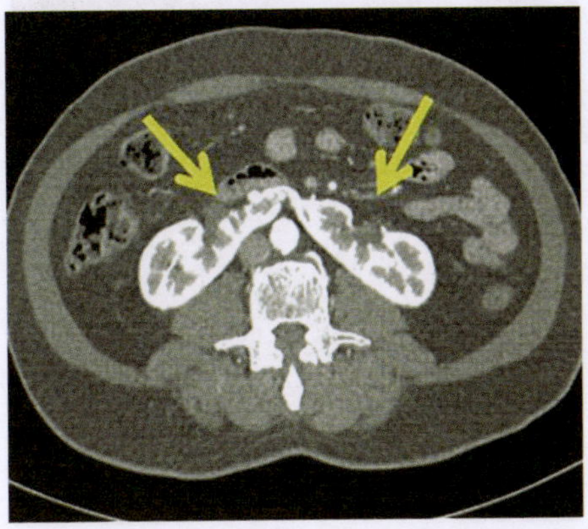

a. Staghorn calculus
b. Horseshoe kidney
c. Crossed fused ectopic kidney
d. Discoid kidney

Ans: b. Horseshoe kidney

92. A neonate presented on day 1 of life with bilious vomiting. X-ray abdomen was done and revealed Double bubble sign. Most likely diagnosis is:

a. Pyloric stenosis
b. Duodenal atresia
c. Esophageal atresia
d. Jejunal atresia

Ans: b. Duodenal atresia

93. A 22-year-old male met with a road traffic accident with injury over his chest and abdomen. He is drowsy with Pulse 110 bpm and BP 90/60 mm Hg. The next step you will tale in this case is:

a. X-ray abdomen
b. CT abdomen
c. e-FAST
d. MRI

Ans: c. e-FAST

94. LINACs are used for production of:

a. Alpha particles
b. X-rays
c. Protons
d. Neutrons

Ans: b. X-rays

95. A 25-year-old male presented with pain and swelling around the knee joint. Diagnosis is:

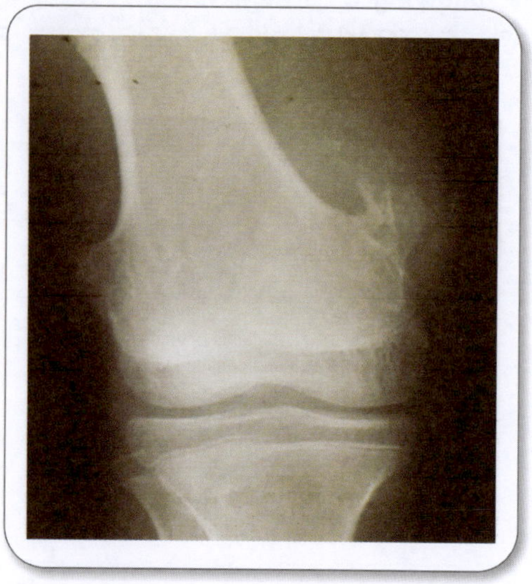

a. Osteochondroma
b. Osteoid osteoma
c. Fibrous dysplasia
d. Ewing's sarcoma

Ans: a. Osteochondroma

96. IOC for parathyroid imaging is:
a. USG
b. CE-CT
c. MRI
d. Sestamibi scan

Ans: d. Sestamibi scan

97. A patient of cervical cancer is being administered a dose of radiotherapy on 5 days of a week followed by a 2 day window period. This type of radiotherapy is known as:
a. Brachytherapy
b. Conventional fractionated radiotherapy
c. Hyperfractionation
d. Hypofractionation

Ans: b. Hyperfractionation

98. What is the gold standard investigation for fistula-in-ano?
a. USG
b. Sinogram
c. CT scan
d. MRI Fistulogram

Ans: d. MRI Fistulogram

FMGE JUNE 2021

99. A child presented with cyanosis and pulmonary hypoplasia. Diagnosis is:

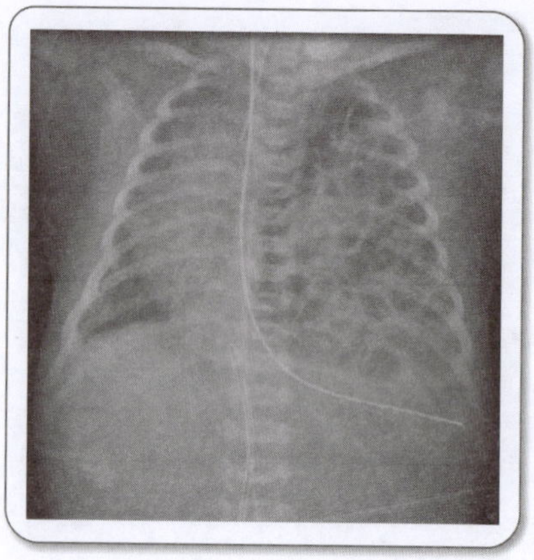

a. CCAM
b. CDH
c. CLE
d. Bronchiectasis

Ans: b. CDH

100. Inferior rib notching is seen in?
a. Coarctation of aorta
b. Marfan's syndrome
c. Rickets
d. SLE

Ans: a. Coarctation of aorta

FMGE DECEMBER 2021

101. A 50-year-old female came with dysphagia and chest pain. A barium swallow study was done. Diagnosis is:

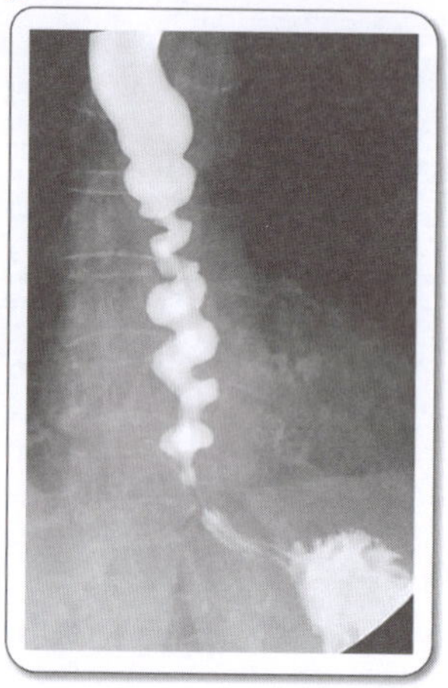

a. Ca Esophagus
b. Achalasia cardia
c. Diffuse esophageal spasm
d. Zenker's diverticulum

Ans: c. Diffuse esophageal spasm

102. Most likely diagnosis in this Popcorn calcification in the lungs is:

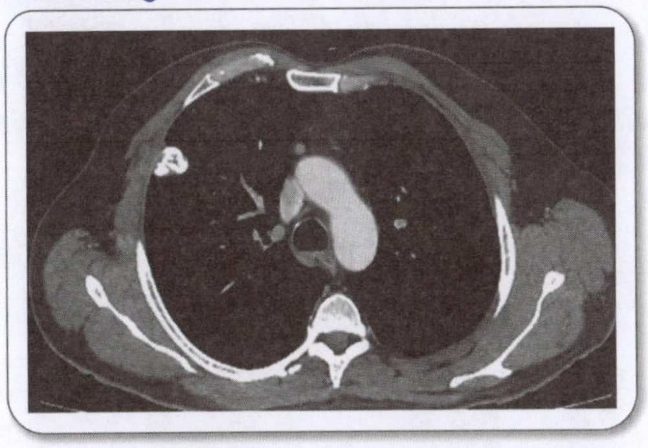

a. Carcinoma b. Hamartoma
c. TB d. Adenoma

Ans: b. Hamartoma

103. The following finding may be seen in:

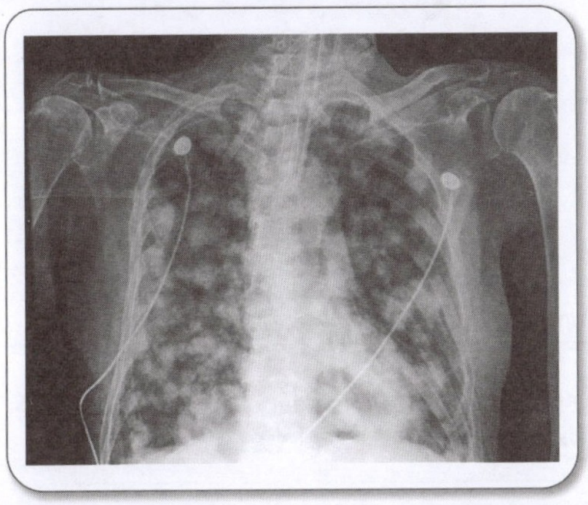

a. RCC b. Choriocarcinoma
c. Endometrial cancer d. All of these

Ans: d. All of these

104. A 35-year-old male presented with pain and swelling around the wrist joint. Diagnosis is:

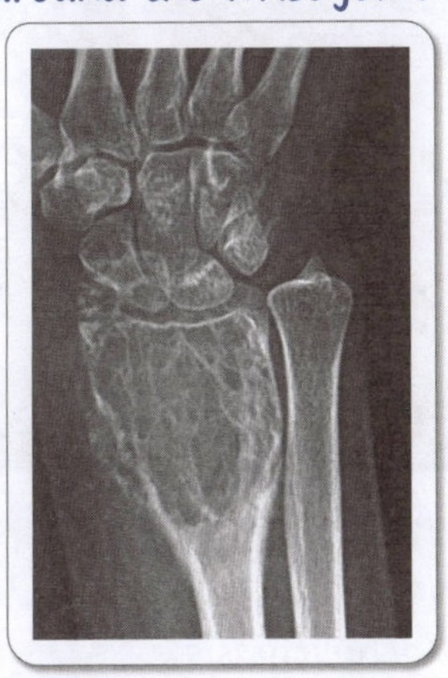

a. SBC b. ABC
c. GCT d. Osteoblastoma

Ans: c. GCT

105. Most radiosensitive organ in the body is:

a. Spleen b. Brain
c. Lungs d. Ovaries

Ans: d. Ovaries

106. A 65-year-old male with h/o MI presents with progressive dyspnea on exertion and pedal edema. A CXR reveals this finding. Diagnosis is:

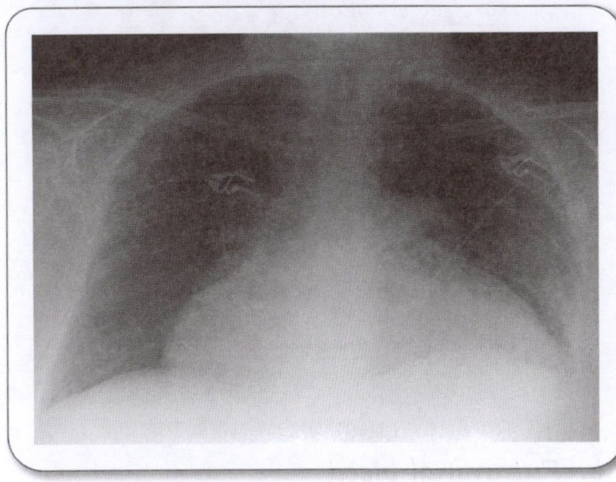

a. Constrictive pericarditis
b. Pericardial effusion
c. Myocardial infarction
d. Congestive cardiac failure

Ans: b. Pericardial effusion

107. A neonate presented with bilious vomiting immediately after birth. A screening abdominal radiograph was obtained and revealed this finding. The most likely diagnosis is:

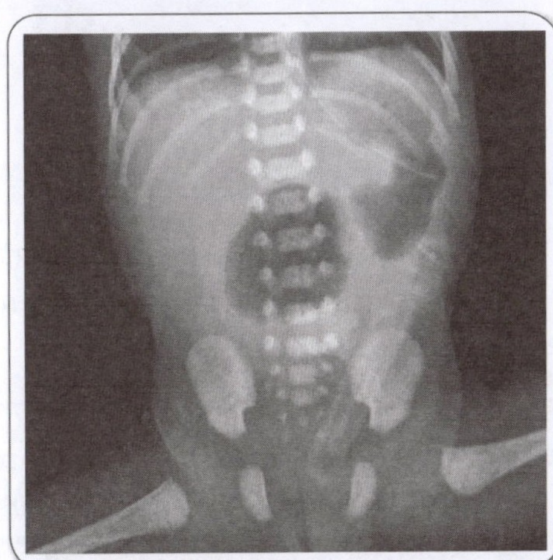

a. Pyloric stenosis
b. Duodenal atresia
c. Tracheoesophageal fistula
d. Biliary atresia

Ans: b. Duodenal atresia

FMGE AUGUST 2020

108. A 60-year-old man on irregular anti-hypertensives presents with altered sensorium and a BP of 220/140 mm Hg. A CT is shown here. Most likely diagnosis is:

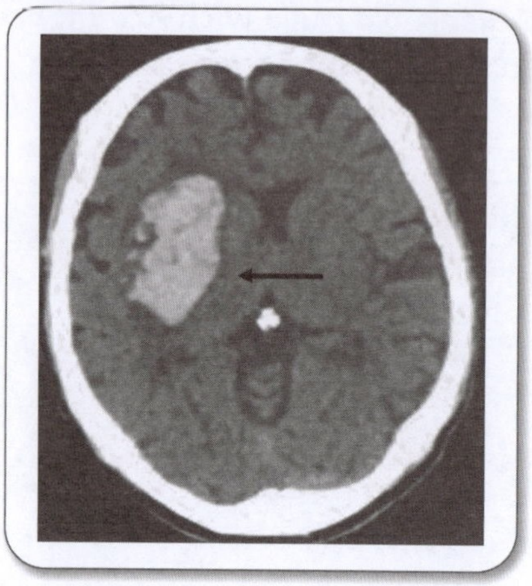

a. Intraventricular hemorrhage
b. Putaminal bleed
c. Pontine hemorrhage d. SAH

Ans: b. Putaminal bleed

109. Diagnosis in this patient on this HSG image is:

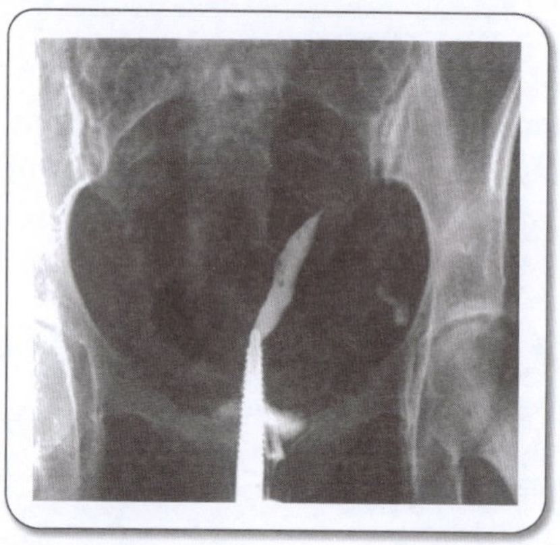

a. Unicornuate uterus b. Bicornuate uterus
c. Didelphys uterus d. Arcuate uterus

Ans: a. Unicornuate uterus

110. Tushar, a 3-year-old child, presented with sudden onset breathlessness and wheezing. Chest X-ray P-A view showed unilateral hyperinflation of the lung. Most likely diagnosis is:

a. Congenital lobar emphysema.
b. Massive consolidation
c. Pneumothorax
d. Foreign body aspiration

Ans: d. Foreign body aspiration

FMGE DECEMBER 2020

111. X-ray of wrist and hand of a child is given as follows. There is prominent cupping and widening of growth plate. What is the diagnosis?

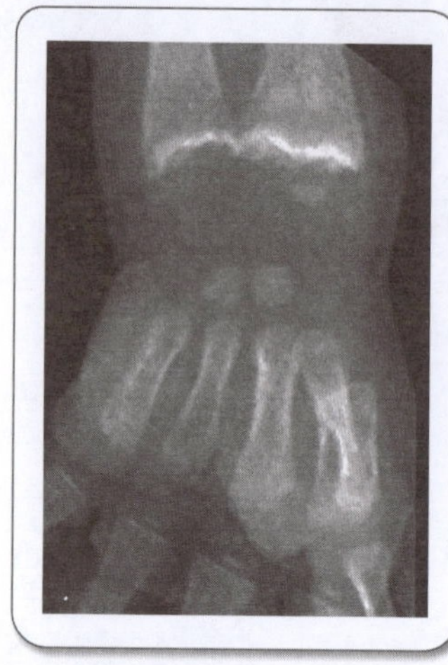

a. Fluorosis
b. Hyperparathyroidism
c. Vitamin C deficiency
d. Vitamin D deficiency

Ans: d. Vitamin D deficiency

112. The following USG image shows which abnormality?

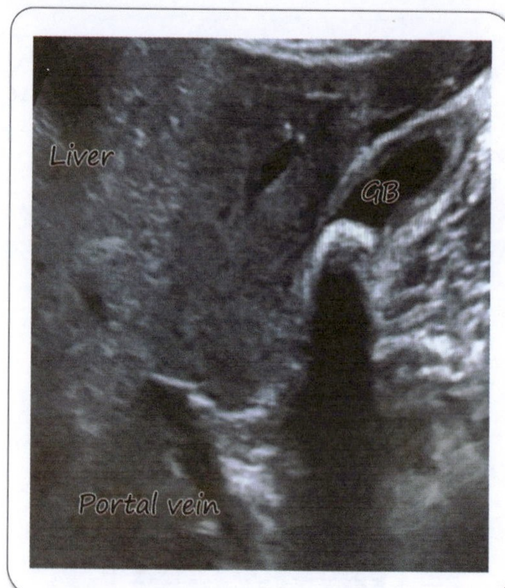

a. GB calculi
b. Choledocholithiasis
c. GB cancer
d. Hydatid cyst

Ans: a. GB calculi

113. Which arterial territory is involved in the following CT scan image?

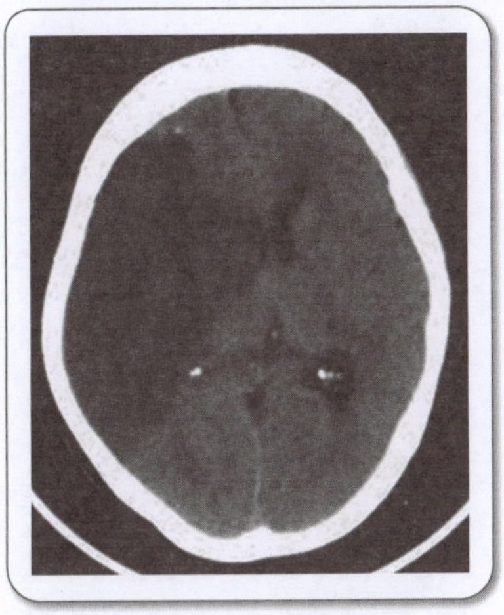

a. Anterior Cerebral Artery
b. Middle Cerebral Artery
c. Posterior Cerebral Artery
d. PICA

Ans: b. Middle Cerebral Artery

114. A 30-year-old Primi c/o vaginal bleeding, pain in abdomen and vomiting. Uterus is enlarged, soft, nontender. Based on the USG, most likely diagnosis is:

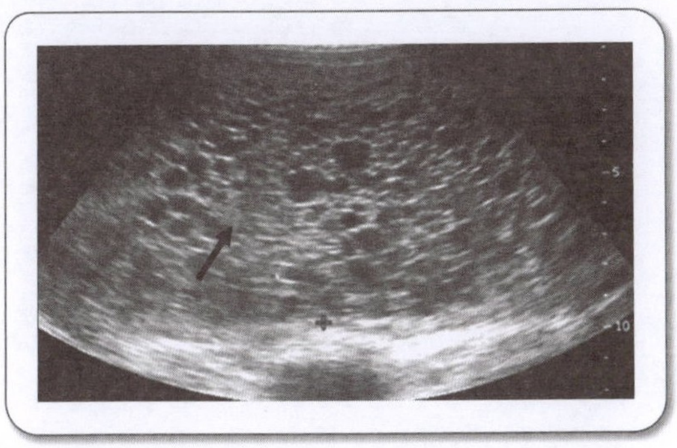

a. H. mole
b. Missed abortion
c. Blighted ovum
d. Ectopic pregnancy

Ans: a. H. mole

115. A patient is evaluated for infertility and HSG is done – which is shown as follows. Most likely diagnosis is:

a. Bicornuate uterus
b. Unicornuate uterus
c. Hydrosalpinx
d. Uterine adhesion

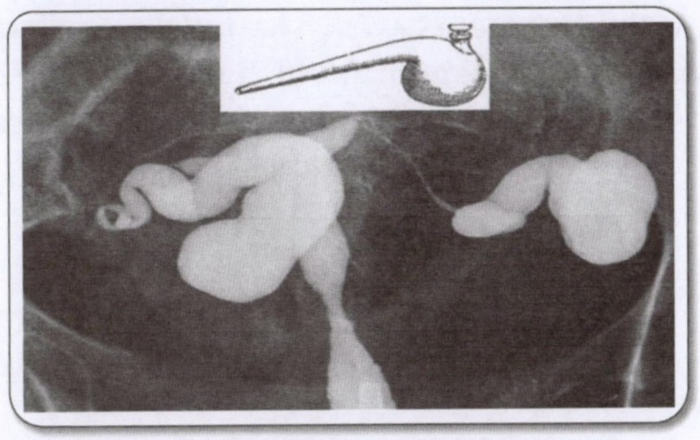

Ans: c. Hydrosalpinx

116. A patient with head trauma is brought to the hospital with altered sensorium. CT shows few petechial hemorrhages but is otherwise normal. Most likely diagnosis is:

a. Traumatic hemorrhagic contusion.
b. EDH
c. SDH
d. Diffuse axonal injury

Ans: d. Diffuse axonal injury

117. Most radiosensitive bone tumor is:

a. Enchondroma
b. Ewing's tumor
c. Osteochondroma
d. Osteosarcoma

Ans: b. Ewing's tumor

118. A patient with recurrent UTI undergoes an IVU study – shown as follows. Can you identify the site of insertion of the ureter arising from the right superior moiety?

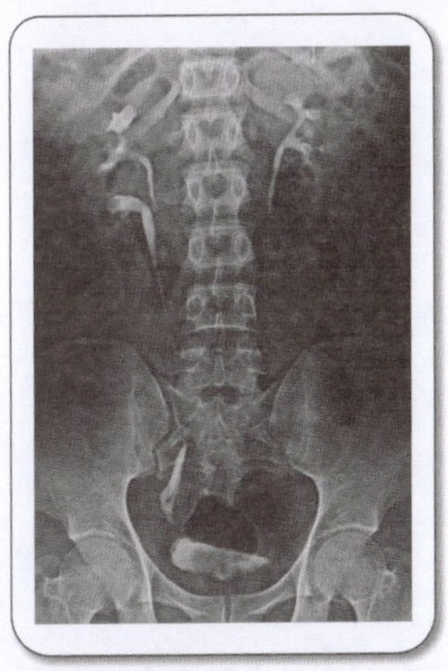

a. Above the trigone
b. Infero-medial to the trigone
c. Penile urethra
d. Perineum

Ans: b. Infero-medial to the trigone

119. A child presents with the following finding on a skull radiograph. All of the following could be the differential diagnoses in this case; except:

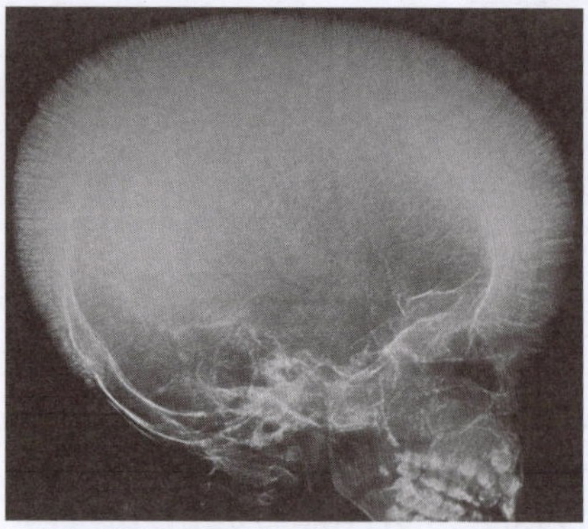

a. Thalassemia
b. Sickle cell disease
c. Hereditary spherocytosis
d. Aplastic anemia

Ans: d. Aplastic anemia

120. A 35-year-old female patient presented with fever, weight loss and elevated ACE levels. A CXR reveals bilateral convex hilar shadows shown as follows. Most likely diagnosis is:

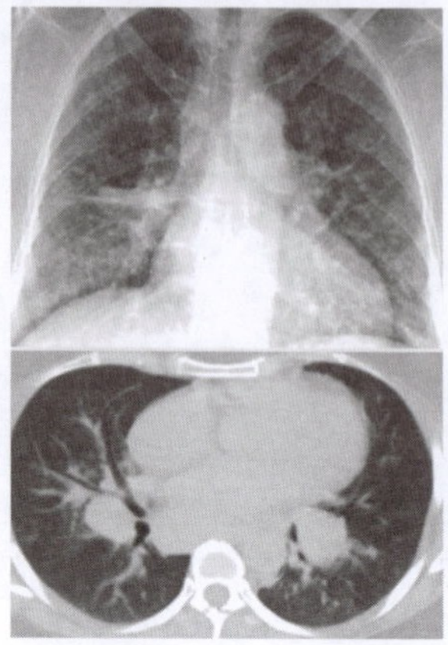

a. TB
b. Silicosis
c. Sarcoidosis
d. Lung cancer

Ans: c. Sarcoidosis